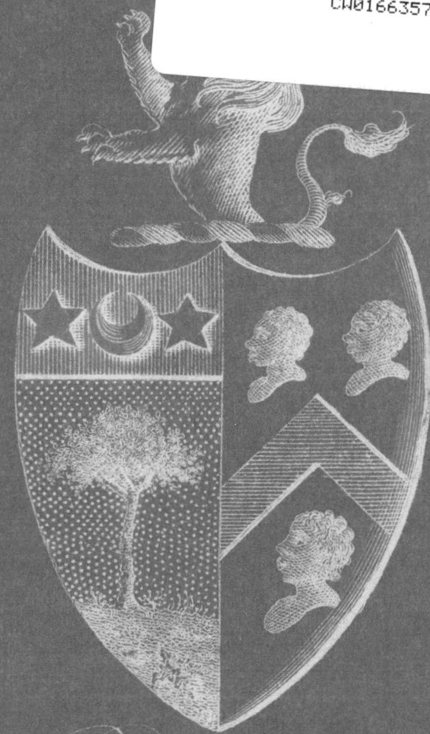

Sir John Silvester. W. Bosanquet

G. De Visme

The French Hospital in England

Its Huguenot History and Collections

In memory of Jacob, 8th Earl of Radnor,
who was elected a director in 1960 and served
as governor from 1971 to 2008

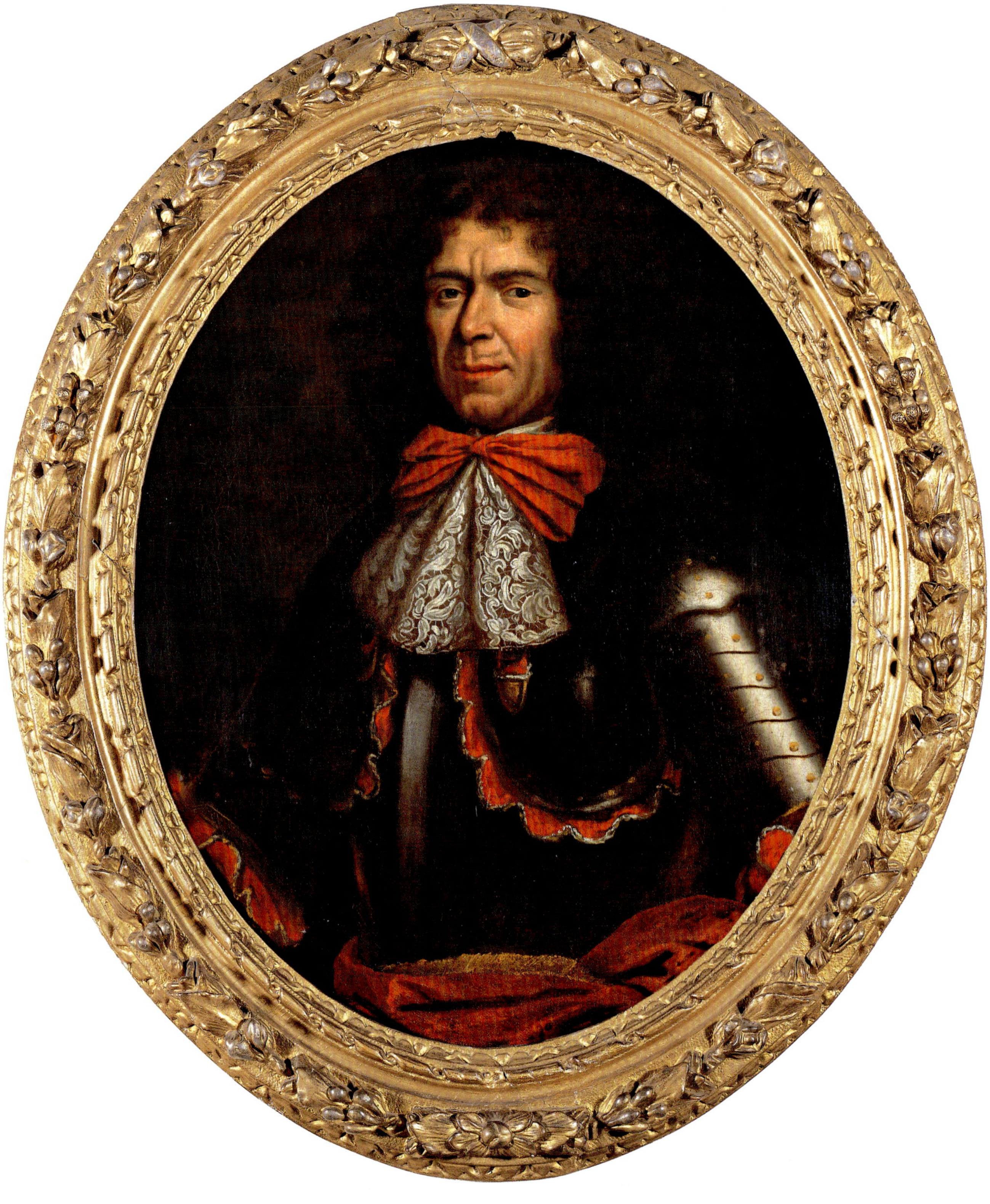

Vostre tres humble
et tres obeissans serviteur
Gastigny

The French Hospital in England

Its Huguenot History and Collections

Tessa Murdoch and Randolph Vigne

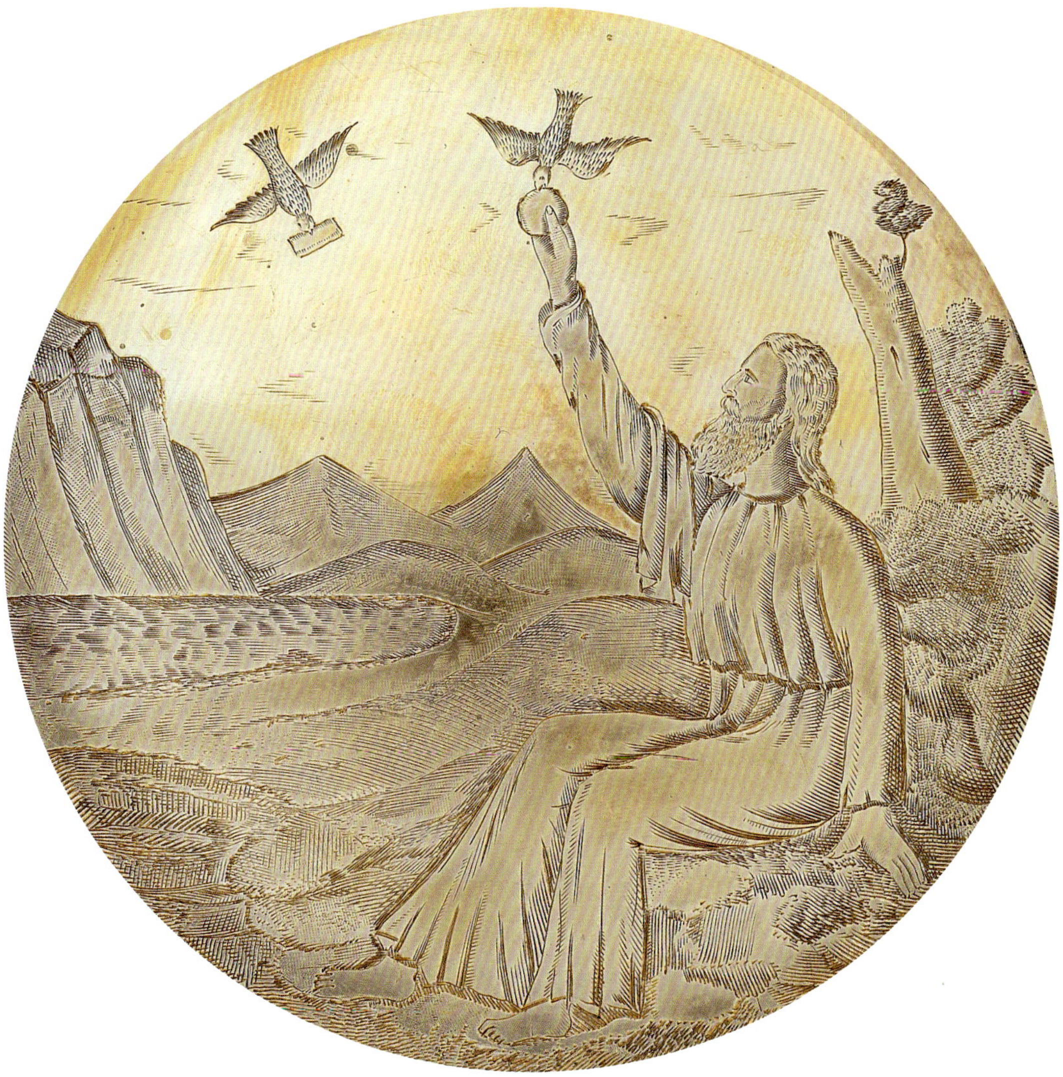

John Adamson
Cambridge, 2009

Support for the publication of this book was provided by
The Idlewild Trust
The Marc Fitch Fund
The Paul Mellon Centre for Studies in British Art

John Adamson,
90 Hertford Street, Cambridge CB4 3AQ, England

Photographs unless otherwise credited were taken by Brenda Norrish.

First published 2009

British Library Cataloguing in Publication Data
A catalogue record for this book is available from the British Library.
ISBN: 978-0-9524322-7-2

Set in Granjon and designed by James Shurmer
Printed on Burgo Larius 150 gsm matt by Conti Tipocolor, Italy

End-papers: Book-plates of directors of the French Hospital, with the year of their first election to the Court given. *Geoffrey Vevers*
Left-hand page, clockwise from top left:
Anthony Chamier (1725–1780), 1780; Lewis Andrew de La Chaumette, 1788; Peter Romilly (1712–1784), 1770; Daniel Josias Olivier (1722–1782), 1765
Right-hand page, clockwise from top left:
Sir John Silvester, FRS, FSA (1745–1822), 1811;
William Bosanquet (1757–1800), 1782; Gerard Devisme, 1788;
Samuel Lichigaray, 1777

Frontispiece (a): Jacques de Gastigny (d. 1708), oil on canvas, circle of Pierre Mignard, c. 1680, in late 17th-century giltwood frame
Jacques de Gastigny bequeathed £500 to build apartments for at least twelve poor, infirm, or sick French Protestant men or women above the age of 50 years. He left a further £500, the interest on which was to provide beds, linen, clothing and other requisites.

Frontispiece (b): Gastigny's signature from a letter. Add MS 83701. *British Library*

Title-page: *Elijah being fed by the ravens*, detail from a silver-gilt alms-dish, maker's mark of George Lambert, London, 1897/8 (see p. 57)

Contents

	Acknowledgements and abbreviations	*page* 6
	Foreword	7
	Introduction	8
1	Jacques de Gastigny's bequest	9
2	The new hospital, the royal charter and the corporation	13
3	Building and furnishing the French Hospital	19
4	Directing and caring at the French Hospital in the eighteenth century	30
5	Waning fortunes in Finsbury	41
6	The French Hospital in Hackney	47
7	Health and heritage: 'The chief Huguenot foundation in this country', 1867–1938	54
8	Under threat, enemy action and evacuation	68
9	Retreat to the country: Compton's Lea, Sussex, 1947–1957	72
10	Retirement in a cathedral city	76
	Directors of the French Hospital: A survey	89
	A list of directors	95
	Huguenot heraldry	102
	Book-plates in the French Hospital and their heraldry	106
	Notes to the Huguenot book-plates illustrated on the end-papers	110
	Inventory of the contents of the French Hospital, 1742	111
	Picture notes	117
	Bibliography	124
	Index	125
	Picture credits	128

Acknowledgements and abbreviations

We owe a huge debt of thanks to Jacob, 8th Earl of Radnor, for his warm encouragement of this project, and are deeply saddened that he did not live to see the book come to fruition. We should like to thank the Idlewild Trust, the Marc Fitch Fund and the Paul Mellon Centre for Studies in British Art for their grants towards the cost of publication. The present officers, in particular the deputy-governor, Peter Duval, and the secretary, Stephen de Crespigny, have provided enthusiastic moral support for the project. Paul Minet, Jeremy Ouvry and Jonathan Ouvry, who are all current directors, have made generous financial contributions. The staff at Rochester has been both welcoming and accommodating to the authors and to other visitors involved, and we are particularly grateful to the clerk, Brigadier J. A. McGregor. Brenda Norrish undertook new photography and we are delighted with her outstanding pictures of the collections at Rochester. Lucy Gwynn, librarian at the Huguenot Library, provided help and advice and kindly arranged the photography of selected items at University College, London. Tim Rawle generously took photographs of the exterior of the French Hospital in Rochester.

We wish to thank Geoffrey Vevers for enthusiastically contributing to the Huguenot book-plate section and Gale Glynn for her good counsel on Huguenot heraldry. We should also like to thank the following: Glenn Adamson, Susanna Avery-Quash, Mark Evans, Susan Foister, Graham Gibbs, Trevor Moore and Paul Williamson. Our special thanks go to Jacob Simon at the National Portrait Gallery, London, for visiting the collection of portraits at Rochester, for commenting on their frames and for assistance in the National Portrait Gallery archives. David Beasley, librarian, and Rosemary Ransome Wallis, curator, at the Worshipful Company of Goldsmiths, and Mrs Ann Wickham were particularly helpful with research into the lives of later directors. Study visits to the French Hospital by members of the Furniture History Society, the Samuel Pepys Club and the Silver Society and the continuous interest of the Friends of La Providence and members and officers of the Huguenot Society of Great Britain and Ireland* have fuelled enthusiasm for the collections at Rochester.

We are delighted at the wide interest shown in this publication around the globe. In North America Huguenot Heritage in New York has been particularly supportive, while in Australia, Robert Nash, secretary of the Huguenot Society of Australia, kindly read the text and made welcome additions. We should also like to express our special thanks to John Adamson for editing and for publishing this book and to James Shurmer for his excellent design.

The study of the Huguenot diaspora and the subsequent contribution made by the Huguenots to the culture of those countries in which they settled have a permanent relevance. This book explores the extraordinary role the French Hospital in England continues to play.

Tessa Murdoch and Randolph Vigne, *October 2008*

Abbreviations

PHS: Proceedings of the Huguenot Society

HSNS: Huguenot Society New Series

HSQS: Huguenot Society Quarto Series

* The Huguenot Society of London, founded in 1885, became the Huguenot Society of Great Britain and Ireland in 1986.

Foreword

Jacob, 8th Earl of Radnor, Governor, 1971–2008

The hospital for poor French Protestants and their descendants residing in Great Britain was incorporated in Finsbury, rebuilt in Hackney in the 1860s, and moved out of London to Sussex after the Second World War. It moved again in 1958 to Rochester, Kent, to provide sheltered housing for elderly people of Huguenot descent. The portrait of Jacques de Gastigny (frontispiece), the founder of the original hospital at Finsbury, still presides over the Court Room where the directors meet monthly at Rochester. This book marks the tercentenary of the hospital's founding bequest in 1708.

I am proud of my family's association with this venerable and worthwhile charity, which continues a much-needed service to the community, while also providing a focus for the rich Huguenot cultural contribution to Great Britain. Earls of Radnor have served successively as governors of this institution since the mid-eighteenth century (figs. 32, 42, 125–7). Its continuing existence bears witness to the tenacity of the descendants of those Huguenot refugees who settled in Britain, encouraged by the freedom to practise their faith. Carefully researched by two current directors, this book is richly illustrated with specially commissioned photographs of the treasures which belong to the French Hospital, including portraits of former directors and officers, as well as silver, furniture, engravings and other memorabilia. Extracts from the early hospital records preserved in the Huguenot Library, illustrate daily life at 'La Providence', as the hospital was affectionately known.

The French Hospital was one of the earliest foundations to cater for London's needy immigrants, and one of the first in Britain to provide sympathetic care for the mentally ill. As a dignified residence for people of Huguenot descent, it sets new standards in meeting both pastoral and physical needs in the twenty-first century. This handsome volume will make the history and continuing existence of this extraordinary charity better known internationally.

Radnor

Introduction

When Henri IV became King of France, the worst of the long and bloody Wars of Religion fought between the royal house and the great Protestant noble families came to an end. Known to the English as Henry of Navarre, he had converted to Catholicism to win the crown and in 1598 signed the Edict of Nantes. This had guaranteed a measure of toleration for French Protestants.

However, Henri IV's grandson, Louis XIV, adhering to a doctrine of 'one faith, one law, one king', instigated a long period of persecution of any of his Protestant subjects who refused to convert to Catholicism. He resorted to such harsh measures as the *dragonnades* (the billeting of troops on Protestant households) and the destruction of their churches. In 1685 he revoked the Edict of Nantes to coerce all remaining Protestants into the Catholic fold or face the consequences of their refusal.

Many of the followers of John Calvin, the reforming Protestant theologian, emigrated from France rather than convert to Catholicism. They were known as Huguenots, a word of uncertain origin used in Geneva where Calvin had settled. The trickle of Huguenots who had left before the Revocation soon turned into a flood. In what was known as the *grand refuge*, a quarter of a million Huguenots fled France at great danger to themselves, leaving behind almost all they owned. Those who endeavoured to escape faced imprisonment, confinement in convents, or were condemned to the galleys; some were even sentenced to death if caught. They found sanctuary in the Protestant nations of Europe especially in German princely states with Calvinist rulers, in Geneva and the Swiss cantons and in Scandinavia. Some forty per cent of the fugitives went to Britain and the Netherlands.

Ever since the Reformation England had welcomed Protestants from abroad and not surprisingly there was considerable sympathy for these victims of Louis XIV's persecution. The Huguenots who came over brought with them the term *réfugiés* which was soon adopted in the English language as 'refugees'. They benefited from the Royal Bounty (fig. 3), a source of funding for Huguenot refugees accumulated through special collections made by every Protestant church in the land. Ordered by Charles II and upheld by later monarchs, the Royal Bounty was controlled by commissioners who were advised by an official English Committee and a Huguenot French Committee consisting of clerical and lay members. The clerical members serviced the churches founded for the needs of the Huguenot community, whereas the lay members distributed alms to those in need whatever their social status.[1]

Most of the able-bodied Huguenot refugees in Britain were soon to contribute to the economy, many becoming prominent and prosperous merchants, soldiers, clerics and skilled craftsmen (especially goldsmiths, clock and instrument makers, and silk weavers).

Nevertheless, there were many who arrived in England destitute and who were too old, too young or too infirm to support themselves. From 1681, a small number of those in the greatest need were cared for in an inadequate hostel in Finsbury, London, managed by the French Committee. A member of this committee, moved by the plight of the inmates, made a handsome bequest in 1708 that set in train the establishing of a major institution for 'poor French Protestants residing in Great Britain'. This was the French Hospital that was to be a forerunner of many health and welfare institutions set up in England in the mid-eighteenth century.

The testator was Jacques de Gastigny (frontispiece). This book is an account of the institution his bequest inspired and helped to found ten years later.

1 Smith, 'Financial Aid', p. 254.

I

Jacques de Gastigny's bequest

Little is known of Jacques de Gastigny (frontispiece).[1] He was appointed Master of King William III's Harthounds and Buckhounds in England in 1689, having served as his master of the hunt in the Netherlands. In England, Gastigny was paid an annual sum of £2,341 for the establishment of the royal hunt – for his sergeant, five horsemen and four foot huntsmen, a servant and a 'brass hunting horn'. This also included his own salary of £500, out of which he was expected to buy horses and pay for servants' lodgings.[2] Gastigny acquired British citizenship by letters patent of 31 March 1690.

Only months later, Gastigny fought as an officer against the French alongside William III at the Battle of the Boyne in Ireland on 12 July 1690.[3] The king sent him as a messenger across the battlefield to halt the charge of Field Marshal Schomberg's mounted squadron, but all in vain as the squadron pressed ahead with heavy losses.

Gastigny was evidently a kind and visionary man and used his influence with King William and Queen Mary to obtain favours on behalf of others in need. He secured a continuing pension for a kinsman of Dumont du Bostaquet, a fellow officer.[4] Queen Mary wrote from Kensington to her lady-in-waiting, Madame d'Obadam, in 1694, about a house of charity at The Hague mentioning Jacques de Gastigny's involvement.[5]

In similar vein Gastigny wrote letters from London to Edward Southwell, Secretary of State for Ireland, in Dublin in 1703, asking him to obtain for his relative 'Monsieur de Fonteine' a lieutenant's commission from the Duke of Ormonde, who was then Lord Lieutenant. Gastigny's request was granted.

Although he had retired in 1701, he maintained a deep interest in military operations. Correspondence between John Churchill, 1st Duke of Marlborough, and Sidney Godolphin, 1st Earl Godolphin, Queen Anne's first minister, throws light upon Gastigny's proposal in 1705 to invade France from Saint-Valéry and take Abbeville.[6] Marlborough was at first sceptical – in his view the plan was 'next to impossible', but after the battle of Oudenarde he wrote, on 12 October 1708, that 'if the war continues for some time it may be attempted but I fear the year is far advanced'.

Marlborough sought to implement what Winston Churchill[7] called 'his greatest strategy'; sending 6,000 troops to France from the Isle of Wight, exactly as

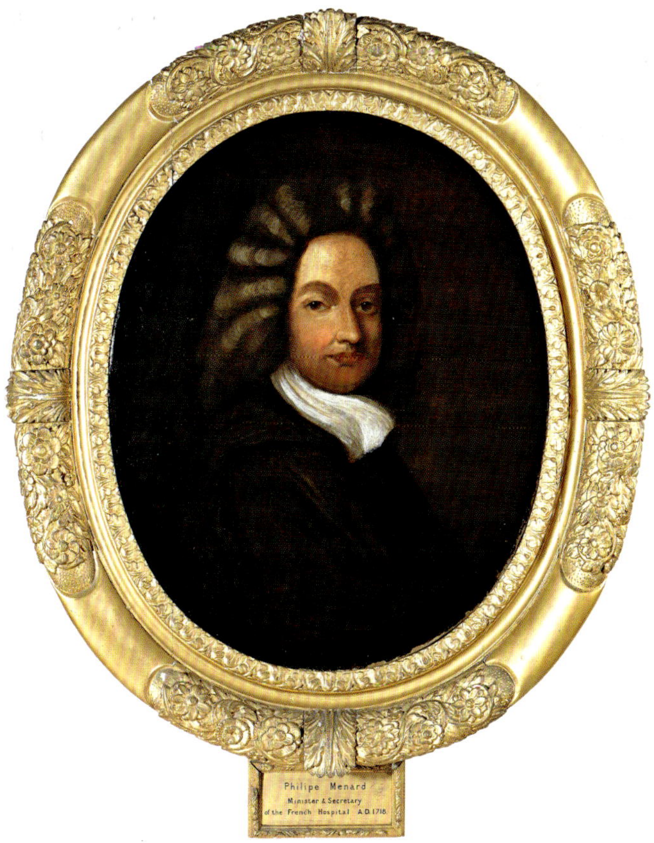
Philipe Menard
Minister & Secretary
of the French Hospital A.D.1718

Fig. 1 Philippe Ménard (d. 1737), oil on canvas, French School, c. 1700

Ménard served as the first chaplain and secretary of the French Hospital from 1718 until his death in 1737. As executor of Gastigny's will, he was the driving force behind the hospital's establishment.

In England from 1700, Ménard was on the clerical committee for administering the Royal Bounty. He launched the first public appeal for the French Hospital and preached the opening sermon in 1718, which, according to the treasurer's accounts, was printed for future reference, although no copy seems to have survived.

Ménard's elder brother Jean was Huguenot minister at Thorney Abbey and a canon of Windsor. He preached the last sermon at the Charenton temple before it was demolished in October 1685. He fled to Holland where he became chaplain to William of Orange.

Gastigny's plan had set out, and taking Abbeville, then joining forces with the combined armies of Marlborough and Prince Eugene of Savoy to defeat France. Yet in June 1709, Godolphin wrote: 'If Mr de Gattigny's thought could bee practicable, this therefore I should think were the proper time to attempt it' as it might take the army 'to the very gates of Paris'.[8] Winston Churchill gave Prince Eugene's unwillingness to support Marlborough as the reason for abandoning Gastigny's plan.[9]

When he retired, Gastigny received a yearly pension of £500 'for the term of his natural life'. He lived for another seven years, dying in November 1708 only three months after writing his will in French. In the will, proved on 2 December 1708,[10] Gastigny left over £3,000 in cash and unspecified goods, the latter to go, with the residue, to his executor, Philippe Ménard (fig. 1). Among the most distinguished Huguenot ministers in Britain, Ménard had served while still in France at the Protestant temple of Saintes (Charente-Maritime), and in exile, first as chaplain to the Calvinist Queen Charlotte Amelia of Denmark in Copenhagen, then as minister of the French Chapel Royal, St James's, London, from 1700. His elder brother Jean had already come to England with William of Orange and was serving as canon of Windsor, having been minister at the great temple of Charenton (fig. 2) outside Paris.

The Ménard brothers received £120 each, with similar bequests going to friends and relatives, many of whom were in the United Provinces. Gastigny left £200 to his servants, including 'Cesar, my *valet de chambre*, Susanne and his little daughter', who also received all his clothes as well as 'other small linen and the three silver mugs and six forks, which are in the ancient mode'. Monsieur de Richosse, who had been Master of the Horse to William III, received £100 as a mark of his friendship. There were bequests for two soup kitchens, La Marmite in Soho and La Soupe in Spitalfields; £100 was left to the Society for the Propagation of the Holy Gospel (founded in 1701); £200 was to be distributed among twenty Huguenot refugee pastors, and a further £200 was for 'the poor of the nation', to be distributed by Ménard. Gastigny's own burial was to take place 'in the nearest churchyard' to his place of death and was to cost no more than £20. Where he is buried is not known.

The balance of £1,000 was specified as follows:

> First, I give £500 to the Pest-house, for to build there some apartments, there to lodge some poor, infirm or sick French Protestants above the age of fifty years, and the woman or maiden the same. My will is that there should be lodgings for twelve poor at least. Moreover, I give the fund of £500, which shall be placed to get thereout the annual revenue, which revenue shall be employed to furnish beds, linen and clothes, and other necessities of the poor French Protestants who shall be in the same place; and the said two £500, making in all £1000, shall be put in the hands of the committee settled for the distribution of the Queen's charity and of the nation, which French Committee shall employ the said sums as it is here above mentioned, and shall give an account thereof to the Messieurs the English commissaries who are, or shall be, settled to receive the other accounts of the said French Committee. And the Executor of this my testament shall take care that the whole be executed according to my intention.

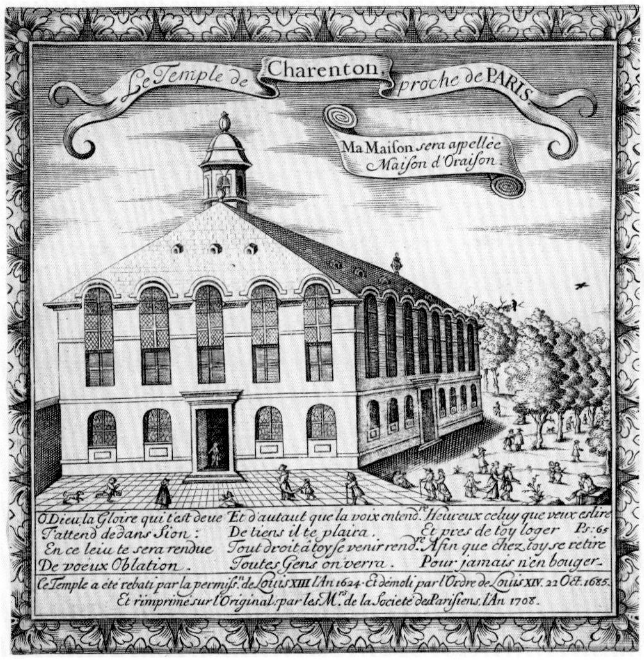
Le Temple de Charenton, proche de PARIS
Ma Maison sera appellée Maison d'Oraison.
O Dieu, la Gloire qui t'est deue
T'attend dedans Sion:
En ce leiu te sera rendue
De voeux Oblation.
Et d'autaut que la voix entend.re
De tiens il te plaira.
Tout droit â toy se venir rend.re
Toutes Gens on verra.
Heureux celuy que veux eslire
Et pres de toy loger Ps: 65
Afin que chez toy se retire
Pour jamais n'en bouger.
Ce Temple a été rebati par la permiss.n de Louis XIII l'An 1624. Et démoli par l'Ordre de Louis XIV. 22 Oct. 1685.
Et rimprimé sur l'Original: par les M.rs de la Societé des Parisiens, l'An 1708.

Fig. 2 The Temple of Charenton, engraving, reprinted in London by members of the Société des Parisiens, 1708

The print bears the words taken from the version of Psalm 65 published by Clément Marot and Théodore de Bèze. The Société des Parisiens was founded in London in 1687 by former members of the Temple of Charenton. Membership was limited to sixty-one, with a joining age between 18 and 41. The applicant had to be of reliable character, sound in mind and body and resident within three miles of Christ Church, Spitalfields. As there were not enough prospective members from Paris it became the Friendly Benefit Society open to Protestants of all nations.

The pest-house referred to in Gastigny's will lay north of Old Street within the parish of St Giles without Cripplegate. This was one of the five London pest-houses to have provided relief during the Great Plague of 1665. For reasons of hygiene, these pest-houses lay beyond the city walls. The Cripplegate pest-house had been built at the time of the plague of 1592 and in 1681 had been handed over to the distributors of the Royal Bounty (fig. 3) for Huguenot refugees from France.

By the late seventeenth century the Royal Bounty had become a considerable resource. William and Mary contributed generously, as did Queen Anne. These funds were further supplemented by parliamentary grants. In the first instance Henry Compton, the Tory Bishop of London and a good friend of the Huguenots, and two other eminent men were made Royal Commissioners. They entrusted the funds to the French Committee, a group of leading Huguenot refugees, for distribution. They were later supervised by the English Committee, worthies from the City of London, who audited the accounts of the clerical division, which had direct responsibility for thirty French Protestant church communities, and the lay division, responsible for the distribution of relief funds. That year a further £40,000 was raised through church and house-to-house collections for the refugees.[11]

The French Committee assumed special responsibility for the upkeep of the Cripplegate pest-house, paying the fees of the visiting doctors and surgeon-apothecary, and the wages of the resident matron and nurse, who cared for the forty to fifty inmates.[12] The chaplain of the pest-house, the Revd Pierre Fontaine, was a cousin of the Revd Jaques Fontaine.[13] Gastigny was a member of the French Committee, regularly attending the weekly meetings. He was also 'a frequent visitor to the Pest House' at Cripplegate. A later director, Arthur Giraud Browning (fig. 59), recorded that 'Gastigny found the house so old and unsuitable and the accommodation it afforded so inadequate that he longed to see his poor fellow-countrymen housed in a building with appointments suited to their French tastes and habits and served by their own kinsfolk'.[14]

Gastigny had attended his last meeting of the committee on 1 September 1708; the following February the committee acknowledged details of the £500 given under Gastigny's bequest and made arrangements for this sum to yield interest for the immediate benefit of the Cripplegate inmates. The French Committee's stewardship of the Cripplegate pest-house was to evolve into responsibility for the French Hospital when it was founded ten years later in 1718. Nine of the 1708 committee's original members became directors of the French Hospital and two served as successive deputy-governors.

The first wave of French-speaking Protestants who had come to Britain and Ireland in the mid-sixteenth century was mostly of Walloons from Spanish Flanders. Five of the sixteen English Committee members in 1705 were of

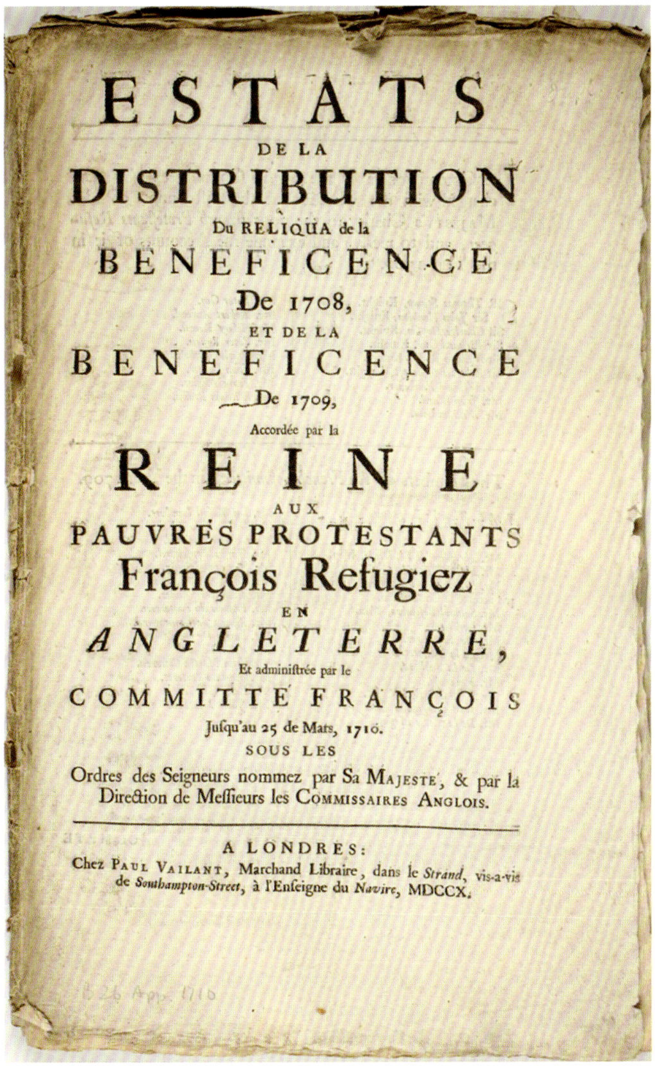

ESTATS
DE LA
DISTRIBUTION
Du RELIQUA de la
BENEFICENCE
De 1708,
ET DE LA
BENEFICENCE
De 1709,
Accordée par la
REINE
AUX
PAUVRES PROTESTANTS
François Refugiez
EN
ANGLETERRE,
Et administrée par le
COMMITTE FRANÇOIS
Jusqu'au 25 de Mars, 1710.
SOUS LES
Ordres des Seigneurs nommez par Sa MAJESTE', & par la Direction de Messieurs les COMMISSAIRES ANGLOIS.

A LONDRES:
Chez PAUL VAILANT, Marchand Libraire, dans le *Strand*, vis-a-vis de *Southampton-Street*, à l'Enseigne du *Navire*, MDCCX.

Fig. 3 (*left*) The Royal Bounty, printed accounts, 1710. *Huguenot Library*

This is the published version of the accounts for the grant of £12,000 made in 1708 and 1709. The accounts were administered by the French Committee and scrutinized by the English Committee. The beneficiaries were listed by social class and the area in which they had settled. The accounts shown here are for the distribution in Brick Lane and Petticoat Lane, Spitalfields. The accounts were published by Paul Vaillant (1671–1739), a Huguenot bookseller in the Strand.

From 1681, the year in which Charles II issued a proclamation offering England as a haven of refuge, the Huguenot refugees were assisted by church collections across the country. A broadsheet of 1688 records that a fund of £40,000 from collections in James II's reign met the needs of some 15,500 refugees of all classes, both in London and the ports where they had landed.

Walloon descent and included Sir John Houblon, James Denew, John Lordell and Sir Peter Delmé. However, the brothers Hilaire and Pierre Reneu had arrived from France in the late seventeenth century and soon made their fortunes in England. Pierre became a founding director of the French Hospital in 1718 and was the recipient of the £100 Gastigny bequest on behalf of La Soupe in Spitalfields. He was the father-in-law of Sir Denis Dutry, a wealthy Flemish merchant of French ancestry.

The Huguenot tradition of self-help and the experience of running the Cripplegate pest-house were valuable factors in its survival. But running costs were hard to meet and disbursements from the Bounty were often very late. Fortunately, the Reneu brothers and Dutry came to the rescue. Gastigny's executor Philippe Ménard, who also served as secretary of the French Committee, husbanded the pest-house bequest carefully. Among the committee members were the army officers Pierre-Jacques du Desert-Dieu and Jacques de La Motte de Blagny, and the successful merchants Jacques Baudouin, Pierre Cabibel the Elder and Philippe Fruchard. Noblemen included Nicolas de Rambouillet, sieur de La Sablière (a kinsman of Henri Massue de Ruvigny, Earl of Galway [fig. 7]) and Guy de Viçouse, baron de La Court of an ancient Languedoc family. The white plume crest of the Viçouse family was said to have been given to an ancestor by Henry of Navarre after the Huguenot victory at the Battle of Ivry in 1590. Navarre's battle cry as recounted in Macaulay's 'Ivry: a Song of the Huguenots' rang out thus:

> Press where ye see my white plume shine, amidst the ranks of war,
> And be your oriflamme to-day the helmet of Navarre.

Viçouse and Cabibel[15] both became governors of the French Hospital and Baudouin its first deputy-governor.

Little is known of the inmates other than their names and dates of arrival as recorded in monthly lists kept by the matron.[16] However, Charles Marmoy sheds some light in his survey of the Cripplegate pest-house as Huguenot refuge, summarizing the 1715/16 report:

> Of the 27 men and 37 women listed 13 were over 70, the eldest being Jean Lemel of Rouen, who was 86; there were four men and three women under 30; Jean Fourreau aged 19 and infirm stayed some six weeks before leaving. Mental illness or senility had brought 15 to the hospital [pest-house] ... In only two cases was there a clue to their past, Edme Boursin of Paris, 72, had been a goldsmith,[17] while Madeleine Boursin of Paris, 78, a jeweller's widow, was *'en enfance'* (as both were inmates ... in June 1716 he could not have been his widow). Two Englishwomen, each married to a Frenchman were among the inmates, as was Elisabeth Haris *'Angloise'*, a cripple who had been a servant in the hospital [pest-house].

As Marmoy shows, the origins of the inmates were widespread: 'from Normandy in the north, La Rochelle and the Île de Ré in the west, from the Cévennes and Languedoc in the south, and from Sedan in the east'.[18] Anne Prestereau had been brought from the Cripplegate pest-house 'affligé[e] en son esprit'; the trauma of fleeing from the Île de Ré in France may have deeply affected her.[19]

1 The only known reference to another member of the Gastigny family in England occurs in the will, proved in 1737, of the Revd Philippe Ménard, Gastigny's executor, in which he left an annuity of £18 to 'Mrs de Fontaine, widow, a relation of the late Mrs Gastigni'. PRO.PROB 11/683 (3 June 1737).

2 J.P. Hore, *History of the Royal Buckhounds* (1898), p. 187.

3 D.W. Ressinger (ed.), *Memoirs of Isaac Dumont de Bostaquet* (*HSNS*, IV, 2005).

4 *Ibid*, p. 235. See J.P. Hore, *History of the Royal Buckhounds* (1898), p. 188.

5 Machtild, Countess Bentinck (ed.), *Lettres de Marie, Reine d'Angleterre ...* (The Hague, 1880), p. 235.

6 Henry L. Snyders, *The Marlborough-Godolphin Correspondence* (Oxford, 1975), vol. 2, *passim*.

7 Winston S. Churchill, *Marlborough, His Life and Times* (1934, 1947 edn), vol. 2, p. 398.

8 Snyders, op. cit., note 6, p. 1277.

9 Churchill, op. cit., note 7, pp. 398–9.

10 PCC Wills PROB 11/505 (2 December 1708). Translation cited by Agnew, pp. 523–4.

11 Smith, *Royal Bounty*, pp. 2–3.

12 The accounts are preserved in the Huguenot Library in London.

13 His memoirs are a classic of Huguenot literature; see D.W. Ressinger, *Memoirs of the Revd Jaques Fontaine*, *HSNS*, II, 1997, pp. 46–7, 202–3. He was not, however, related to Captain Benjamin Elias Fontaine, Gastigny's kinsman.

14 Browning, 'Origin and Early History', p. 44. No source stated.

15 Cabibel was in the silk trade and his grand-daughter, Anne-Rose, was to marry Jean Calas of Toulouse, broken on the wheel on a trumped up charge in 1762, which led to Voltaire's great crusade for religious toleration (see figs. 35–6).

16 Madame Madeleine Liège was succeeded by Madame Anne Bachelier and later by 'Sr Nissole et sa soeur Mme de La Prade'.

17 Murdoch, *Beyond*, p. 120.

18 Marmoy, 'Pest House', p. 397.

19 Robert Nash, in a personal communication, May 2008, citing Marmoy, *Inmates and Applicants*.

2

The new hospital, the royal charter and the corporation

After the Great Fire of London of 1666 several almshouses were rebuilt by City of London guilds and at the same time new almshouses were founded. Many of these were situated where Huguenot refugees had settled to the east of the city. In 1692, Robert Aske founded almshouses for the Haberdashers' Company at Hoxton,[1] while Lady Mico founded those for the Mercers' Company at Stepney. Trinity Almshouses in Mile End Road opened in 1695 at the behest of the Corporation of Trinity House for '28 decayed Masters and Commanders of Ships or ye widows of such as are maintained' (fig. 4). From the 1703 bequest of Sir Robert Geffrye the Ironmongers' Company created almshouses at Kingsland Road, Dalston.[2]

There was already growing commitment to improving the welfare of the needy. But the challenge for Philippe Ménard as Gastigny's executor in 1709 was not to provide almshouse accommodation but to better the living conditions of the inmates of Cripplegate pest-house. This entailed building an extension of 'apartments' funded by Gastigny's bequest. Having tried in vain to persuade the Corporation of the City of London to lease the land adjoining the pest-house, Ménard invested the bequest

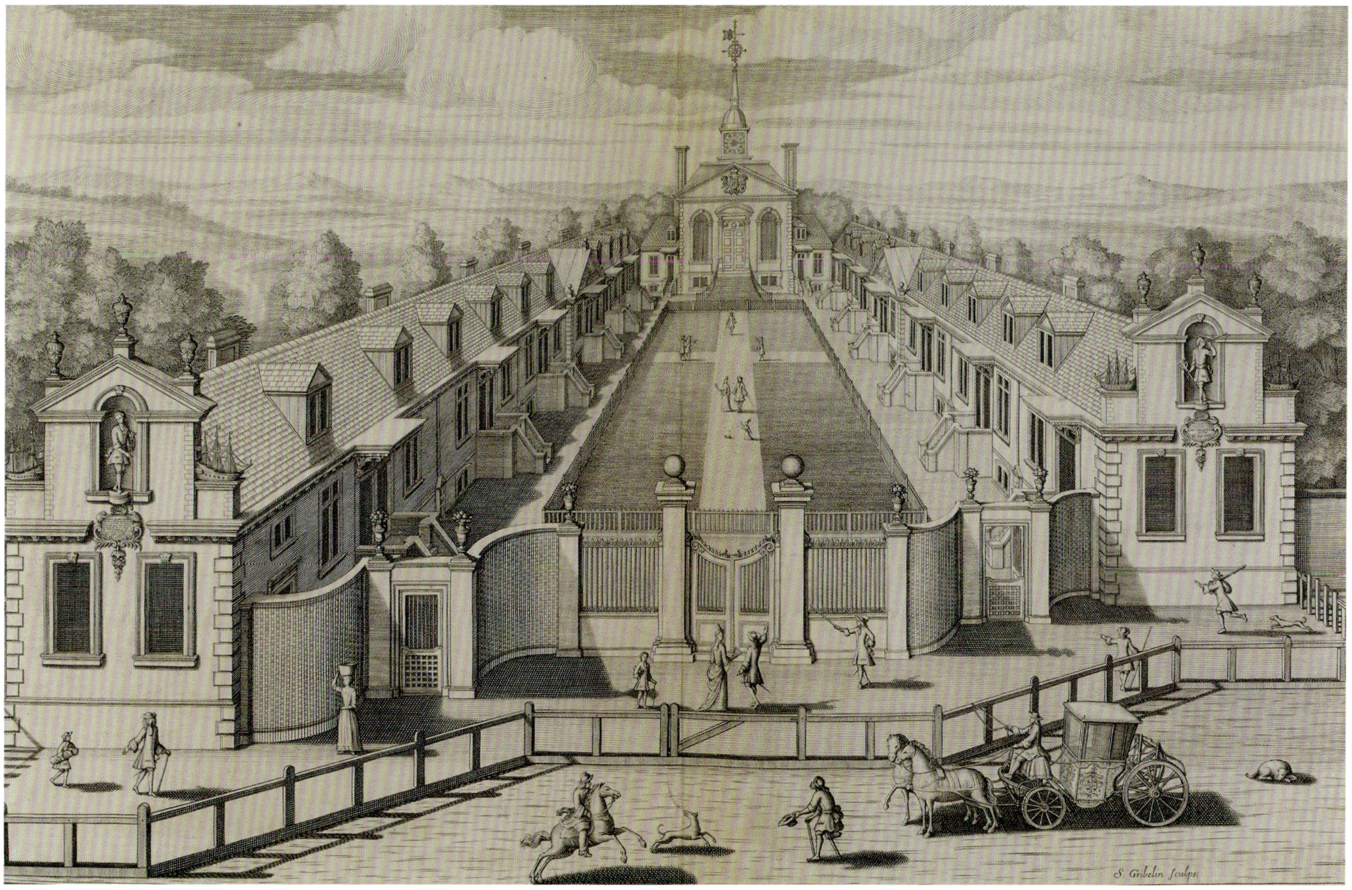

Fig. 4 *Trinity Almshouses at Mile End*, engraving, Simon Gribelin, 1696. *British Museum*

Built in 1695 for masters or commanders of ships or their widows on land provided by Captain Henry Mudd, the cottages are grouped around a chapel. These and other similar almshouses founded by London institutions inspired the foundation of La Providence and the French Almshouses in Black Eagle Street, Spitalfields. Gribelin came from a leading Huguenot family of watchmakers and engravers from Blois and by 1681 had settled in London.

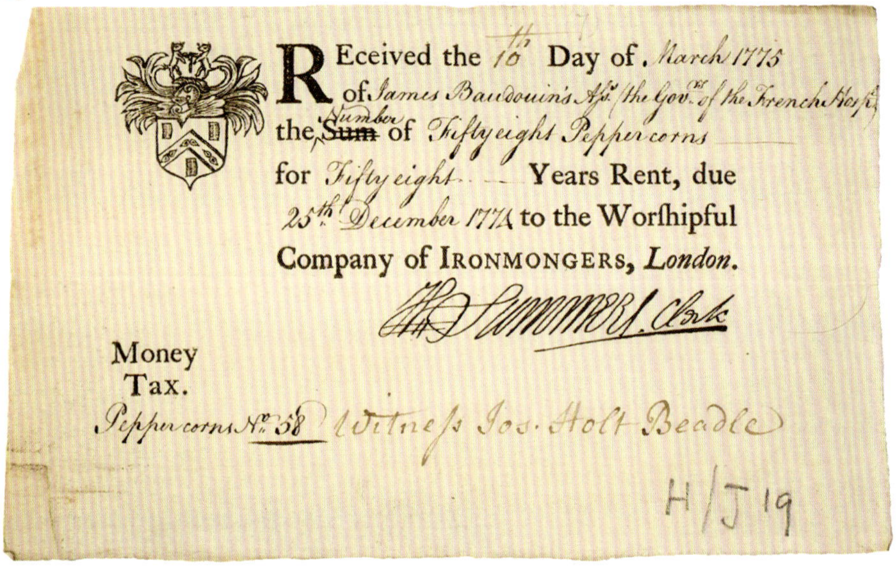
Received the 10th Day of. March 1775
of James Baudouin's Ass. the Gov. of the French Hosp.
the ~~Sum~~ Number of Fiftyeight Peppercorns
for Fiftyeight ... Years Rent, due
25th December 1774 to the Worſhipful
Company of IRONMONGERS, *London*.
[signature] Clerk
Money
Tax.
Peppercorns No. 58 Witness Jos. Holt Beadle
H/J 19

Fig. 5 Receipt for 58 peppercorns representing the rent due to the Worshipful Company of Ironmongers for the lease of the land on which the French Hospital was built, 1774. *Huguenot Library*

This nominal rent was received by the Clerk and Beadle of the Ironmongers' Company from James [Jacques] Baudouin's representative. Baudouin had served as deputy-governor of the French Hospital from 1718 to 1720 when the lease was first taken out.

money and the interest helped alleviate immediate financial pressures.

Luckily another plot of land, known as the Golden Acre, became available south of the pest-house. Its owners, the Ironmongers' Company, agreed to sell the 990-year lease for a peppercorn rent (fig. 5) and the lease was signed on 25 March 1716 by Jacques Baudouin on behalf of the French Committee.

The ensuing appeal was endorsed by the Revd Louis Saurin, brother of the more famous Revd Jacques Saurin (fig. 6), but nevertheless one of the most distinguished of the refugee pastors,[3] as *modérateur,* and Philippe Ménard as *secrétaire*. Donations ranging from one guinea to £100 were made by almost sixty subscribers and came to a grand total of £474 9s. Even more gifts were to follow so that by November 1718 £2,372 16s had been collected.[4]

All told, there were some 600 subscribers to the appeal, the most generous of whom were Jacques Baudouin (£100), Benjamin Baronneau, Paul Dufour and Louis de Tudert (each £50), the marquise de Gouvernet (£52 10s), Lord Galway (£40) (fig. 7), and the duchesse de La Force (£20), the merchants Moreau (£50), Le Coq and Le Bas (£40 each).[5] Louis de Tudert had already shown his generosity when he presented the French congregation at Hoxton with a paten (fig. 8).[6] The largest donation of £150 came from the Revd Jean Ménard, Philippe Ménard's brother. The Francophile Duke and Duchess of Kingston were among the handful of English donors as was George I's first minister, Charles Spencer, Earl of Sunderland.

So much funding was made available that the ambition

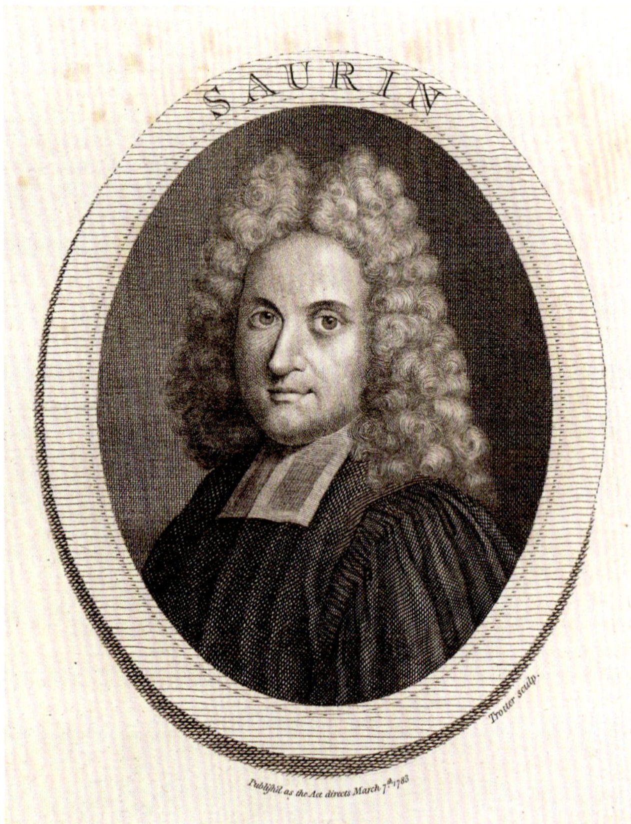

Fig. 6 Revd Jacques Saurin, engraving, Thomas Trotter, 1787

Jacques Saurin came from Nîmes. He was elected minister of the French Church of London in 1701, a post he held until 1706 when he sought permission to leave on grounds of ill health. Saurin went on to the Netherlands. His brother Louis, also a distinguished minister, presided over the meeting of the French Committee for the distribution of the Royal Bounty on 3 March 1716 at which it was proposed to purchase land and invite subscriptions for the building of a hospital.

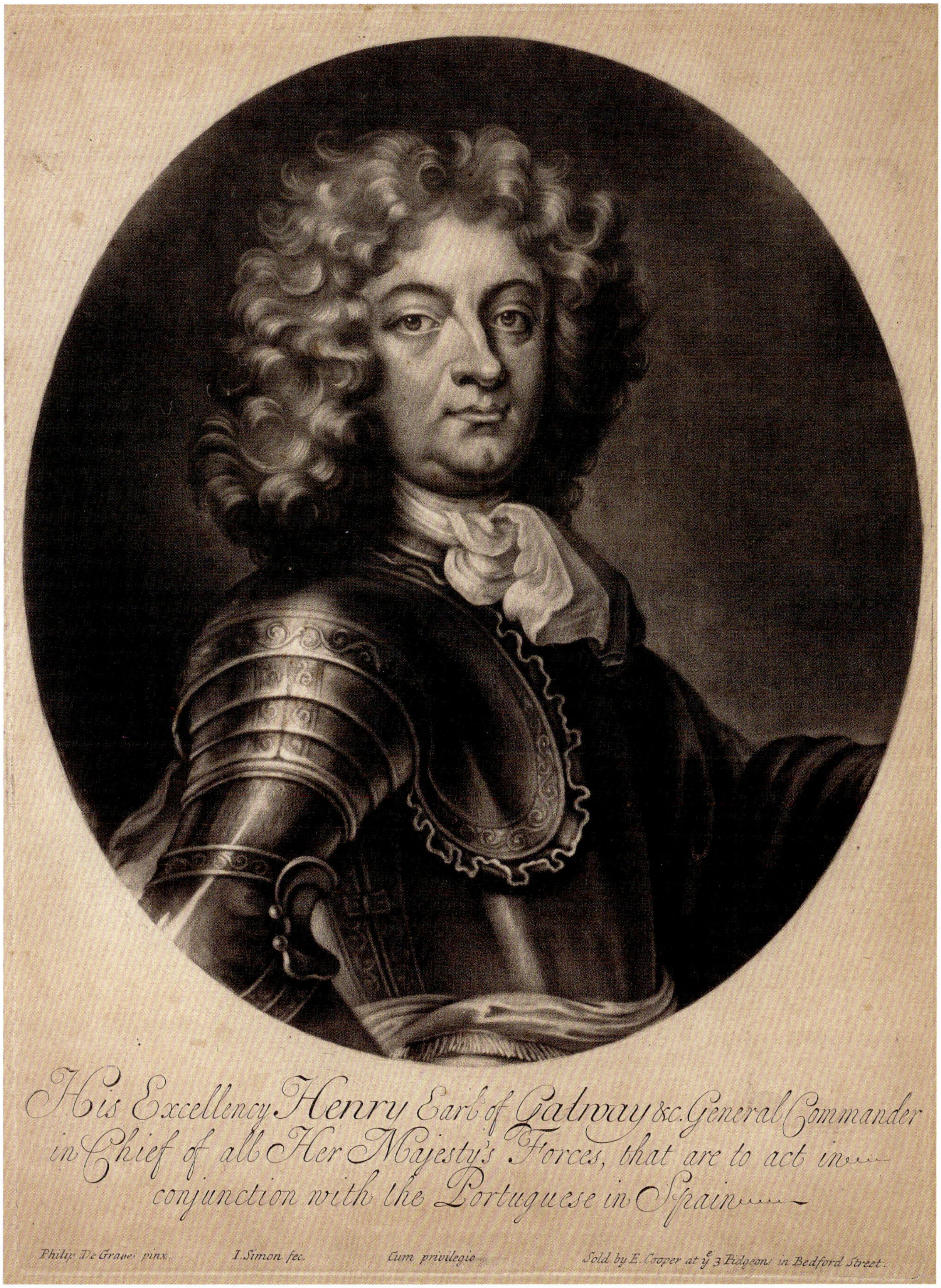
His Excellency Henry Earl of Galway &c. General Commander
in Chief of all Her Majesty's Forces, that are to act in
conjunction with the Portuguese in Spain
Philip De Graves pinx.
I. Simon fec.
Cum privilegio
Sold by E. Cooper at ye 3 Pidgeons in Bedford Street.

Fig. 7 Henri de Massue de Ruvigny, Earl of Galway (1648–1720), mezzotint, John Simon, c. 1705

Galway fought at the Battle of the Boyne and founded the military refugee community at Portarlington. He served as Commander-in-Chief of the English Forces in Ireland and twice as ruling Lord Justice. On the accession of George I, Ruvigny presented the new king with an address on behalf of the Huguenot community in London congratulating him on establishing the Protestant succession.

of the French Committee grew from merely building an extension to the Cripplegate pest-house to building a brand new hospital. Plans were drawn and building began even before a royal charter of incorporation had been obtained. On behalf of the French Committee, the Earl of Galway petitioned George I. In the deed the committee members are dubbed 'Refugees Naturalized in behalfe of themselves and severall French Refugees who have the happiness of being Your Majesty's Subjects'. The petition recalled Gastigny's bequest 'towards the building of an Hospitall … which has induced your humble Petitioners to begin building an Hospitall for lodging or subsisting a small number of the Poorest Sort of their Nation.' It went on to say:

> This Charitable design hath met with great encouragement from Severall pious Souls who have Cheerfully Contributed towards it and your humble Petitioners hope to bring it to a happy Conclusion Trusting under God Almighty that it will bee attended with such Usefull and happy Effects as to bee hereafter maintained and supported by all Good and Charitable Christians.

The petition recalled the purchase of the Golden Acre, provided for a governor, Henry [Henri], Earl of Galway, a deputy-governor, James [Jacques] Baudouin, and thirty-seven directors with the power to institute by-laws and pass resolutions, to elect also a treasurer and a 'Minister … of the Church of England' and to commission a Common Seal.[7] The supporting document to the petition for the building of the French Hospital states that Gastigny's £1,000 legacy 'not being Sufficient to Carry on and Compleat the building of the said Hospitall', a further £1,500 had been raised.[8]

When the petition was referred to the Attorney-General, Sir Edward Northey, MP, he certified that 'the Design of the Petitioners [was] very just and Charitable' and raised no objection to the incorporation. It was agreed that it should be called the 'Hospital for Poor French Protestants and their Descendants Residing in Great Britain'. It was further agreed that 'the Capacity of Purchasing Land be Restrained to a certain Annual Value' and that the hospital 'relieve' only 'French Protestants or their descendants resident in Great Britain for six months or more' and 'who shall take the Oaths of Allegiance and Supremacy and the Abjuration Oath before the Governor and Directors or any three or more of them.'[9] The French Hospital was incorporated under the Great Seal by letters patent signed by Charles Cocks, Clerk of the Patents, and dated 24 July 1718.[10]

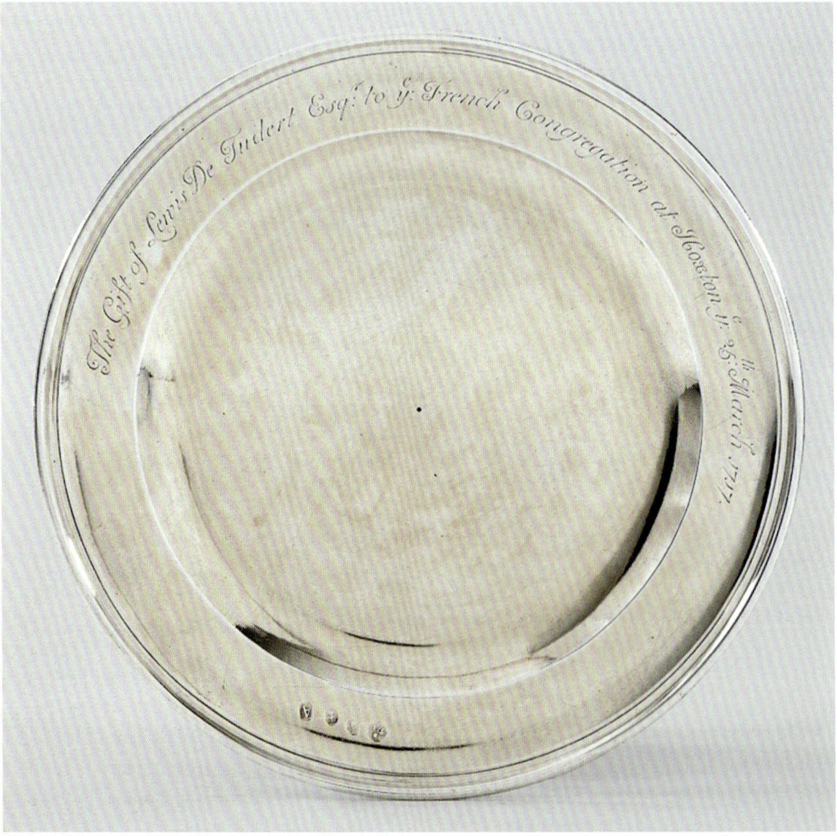
The Gift of Lewis De Tudert Esq.r to y.e French Congregation at Hoxton y.e 25 March 1717

Fig. 8 Paten, silver (Britannia standard), maker's mark of Robert Hill, London, 1716/17, given by Louis de Tudert to the French congregation at Hoxton, 1717

Louis de Tudert acted twice as guarantor to inmates of the hospital; in 1719 to Marie Vautier and in 1727 to Magdeleine Fauchet. Marie Vautier 'na Rien aporté que Ce quelle avoit sur son corps'. He paid 2 shillings 6 pence per week for her maintenance, but did not contribute to the cost of her funeral five years later. For Magdeleine Fauchet he made a weekly contribution of 1s 6d and 6s 3d towards the cost of her funeral in 1729. When he died in 1739 and was buried in the Dutch church, Austin Friars, he left bequests of £100 each to the French Hospital and the Spitalfields 'Soupe' as well as £25 to the Swiss Society; £250 to the hospital in Geneva and £100 for the fortifications of Geneva. See Marmoy, *Inmates and Applicants*, I and II.

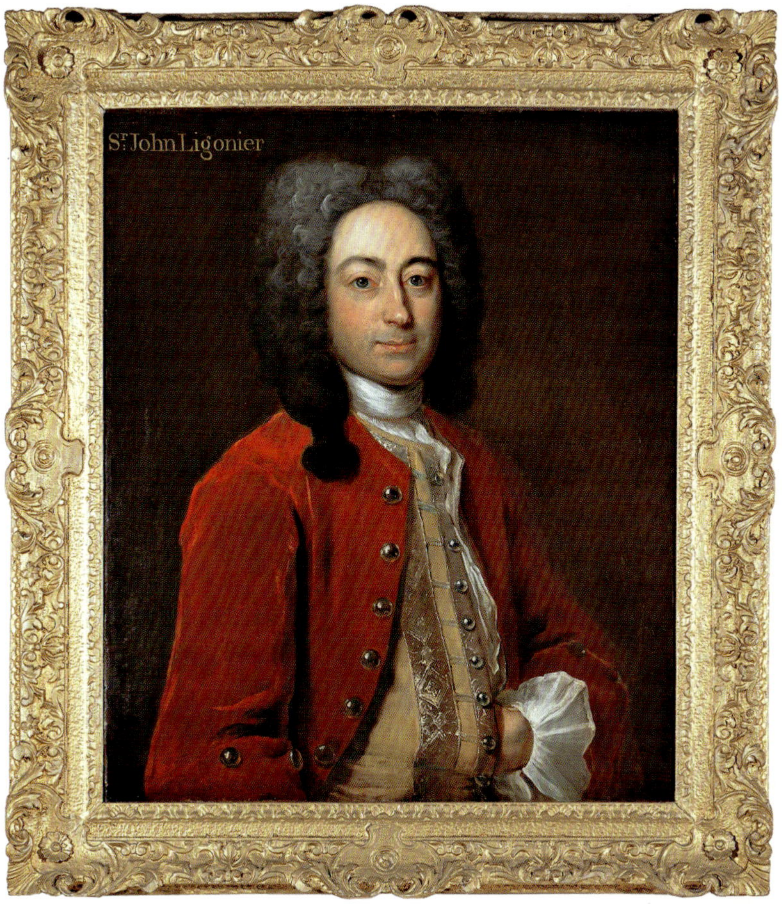

Fig. 9 Sir John [Jean-Louis] Ligonier, later Field-Marshal Earl (1680–1770), oil on canvas, Philip Mercier, c. 1738, in contemporary giltwood frame

Sir John (later Earl Ligonier) was governor of the French Hospital from 1748 to 1770. The son of Louis de Ligonier from Castres, he left France under an assumed name at the age of seventeen, settling initially in Dublin in 1697. He joined the army in the reign of William III and served under John Churchill, 1st Duke of Marlborough, from 1702 in the Wars of the Spanish Succession. He was Commander-in-Chief of the British Army and Master General of the Ordnance during the Seven Years' War, 1756–1763.

The son of a Huguenot tapestry weaver, Philip Mercier was born in Berlin. He studied there under the painter Antoine Pesne, and toured Italy and France, before settling in London in 1716, where he worked as a dealer and artist. In 1729 he was appointed Principal Painter and Library Keeper to Frederick, Prince of Wales.

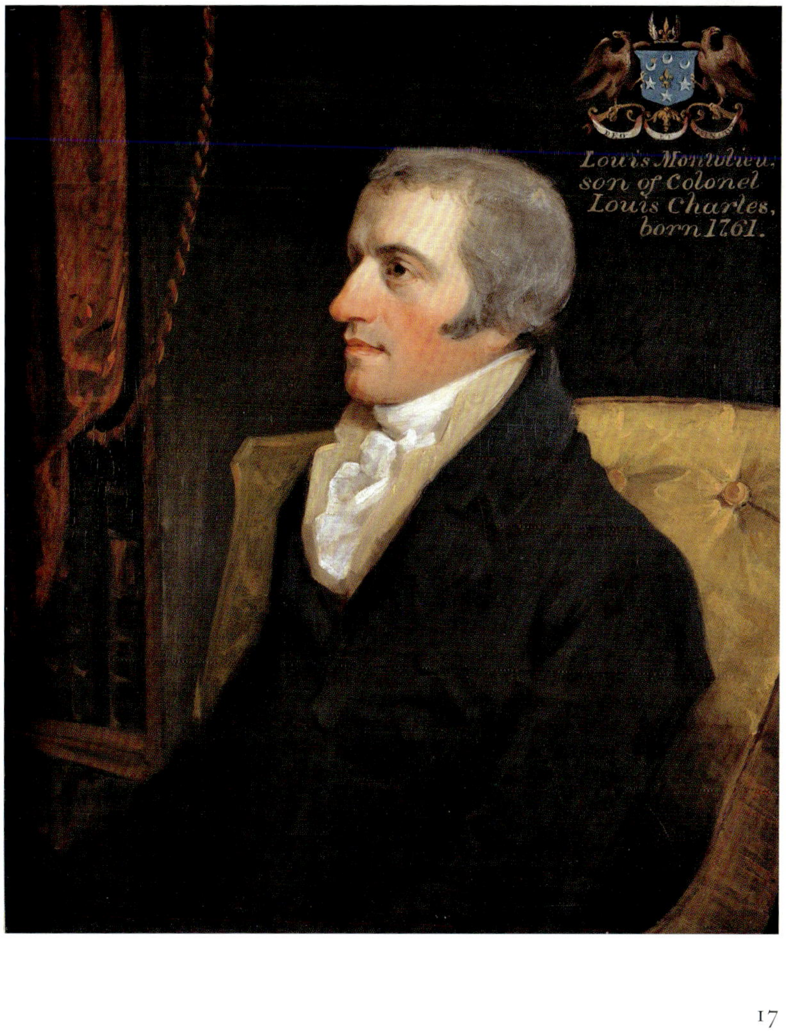

Fig. 10 Louis Montolieu, baron de Saint-Hippolyte (c. 1761–1822), oil on canvas, Joseph Clover, 1806

Louis Montolieu was the son of Colonel Louis Montolieu who became a director in 1759 and was lieutenant-colonel, 2nd Troop of Horse Guards. He married Elizabeth, the daughter of Peter and Clara Le Heup (figs. 77 and 78). He was a kinsman of David Montolieu de Saint-Hippolyte and two of his maternal uncles were directors; Jacques Molinier elected in 1721 and Charles Molinier in 1756.

Joseph Clover (1779–1853) was a portrait painter working in London and Norwich.

The royal charter of incorporation recalled Gastigny's bequest, granted royal sanction, named the Earl of Galway and the thirty-seven founding directors and duly granted them and their successors incorporation with all that entailed. It allowed a 'Common Seal for the Affairs and Business of the said Corporation' to be used 'forever hereafter'. They could own buildings and land, appoint and re-elect officers, make by-laws, make decisions with a quorum of ten, and pass resolutions after the giving of three days' notice by the secretary.[11] In the *Ordres et Règlements*,[12] known today as the 'Blue Book', the governors, the other directors and officers are listed with their dates of election.[13] A thousand copies of the first edition were published in French in 1723.[14] An English translation was also included.

From very early on, the inmates called the institution La Providence. It was named thus in wills in the 1720s, perhaps inspired by the choice of Elijah being fed by the ravens (1 King's 17:6) as the corporation's own seal. At the Court meeting in November 1718, a director, Pierre Marchant, was asked to order the seal from a die maker. As a working jeweller Marchant was well placed to do so.[15]

The directors were prosperous merchants, professional men, clergy and master craftsmen. Some were distinguished soldiers, among them Galway (fig. 7), Ligonier (fig. 9), Montolieu, baron de Saint-Hippolyte (fig. 10), Louis de Jean (fig. 11), the Montresor family, and Generals John Carnac and William Anne de Villettes.

The Huguenot community in London had founded an institution that was financially independent. Amidst orchards and market gardens the buildings of the French Hospital were already rising. There the community would house fellow Huguenots in need.

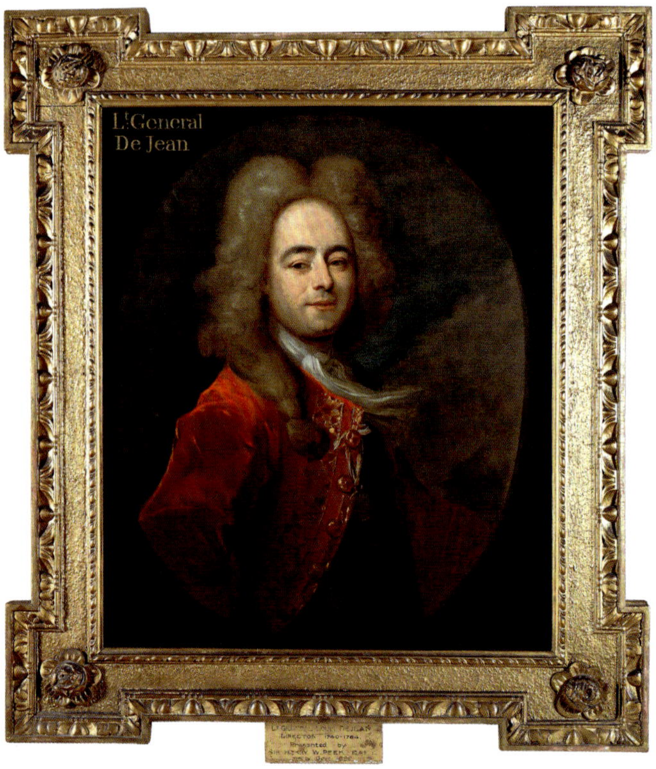

Fig. 11 Lieutenant-General Louis de Jean (1706–1764), oil on canvas, formerly attributed to Philip Mercier, 1730s, in contemporary carved and gilt frame

De Jean is shown as a lieutenant-colonel in the Grenadier Guards. He became a colonel in the 14th Light Dragoons in 1752 and 6th Dragoon Guards in 1757. He was second in command to General Wade during his campaign in the Scottish Highlands. Lieutenant-General de Jean was a director of the French Hospital from 1740 and proposed his friend and comrade Sir John Ligonier as a director. De Jean died in Dublin in 1764.

1 P.H. Ditchfield, *The City Companies of London and Their Good Works, A Record of Their History, Charity and Treasure* (1926), pp. 27, 30–1, 120–1, 143, 155–6; Ben Weinreb and Christopher Hibbert, *The London Encyclopaedia* (1983), p. 890.

2 Now the Geffrye Museum.

3 By 1716 the Revd Jacques Saurin was serving as a French Protestant minister at The Hague.

4 Browning, 'Origin and Early History', Appendix 2, pp. 61–2. Browning's National Archives reference for his Appendices 2, 3 and 4 is Home Office Law Papers, vol. 2, now catalogued as SP 35. See SP35/14 for an advertisement relating to a fund for the relief of poor French refugees.

5 For Le Bas, see T. Murdoch, 'A Brass Inlaid Jewel Chest on Stand made for Rebecca, Viscountess Harcourt,' *Furniture History*, XXXIII (1997), pp. 104–8.

6 This is now in the French Hospital collection.

7 Browning, 'Origin and Early History', Appendix 3, pp. 63–4.

8 *Ibid.*, Appendix 3, pp. 66–7.

9 *Ibid.*, Appendix 3, pp. 65–6.

10 Illustrated in Murdoch, p. 83.

11 Browning, 'Origin and Early History', Appendix 4, pp. 70–3.

12 Known as *Charter and By-laws* from 1860.

13 The 'Blue Book', first published in 1723, has run to ten editions, the latest published in 2000.

14 As recorded in the French Hospital Court Minutes for 3 July 1723.

15 He was almost certainly related to a Pierre Marchant who was received into the Paris Goldsmiths' Company as the son of a master in 1659 (Murdoch, *Beyond*, p. 126). By 1689, the list of Paris goldsmiths states that this Marchant was in England, where he was recorded as a goldsmith in 1694 and a 'Marchand Jouaillier' in 1698. By 1699, he was in the parish of St Anne's, Porter Street (Joan Evans, 'Huguenot Goldsmiths in England and Ireland', *PHS*, XIV, 4 (1933), p. 545).

3

Building and furnishing the French Hospital

The only records to survive of the original building works at the Golden Acre site[1] are eighteen receipts for payments on account and the final statement signed by the contractor, Peter Legrant.[2] The receipts are dated from 11 July 1716 to 19 December 1718 and the final statement totalling £2,750 was settled on 12 March 1719.

The largest component was £1,741 3s 4d paid for '35 square and 82 foot 4 inches of building at £50 per square', and a further £740 for building the kitchen, chapel and gallery, 'nine roomes for the Madd Pepell', closets, wells, 'kirbs', doors, windows, the 'Beare Seller'and 'straw Houses'. The £101 remaining paid for beds and pillows, 'closase stooles', 'presses', door-cases, locks, hinges, much bricking up of doors and windows of the abandoned pest-house on the northern border of the hospital's grounds, and for 'mending the plastring of the Ould House'.[3]

Forty of the hospital's first sixty inmates moved from the Cripplegate pest-house with the steward, Nissole, as well as his sister and the indoor and outdoor servants. Nissole found the challenge of the move too much and in 1720 was succeeded by Jean Chaboussant, one of three French Committee members of the Royal Bounty not to become directors of the French Hospital.[4]

A preliminary meeting of the governor and directors of the French Hospital was held on 3 September 1718. Ménard was elected secretary, Louis Royrand des Clouseaux (a cousin of Madame Ménard) treasurer and the Revd François Duplessis, who had succeeded Pastor Fontaine at

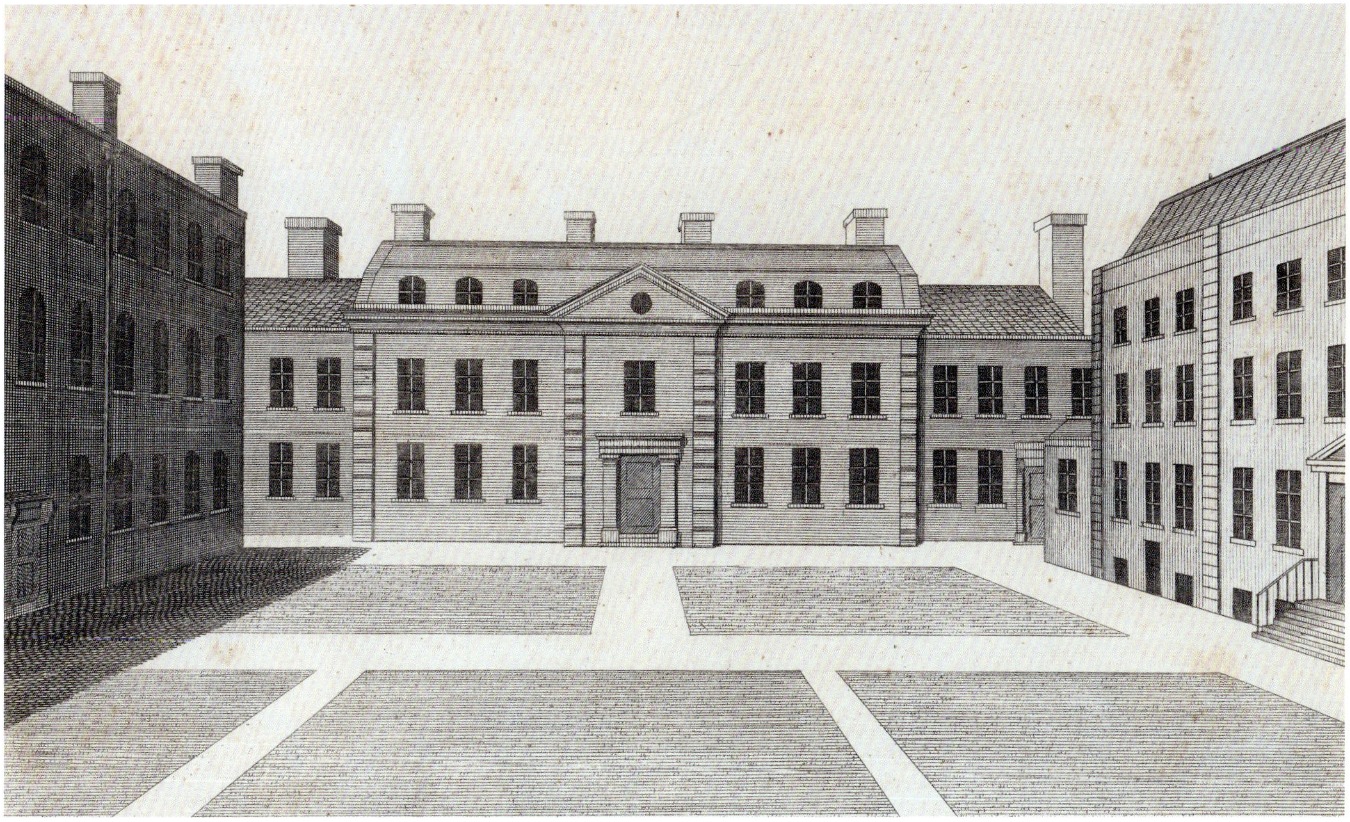

Fig. 12 *The French Protestant Hospital, near Old Street*, engraving by B. Cole from Maitland's *History of London*, 1756
This shows the western quadrangle situated on the other side of Pest House Row from the Peerless Pool. To the east of the hospital, French Alley led to St Luke's Church, completed in 1733 to the designs of John James and Nicholas Hawksmoor.

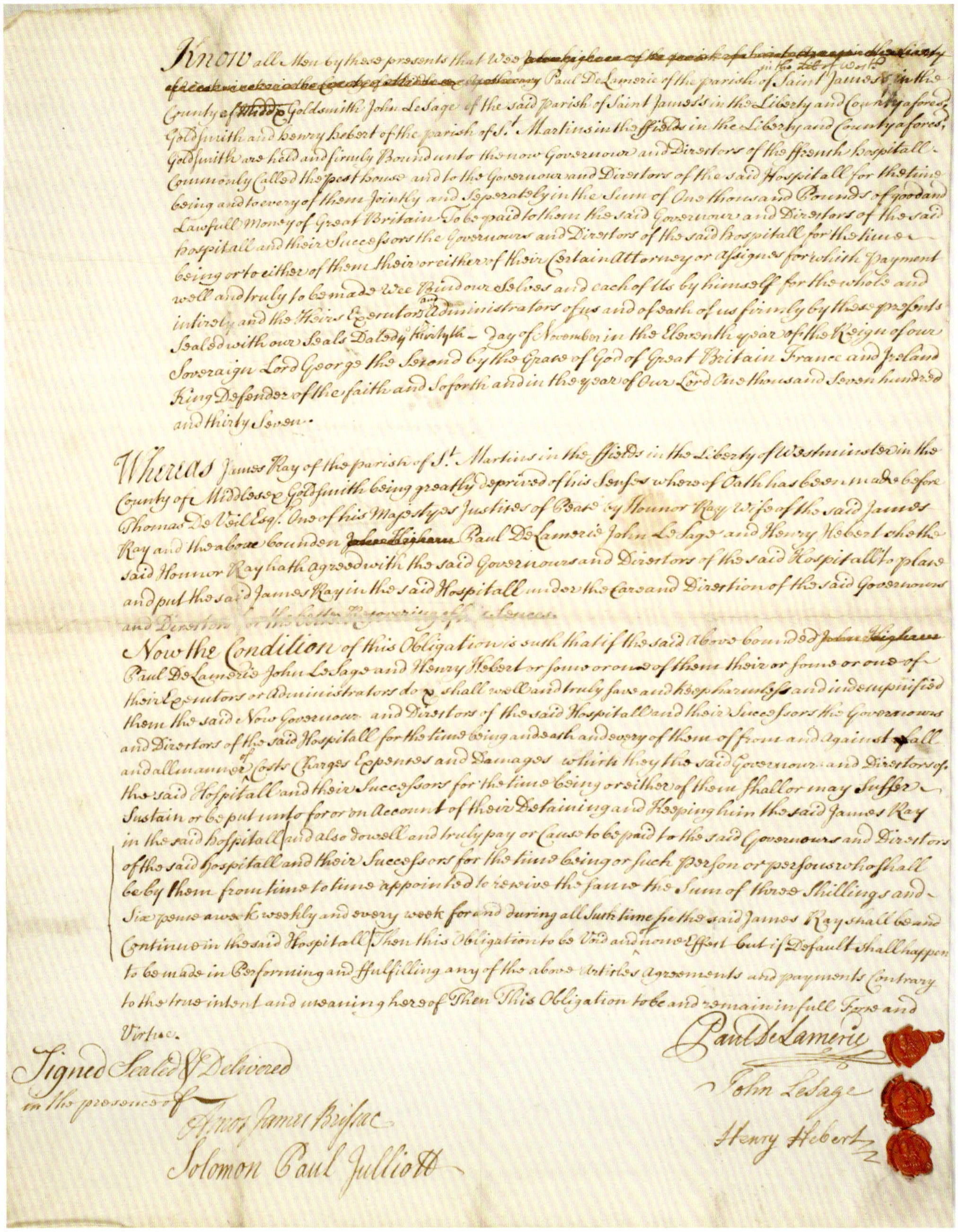

Know all Men by these presents that Wee [illegible] in the Lib of Westm Paul De Lamerie of the parish of Saint James's in the County of [illegible] Goldsmith John LeSage of the said parish of Saint James's in the Liberty and County afores. Goldsmith and Henry Hebert of the parish of St. Martins in the ffields in the Liberty and County afores. Goldsmith are held and firmly Bound unto the now Governour and Directors of the ffrench Hospitall Commonly Called the pest house and to the Governour and Directors of the said Hospitall for the time being and to every of them Jointly and Seperately in the Sum of One thousand Pounds of good and Lawfull Money of Great Britain To be paid to them the said Governour and Directors of the said hospitall and their Successors the Governours and Directors of the said hospitall for the time being or to either of them their or either of their Certain Attorney or Assignes for which Payment well and truly to be made Wee Bind our Selves and each of Us by himself for the whole and intirely and the Heirs Executors and Administrators of us and of each of us firmly by these presents Sealed with our Seals Dated ye thirtyth day of November in the Eleventh year of the Reign of our Sovereign Lord George the Second by the Grace of God of Great Britain France and Ireland King Defender of the faith and So forth and in the year of Our Lord One thousand Seven hundred and thirty Seven.

Whereas James Ray of the parish of St. Martins in the ffields in the Liberty of Westminster in the County of Middlesex Goldsmith being greatly deprived of his Senses whereof Oath has been made before Thomas De Veil Esq. One of his Majestyes Justices of Peace by Honnor Ray Wife of the said James Ray and the above bounden [illegible] Paul De Lamerie John LeSage and Henry Hebert or the said Honnor Ray hath agreed with the said Governours and Directors of the said Hospitall to place and put the said James Ray in the said Hospitall under the Care and Direction of the said Governours and Directors for the better Recovering of his Senses.

Now the Condition of this Obligation is such that if the said Above bounden [illegible] Paul De Lamerie John LeSage and Henry Hebert or some or one of them their or some or one of their Executors or Administrators do or shall well and truly save and keep harmless and indempnified them the said Now Governour and Directors of the said Hospitall and their Successors the Governours and Directors of the said Hospitall for the time being and each and every of them of from and against all and all manner of Costs Charges Expenses and Damages which they the said Governour and Directors of the said Hospitall and their Successors for the time being or either of them shall or may Suffer Sustain or be put unto for or on Account of their Detaining and Keeping him the said James Ray in the said hospitall and also do well and truly pay or Cause to be paid to the said Governours and Directors of the said hospitall and their Successors for the time being or such person or persons who shall be by them from time to time appointed to receive the same the Sum of three Shillings and Six pence a week weekly and every week for and during all Such time as the said James Ray shall be and Continue in the said Hospitall Then this Obligation to be Void and of none Effect but if Default shall happen to be made in Performing and ffulfilling any of the above Articles Agreements and payments Contrary to the true intent and meaning hereof Then This Obligation to be and remain in full Force and Virtue.

Signed Sealed & Delivered in the presence of
Amos James Brissac
Solomon Paul Julliott

Paul De Lamerie
John LeSage
Henry Hebert

Fig. 13 Affidavit signed by Paul de Lamerie for James [Jacques] Ray, 1737. *Huguenot Library*

The celebrated goldsmith Paul de Lamerie and the goldsmiths Henry [Henri] Hebert and John [Jean] Le Sage, served as guarantors against the costs of any damages caused by the goldsmith Jacques Ray when he became an inmate of the hospital. No longer able to cope with the daily demands of his trade, Ray had taken to wandering the streets crying 'Oranges and Lemons'.

the Cripplegate pest-house, 'Minister and Chaplain'. The second meeting or Court, held the following month, adopted the by-laws, many of them unchanged to this day. On 12 November the hospital and the chapel were dedicated 'after the Rites of the Church of England' and a sermon was preached by Philippe Ménard 'in the midst of a great concourse of refugees and their families'.[5]

The earliest known view of the hospital buildings put up by Peter Legrant is the engraving by B. Cole in Maitland's *History of London* (1756, fig. 12). It shows the seven-bay centre block of the ultimately H-shaped range of buildings, built on two quadrangles with the two later wings forming the front quadrangle added in 1732–3 by Thomas du Bisson.

Du Bisson was clerk of works at Winchester Palace, Southwark, and had been clerk of works at Stanmer Park, near Brighton, under Nicholas Dubois. He was surveyor of the London property of the Earl of Guilford, and may have worked with Dubois on the houses of Hanover Square.[6]

The later wings at the French Hospital contained a ground-floor kitchen and two refectories, one for the men and one for the women, with rooms and infirmaries on two floors above. The directors' Court Room was probably adjacent to the men's refectory.

Du Bisson's extensions included better accommodation for the mentally ill. Their small cells, known as 'les petites maisons', were rebuilt to his design and two 'warming rooms' fitted with 'warm air machines' were also provided.

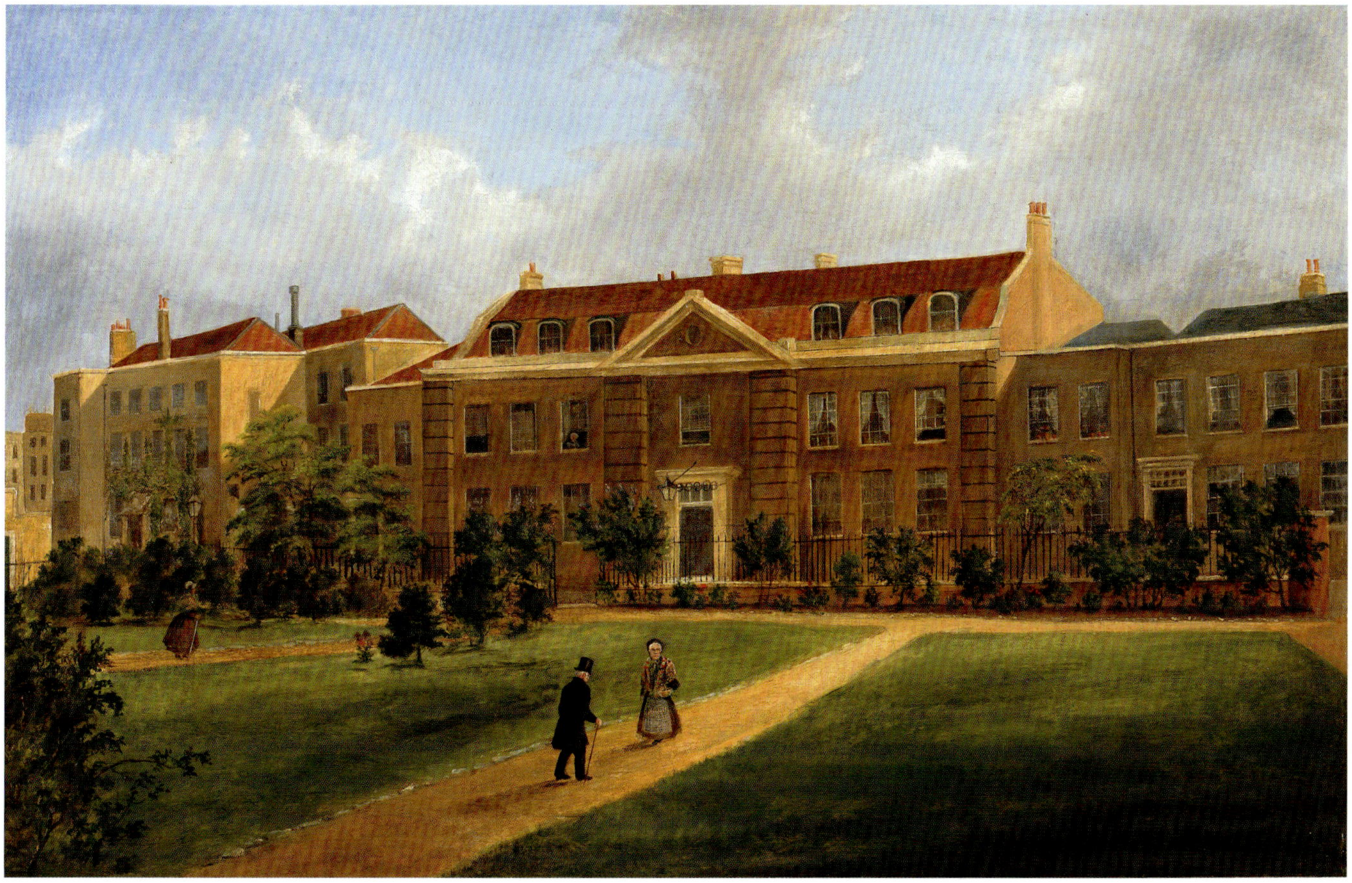

Fig. 14 *The French Hospital, Old Street, Finsbury*, oil on canvas, artist unknown, c. 1860

The main pedimented building housed the refectory to the left with kitchens beyond and the directors' Court Room to the right. The door on the left opened into the chapel. The wash-house, larders and stores were in the adjoining building at the far left. There is still a Galway Street on the site today commemorating the first governor.

This building also housed a five-foot-deep cold-water cistern 'constructed like the one at Bedlam'. Yet, unlike Bedlam, the French Hospital saved the mentally ill from the indignity of public viewing. The goldsmith, Jacques Ray, admitted to the French Hospital in 1737 with the backing of his celebrated colleague in the trade, Paul de Lamerie, would have benefited from the improvements to these facilities (fig. 13).[7]

The cost of building the extensions turned out to be below the estimate and Du Bisson wrote on his receipt: 'I have made a present of the amount of this bill to the Corporation'.[8]

In 1763 the bakehouse wing was rebuilt following a successful appeal and a new brewery erected in 1765, both designed by a new architect, Boulton Mainwaring. Starting as an apprentice joiner in Cheshire, Mainwaring later worked as an architect in London and Middlesex, His most notable achievement was his London Hospital building of 1757 still standing in the Whitechapel Road.

The French Hospital was among the first of the London hospitals in the modern sense to be founded in the eighteenth century. The earlier foundations of Les Invalides, Paris, the Royal Hospital, Chelsea, and the Royal Hospital, Kilmainham, near Dublin, may have been an added source of inspiration. A hospital for retired seamen had been established at Greenwich, to the east of London and by 1704 the Royal Naval Hospital, Greenwich, was ready to receive the first 42 residents and by December 1708 the number had risen to 350.[9] After the French Hospital's incorporation in 1718, Westminster followed in 1720; Guy's in 1721; St George's in 1733; the London Hospital in 1740; and the Middlesex in 1745. The French Hospital also anticipated other London charitable institutions with special philanthropic purpose: the Foundling Hospital of 1739; the Magdalen Hospital (for penitent prostitutes) of 1758; the Marine Society (which trained homeless boys for the sea); and the Asylum for Female Orphans.[10]

The French Hospital also took in soldiers and sailors who had served in the British army and navy. Pierre Le Blond was admitted in 1750 as a hapless sailor aged 34 who had been totally blinded in a cannon accident on board ship. He apparently took to drink. Pierre Rousset had been admitted in 1746 having served as a sergeant in Portugal, and François Rondelet in 1750 having spent his life in the army.[11]

The French Hospital accounts record improvements to the extensive grounds, including the planting of seventeen trees in the courtyard in April 1719. Then in 1738, after thirty years of refusal to co-operate, the Corporation of London's Land Committee sold the Cripplegate pest-house site to the French Hospital on a 970-year lease for a rent of £400 10s per annum.[12] When the old pest-house was demolished that same year, this site was also made over to gardens. The following year an orchard of 180 fruit trees was planted comprising 'mulberries, peaches, quinces, nectarines and vines, as well as plums, cherries and pears ('Beurre de Roi', 'Bonchrétienne', 'Doyanné de Comice', 'Saint-Germain' and other varieties recorded by the gardener Fonteneau)'.[13]

The earliest known painting of the French Hospital dates from the nineteenth century (fig. 14), and the only published descriptions of its buildings date from their last days, when the surroundings had changed beyond recognition. Nevertheless, the applications for admission recorded from 1718 paint an extraordinary picture of the circumstances of those admitted. The diary kept by the steward Adam Roumieu from 1742 to 1769, gives a glimpse of day-to-day housekeeping and the lives of the inmates and the inventories of 1742 (see pp. 111–16) and 1766 provide detailed listings of the hospital's contents and equipment.[14]

As Charles Marmoy, the compiler of the alphabetical directory of applications for admission, has noted, 'The ordeals which so many had endured had proved too much for some',[15] and cites the case of David Coste, who had been a clandestine pastor in France and had gone mad after escaping to England. The suffering of those who escaped from France, some undergoing imprisonment, torture or maltreatment, some losing kith and kin or friends, was extreme. The stress of being a refugee combined with the uncertainties of daily life of the urban poor was more than some of them could bear. Some of those who had suffered were admitted to the French Hospital. Pierre Tartas (1730), David Couderc (1733), Jean Lardant (1733) and Isaac Raymond (1757) were all inmates who in France had been condemned to the galleys for their faith.[16] Several inmates had been imprisoned, including Jean Desmarets (1730), who had 'beaucoup souffert en France', and Abraham L'Houmeau (1749), who had escaped from prison in France, having been arrested for attending a religious assembly, and had been forced to leave behind a wife and four children.[17]

The detailed information about the inmates in the registers, medical and funeral accounts as well as in the stewards' reports provides a rare insight into their lives before and after admission.[18] The great majority were penniless and infirm. Marie Caillon of Spitalfields, was 'très infirme et hors d'état de gagner sa vie'; Jaques Goudemay, 51, originally of Picardy, was 'affligé d'Asthme et Hydropisie', in 1758, and François Rossignol from Babre in the Languedoc (Barre, Lozère?), 70, 'très pauvre et affligé de Goute & Rhumatisme qui le mettent entierement hors d'Etat de travailler', in 1763. Poor Rossignol was placed in the Petites Maisons, which was the section of the hospital for the mentally ill, until a bed could be found for him 'dans la maison', with inmates of sound mind. He left in 1767, having married Madeleine Ganeron, who had been living in the Petites Maisons until 'cured'. Her return as a widow was accepted in 1770 since she was 'très destistuez et incapable de travailler' but 'on ne la trouve pas'.

La Providence provided both for the sick, like Jaques Goudemay, noted on arrival as 'maintenant Malade au Lit' and also for the old, one of whom was described simply as 'très infirme et incapable de gagner sa vie' and another 'entierement sourd et fort pauvre'. From 1718 onwards, applicants had to be so ill or infirm that they could no longer work. Physical conditions at the hospital were perhaps superior to their own homes or better than those other members of their family could provide. Thus inmates were allowed considerable dignity in their old age.[19] The young were also accepted as inmates despite Gastigny's stipulation to help those 'over fifty years'. There was Jean-Jaques Pennel (or Pesnel) , 15, who was admitted with an ulcerated broken leg and left cured seven months later,[20] or the deranged Nathanael Bobin, 10, admitted in 1731 and who remained in the Petites Maisons until his death twenty-nine years later. Like Guy's Hospital, founded in 1720, the French Hospital cared for many such who were *aliénés* or insane, whether victims of depression or 'furiously mad' and 'dangerous'. Marie L'Heureux, admitted in 1744 and aged about 40 (one of thirteen inmates or applicants of that name between 1725 and 1819), was moved to Guy's in 1745, where she died in 1750, her burial paid for by the corporation.[21]

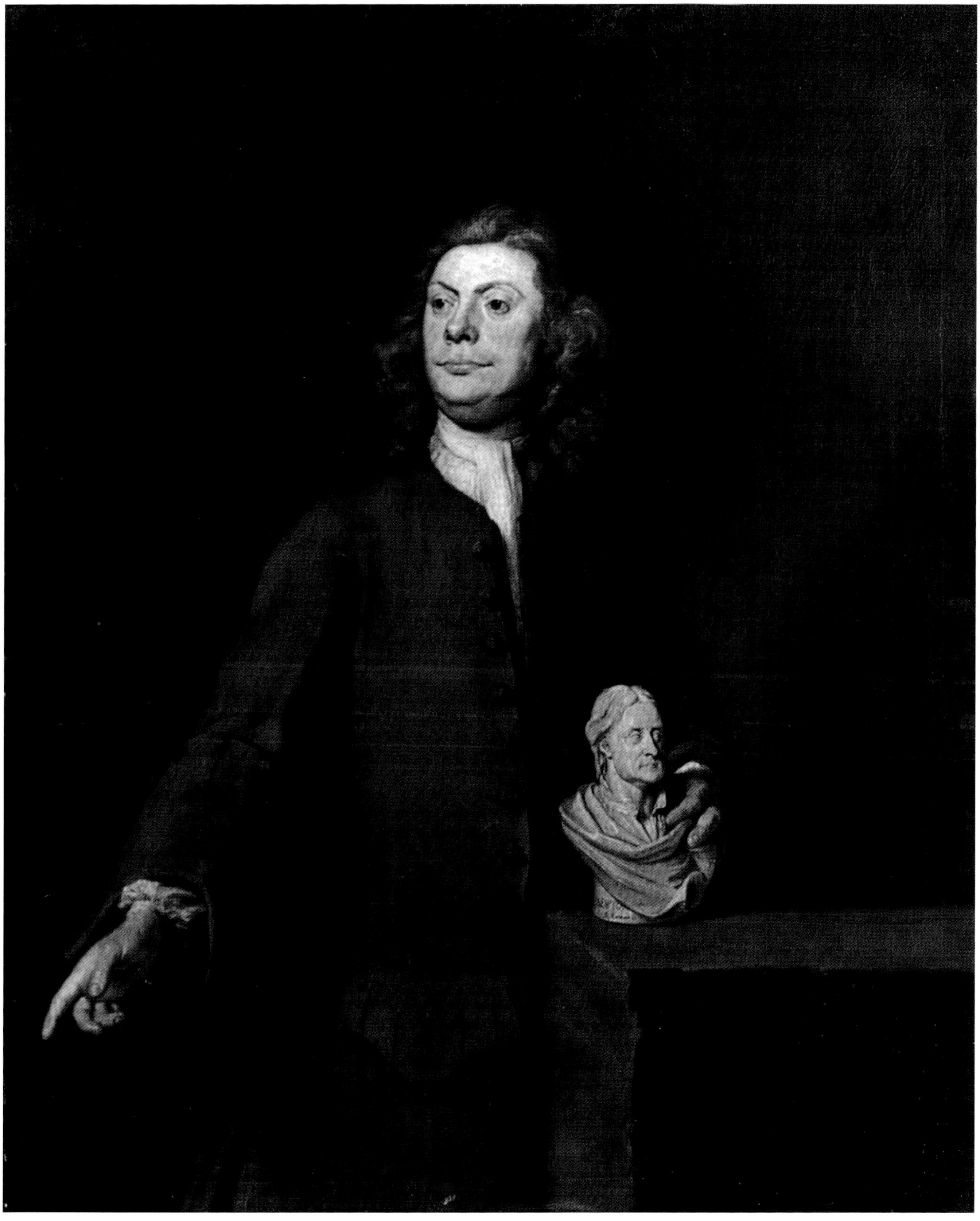

Fig. 15 David Le Marchand (1674–1726), oil on canvas, Joseph Highmore, c. 1723. *National Portrait Gallery*

Trained in Dieppe as an ivory carver, Le Marchand opened a shop in Edinburgh in 1696 and later settled in London, where he specialized in portrait medallions. He died at the French Hospital on 17 March 1726. He is shown here with his ivory bust of Sir Isaac Newton.

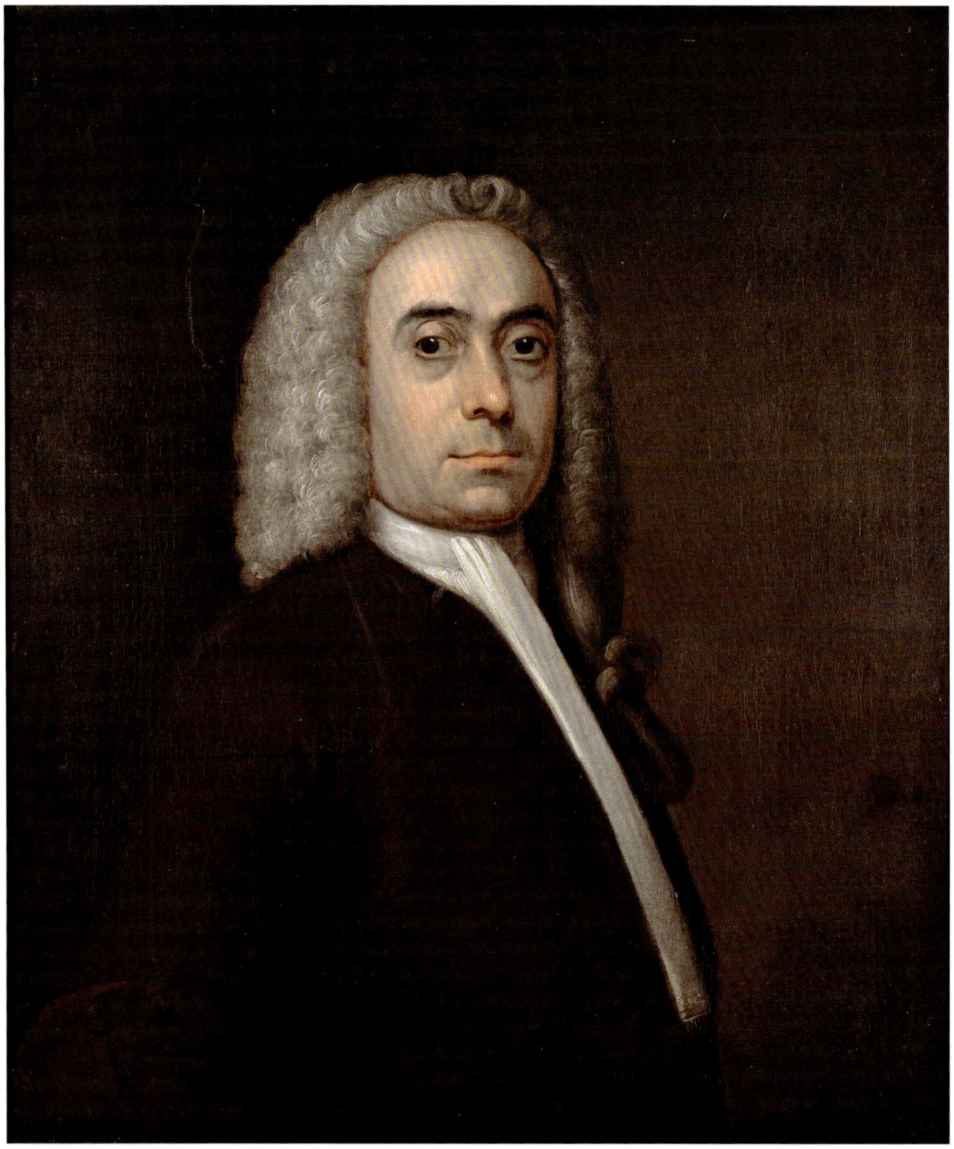

Fig. 16 (*left*)
Jean-Henri Guinand (1686–1755), oil on canvas, circle of John Theodore Heins, c. 1735

Serving as a director from 1721, then as deputy-governor from 1739, Guinand ensured financial support for needy Huguenots during the very severe winter of 1739–40. An elder of the French Church, Threadneedle Street, and a merchant in partnership with Marchant and Desmaretz, Guinand commissioned the inventory of the French Hospital for the new steward Adam Roumieu in 1742 (see the transcription of the inventory on pp. 111–16).

Fig. 17 (*below*)
Francis Calvert's bill for oil, 1743. *Huguenot Library*

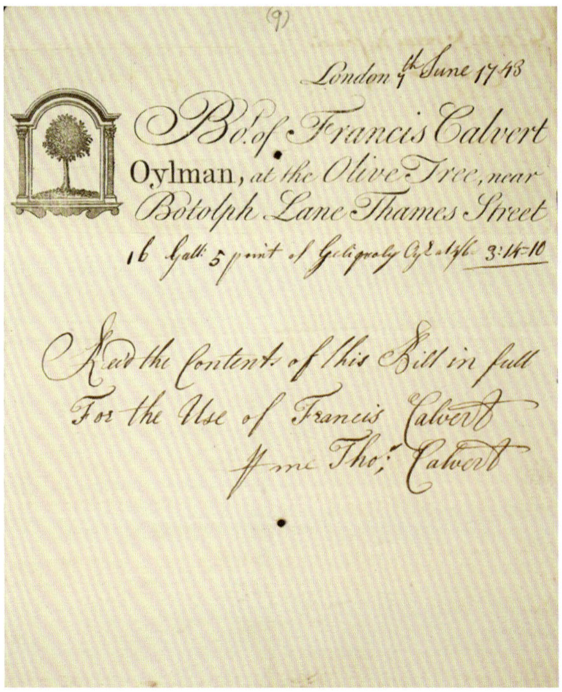

(9)

London 7th June 1743

Bo.t of Francis Calvert
Oylman, at the Olive Tree, near
Botolph Lane Thames Street

16 Gall. 5 pint of Galipoly Oyl @ 4/6 3:14:10

Rec.d the Content of this Bill in full
For the Use of Francis Calvert
p me Tho: Calvert

The most distinguished amongst the early inmates was the sculptor David Le Marchand, 'an ingenious man for working in ivory', who was admitted to the hospital in 1725 and died there a few weeks later (fig. 15).

Life at the hospital was not uneventful. Those who stayed out, stole food, or missed meals, or came home intoxicated incurred some form of punishment. One old lady was said to have hidden half a hundredweight of coal under her bed! Former hospital staff often retired as residents there, although sometimes their behaviour also left much to be desired. The staff listed in the 1742 inventory include the gardener Fonteneau and his wife, the caretakers of the Petites Maisons, Antoine Colin and his wife, and their nineteen-year-old son Jean, who was admitted in June 1743 and died there the following month. By 1744, Daniel Aubertin, 'Domestique dans la maison pendant 9 ans', was no longer able to perform his duties and was admitted as a resident. The following year he was

Fig. 18 (*right*) Joseph Kilpin's bill for sugar, 1743. *Huguenot Library*

Fig. 19 (*bottom*) Benjamin Knott's bill for linen, 1741. *Huguenot Library*

Fig. 20 (*bottom, right*) J. Perchard's bill for pewter, 1739. *Huguenot Library*

Perchard supplied pewter plates, porringers and spoons for the dining tables, chamber pots and stool pans for bedroom use, and exchanged a 'Communion pott' for the Chapel. He received old pewter in exchange for new.

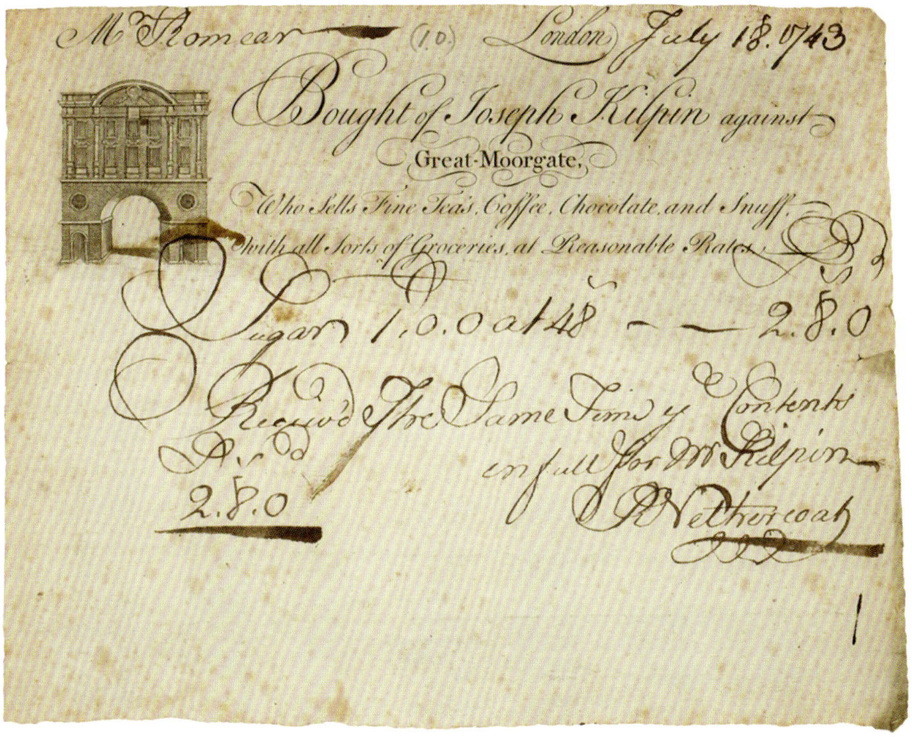
Mr Romcar (10) London July 18. 1743
Bought of Joseph Kilpin against
Great-Moorgate,
Who Sells Fine Teas, Coffee, Chocolate, and Snuff,
With all Sorts of Groceries, at Reasonable Rates
Sugar 1.0.0 at 48 — — 2.8.0
Received The Same Time ye Contents
in full for Mr Kilpin
2.8.0
R Nethercoat

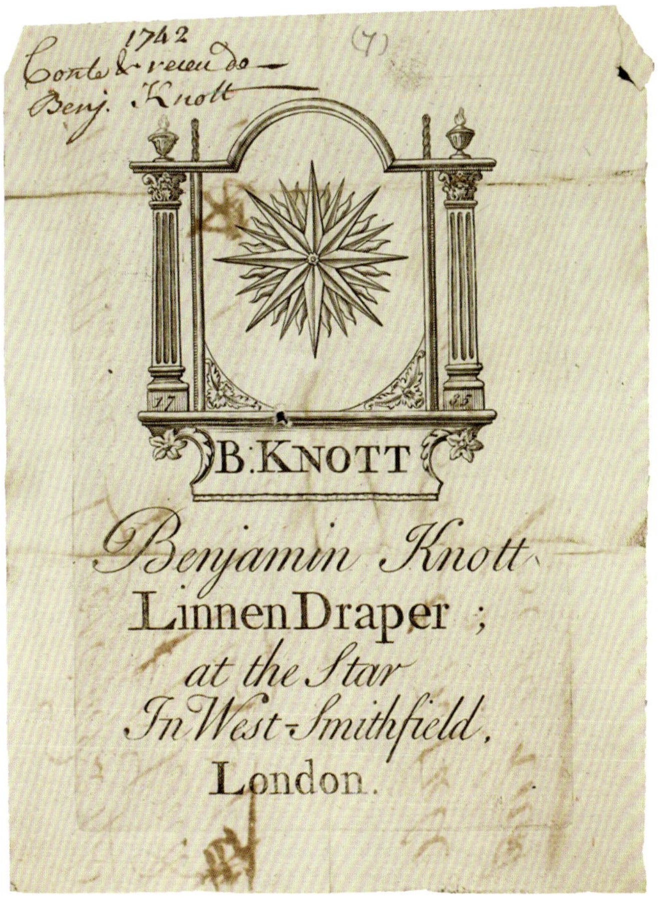
1742
Conte & recd do
Benj. Knott (7)
B.KNOTT
Benjamin Knott
Linnen Draper;
at the Star
In West-Smithfield,
London.

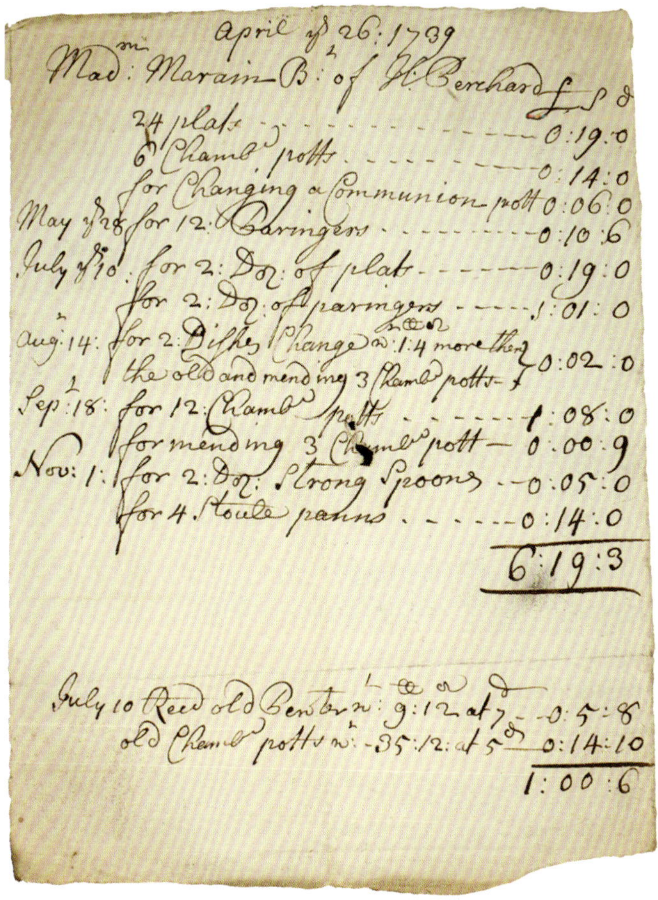
april ye 26: 1739
Madm: Marain Bt: of J. Perchard £ s d
24 plats — 0:19:0
6 Chamb potts — 0:14:0
for Changing a Communion pott 0:06:0
May ye 28 for 12 Paringers — 0:10:6
July ye 10: for 2: Dz: of plats — 0:19:0
for 2: Dz: of paringers — 1:01:0
Aug: 14: for 2 Dishes Change wt 1:4 more then the old and mending 3 Chamb potts 0:02:0
Sep: 18: for 12 Chamb potts — 1:08:0
for mending 3 Chamb pott — 0:00:9
Nov: 1: for 2: Dz: Strong Spoons — 0:05:0
for 4 Stoule panns — 0:14:0
6:19:3
July 10 Recd old Pewter wt: 9:12 at 7 — 0:5:8
old Chamb potts wt: 35:12 at 5 — 0:14:10
1:00:6

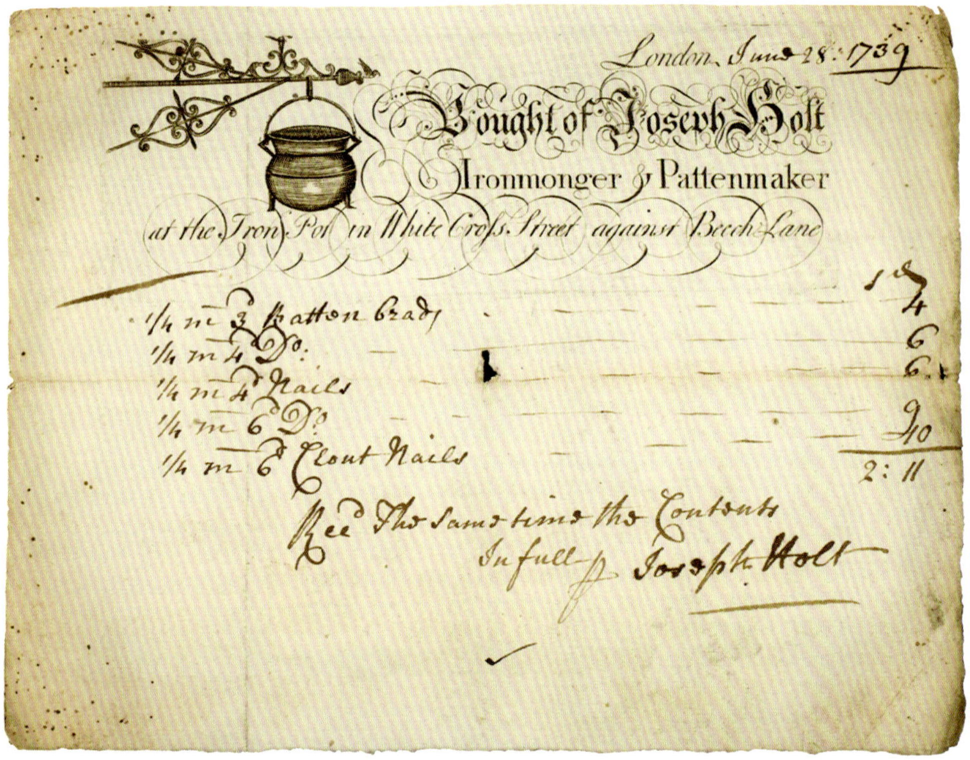
London, June 28: 1739
Bought of Joseph Holt
Ironmonger & Pattenmaker
at the Iron Pot in White Cross Street against Beech Lane

1/4 m 3 Batton brads	1 4
1/4 m 4 Do:	6
1/4 m 4 Nails	6
1/4 m 6 Do	9
1/4 m 6 Clout Nails	10
	2: 11

Recd the same time the Contents
In full p Joseph Holt

Fig. 21 (*left*) Joseph Holt's bill for ironware, 1748. *Huguenot Library*

This bill is for the supply to the French Hospital of nails, among them batten brads and clout nails.

Fig. 22 (*bottom*) Trade card of Elizabeth and Martha Baker, 1757. *Huguenot Library*

Trading at the sign of the China Jar, near the post-office in Lombard Street, they sold 'China, Glass, Stafford Shire and the best Earthen Wares &c at the Lowest Prices'. In 1755 they supplied the French Hospital with '3 dozen: wine glasses a 6/- a dozen and two stone Chamber pots at one shilling each'.

reprimanded for breaking the rules, and in 1751, he came home drunk after the meal and was rude to the steward and his wife, M. and Mme Roumieu. He was asked to leave within a month.[22]

The inventory of 1742 was taken by Jean-Henri Guinand, a director from 1721 and deputy-governor from 1739 (fig. 16), in partnership with his fellow director Claude Desmarets and provides further insight into the way of life of the inmates, staff and directors at the hospital. Contemporary tradesmen's bills shed light on the geographical location of suppliers, the quality of bedding and on the diet of the residents. It is clear that the inmates of the French Hospital were well fed. They had ample meat, bread, beer and butter.[23] Wine and olive oil were provided by Messrs Leglive & Ardouin and Francis Calvert (fig. 17); sugar was supplied by Joseph Kilpin (fig. 18); Samuel Hayward at the Star at the corner of Milk Street in Cheapside provided flaxen sheeting as did Benjamin Knott, 'Linnen Draper' (fig. 19). J. Perchard provided pewter in 1739 (fig. 20); Joseph Holt, ironware in 1748 (fig. 21). Elizabeth and Martha Baker provided glass and ceramics in 1757 (fig. 22).

The 1742 inventory (see pp. 111–16) brings to life the circumstances in which the inmates and staff lived. The gardener M. Fonteneau lived with his wife in some comfort.

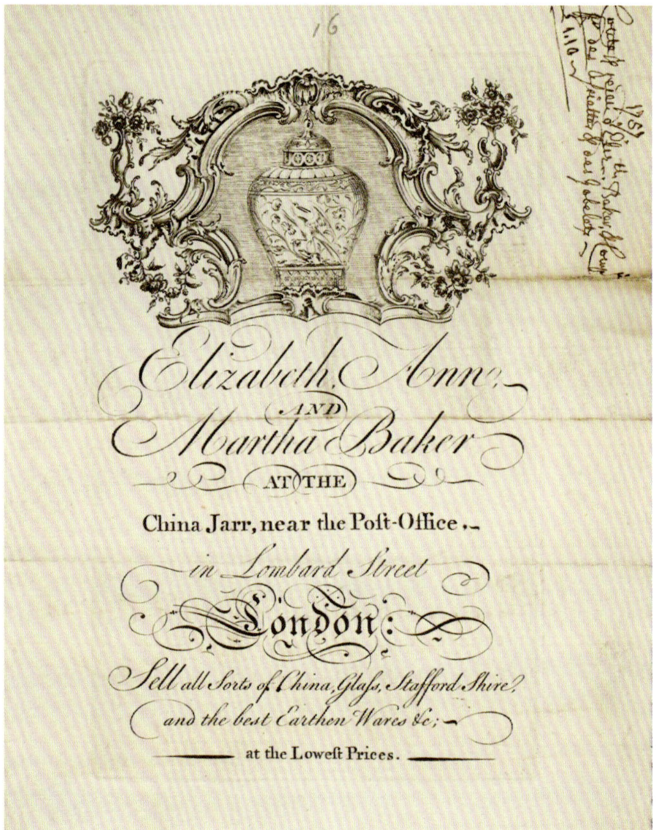
16
Elizabeth, Anne,
and
Martha Baker
at the
China Jarr, near the Post-Office
in Lombard Street
London:
Sell all Sorts of China, Glass, Stafford Shire
and the best Earthen Wares &c:
at the Lowest Prices.

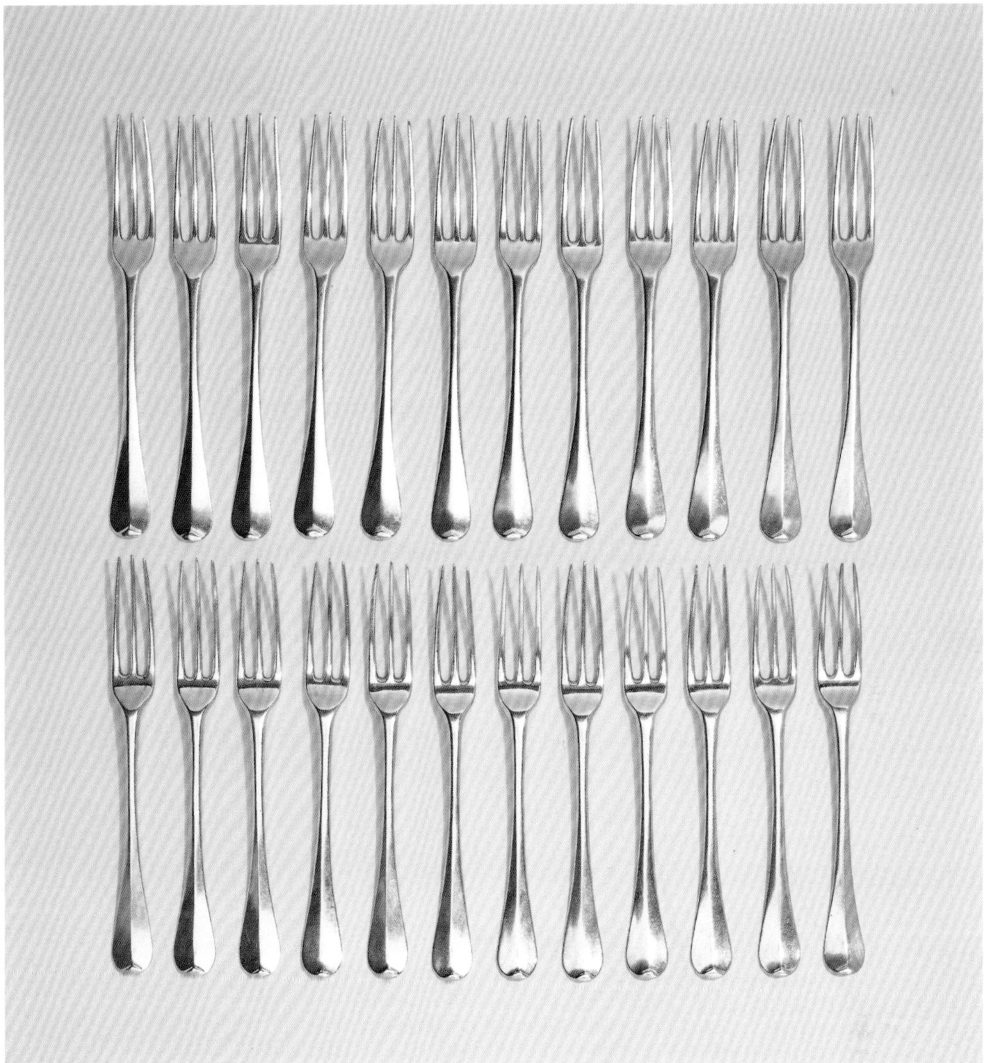

Fig. 23 Set of three-pronged forks, sterling silver, maker's mark of William Scarlett, London, 1722/3, each inscribed: 'French Hospital'

The inventories for 1742 and 1766 list the silver cutlery used by the directors. This included this still complete set of 24 silver forks as well as 24 soup spoons, 2 larger soup spoons, 22 smaller spoons and 6 salt spoons for salt and mustard. The '24 Couteaux a manches d'ivoire' were listed as the responsibility of Daniel Aubertin, one of the domestic servants. The directors ate from pewter plates.

Their bed was hung with green curtains; they had a cupboard and two chests in which to store their possessions. Six rush-bottomed side chairs and an elbow-chair with two tables, two looking-glasses, three brass chandeliers, and a tea urn implied that they were able to entertain their neighbours in some style. But although staff had married quarters, only single people, widows and widowers were admitted to the hospital as inmates. The grandest resident in 1742 was Mlle Constance Buissiere. When she died in 1746 she left the extremely valuable contents of her wardrobe, augmented by the belongings of her sister Jane, who had died in 1740, to one of the hospital servants, Marie Latour. Mlle Buissiere's damasks, satins and silks were in stark contrast with the mundane hats and stockings and shirts which Widow Carcin distributed to other inmates on demand. Constance Buissiere had been resident in the hospital since 1728, following a referral by her uncle, the surgeon Paul Buissiere. Among her luxury goods, Constance had japanned toilet boxes and two snuff-boxes and even her book of psalms was mounted with silver. Marie Latour, who had provided nursing care for Constance Buissiere, may be identified with the Marie Latour who became an inmate of the hospital in 1755. She had previously served as a nurse at the Foundling Hospital.[24]

Jeanne Harpin, like Constance Buissiere was rather well-to-do, but sadly, on the recommendation from two doctors and an apothecary, was admitted with 'l'esprit fort Derrangé'. She had been lodging with Jean Vitrac and was connected with L'Église des Grecs in Hog Lane, since M. Fougeron, the porter at that church, delivered her furniture and silver to the French Hospital in 1736. The 1742 inventory includes a list of her silver, which was entrusted to Mme Marin, the steward at that time. On

Jeanne Harpin's death in 1743, her silver soup spoons and teaspoons were kept for the use of the directors, but the rest was sold and the proceeds given to the hospital. Although a number of the inmates brought with them small items of silver, mostly teaspoons, the hospital provided pewter vessels and cutlery for the daily meals. The 1742 inventory demonstrates the quantities of butter and Cheshire cheese consumed. It is perhaps more surprising that pewter was also used for communion. In 1742 the communion tablecloth, napkins, flagon, two cups and two plates were the responsibility of Widow Carcin. The chaplain was Jacques Duplessis. He had lived in Leiden until 1742 when he accepted the post in London.

In contrast to the inmates, the directors ate with silver cutlery, and the set of 24 three-pronged forks, hallmarked 1722/3 (fig. 23), is still in regular use at directors' lunches in Rochester. The castors by the Huguenot goldsmith Thomas Bevault (fig. 24), hallmarked in 1714/15, were described as 'sucriers' in both the 1742 and 1766 inventories. According to the 1742 inventory the directors' Court Room was furnished with 5 tables and 38 red-leather chairs and the walls were hung with portraits, engravings and a looking-glass[25] given by an anonymous benefactor in 1733 (fig. 25). A wall panel recorded the apprentices whose premium was paid from the charity. A cupboard housed the hospital records; a chest contained further archives, and a large pewter chamber pot completed the comfort offered to the directors at their monthly meetings.

Medical needs were attended to by the visiting surgeon-apothecary, whose room had been fitted out with great care

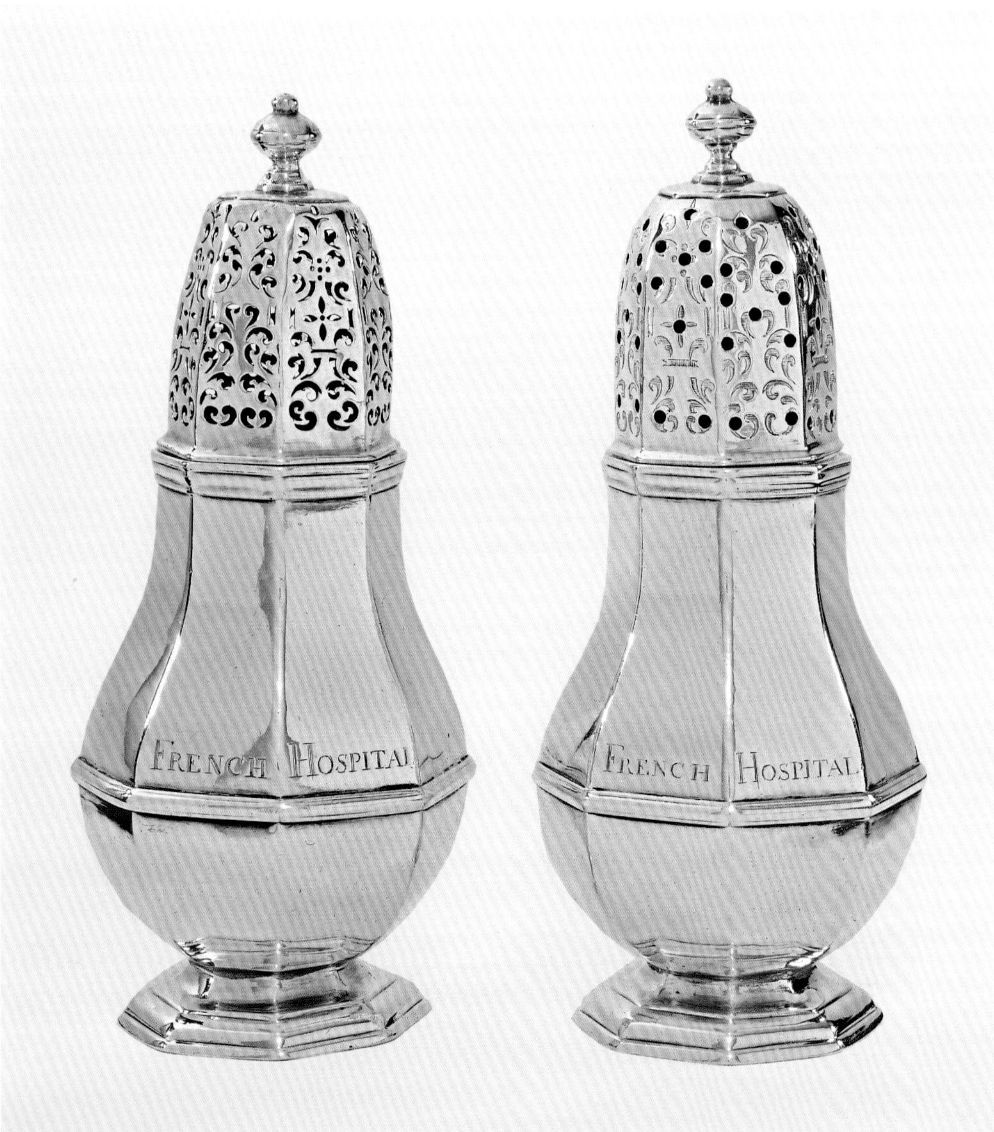

Fig. 24 Pair of sugar castors, silver (Britannia standard), maker's mark of Thomas Bevault, London, 1714/15]

These castors were listed in the 1742 inventory as in the care of Widow Carcin, and in the 1766 inventory as 'sucriers' amongst silver used by the directors. Thomas Bevault registered his own maker's mark in 1712, when he was living in Foster Lane in the City of London, adjacent to the hall of the Worshipful Company of Goldsmiths.

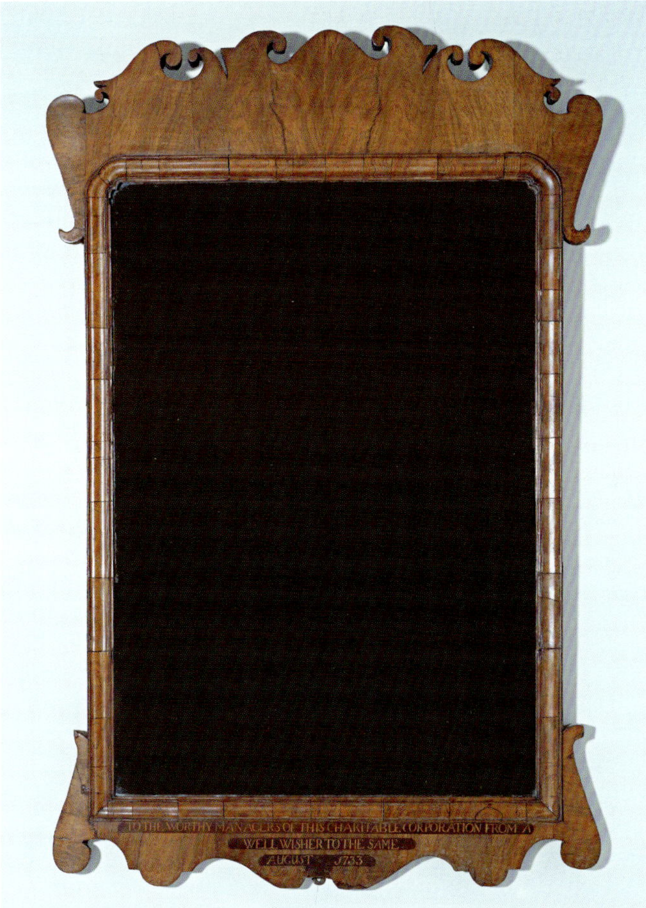
TO THE WORTHY MANAGERS OF THIS CHARITABLE CORPORATION FROM A
WELL WISHER TO THE SAME
AUGUST 1733

Fig. 25 Looking-glass, walnut, c. 1733

Listed in the 1742 and 1766 hospital inventories as being in the 'Salle des Directeurs', it was one of several looking-glasses recorded in the hospital in 1742. Others were in Widow Carcin's room and one of the maids' rooms, the latter perhaps a bequest from one of the inmates. By 1766, there was also a looking-glass in the surgeon's room.

in 1739. By 1766 the 'Chirurgie' was furnished with six chairs, a table and a looking-glass and the fireplace offered warmth and comfort. Jacques Demedis, who recommended Jeanne Harpin for admission, served as surgeon-apothecary to the hospital for nearly fifty years from 1718 to 1766.[26]

Linguistically, the 1742 inventory is a fascinating document. Although written in French, there are already signs of the influence of English on the compilers' use of language. One amusing instance is the use of the word 'mogue' for 'mug'.

1 Named after the Peerless Pool adjoining the street to Islington, where bathing by local people was allowed.

2 *HSQS*, LVI (1983), p. 59.

3 Huguenot Library (HL) H. F2.1. See also Browning, 'Origin and Early History', Appendix 7, pp. 75–8.

4 The others were a silk merchant, Jean Montand, bankrupt in 1717, and the superannuated François Le Coq de Saint-Leger, described by John Evelyn in 1697 as 'a French refugie who left great Riches for Religion, a very learned civill person' (John Evelyn, *Diary,* ed. E.S. de Beer [Oxford, 1955], p. 549).

5 Browning, 'Origin and Early History', p. 56.

6 Howard Colvin, *A Biographical Dictionary of British Architects, 1600–1840* (1975), p. 323.

7 HL H.D8.5.

8 HL H.F2.2.

9 Royal Hospital Books 1684–1707, Dublin Record Office; Geoffrey Beard, *Sir Christopher Wren*, Edinburgh (1982), pp. 44–5, figs. 56–8; C.G.T. Dean, *The Royal Hospital, Chelsea*, London (1950).

10 Roy Porter, '"Every Human Want": The world of eighteenth-century charity' in *Enlightened Self-interest: The Foundling Hospital and Hogarth*, The Thomas Coram Foundation for Children, London (1997), pp. 12–15.

11 Marmoy, *Inmates and Applicants*.

12 HL H.E5.1.

13 This is presumably André Fonteneau who entered the French Hospital as a resident in 1736; his entry is endorsed thus: 'en lui payer gage comme Jardinier'. His wife Anne was admitted as a resident in 1752, aged 77. The family came originally from Saintonge. See Marmoy, *Inmates and Applicants*, vol. 1.

14 *Livre d'Adam Roumieu, oeconome d'Hôpital François.* HL H.C.1/3.

15 Marmoy, 'La Providence', p. 342.

16 *Les Galères de France et les galériens protestants*, Gaston Tournier, Les Presses de Languedoc, 1984.

17 Robert Nash, in a personal communication, May 2008.

18 Marmoy, *Inmates and Applicants*, pp. 52–3.

19 Robert Nash, in a personal communication, May 2008.

20 1752.

21 Marmoy, *Inmates and Applicants*, pp. 52–3.

22 Marmoy, *Inmates and Applicants.*

23 Robert Nash, in a personal communication, May 2008, citing Marmoy, 'French Hospital', p. 242.

24 Marmoy, *Inmates and Applicants*, vol. 2.

25 It now hangs in the lobby at the French Hospital in Rochester.

26 Murdoch, p. 84.

4

Directing and caring at the French Hospital in the eighteenth century

The numbers of inmates rose steeply: from 80 in the first few years to 125 in 1729, to 230 by 1760. Admissions were fairly evenly spread between the City of London, the West End (including Soho) and the East End (mainly Spitalfields). The ensuing steep rise in expenditure was met by generous donations and legacies from the Huguenot community as well as continuing grants from the Royal Bounty.

When Ruvigny, Earl of Galway, the founding governor, died in 1720, he left £1,000 to the hospital. His successor was Philibert d'Hervart, baron d'Huningue. D'Hervart's father had been the great Huguenot finance minister under Cardinal Mazarin whose private wealth had secured Alsace for Louis XIV. D'Hervart, who died only six months after taking office, bequeathed to the hospital £4,000, being the share of his estate that would have gone to a son who predeceased him.[1]

Following the example of Gastigny's original bequest in which he stipulated that half the money should be invested to provide further income for the hospital, the directors decided that they should do likewise and invest some of the gifts received. The purchase of Bond's Court in Walbrook for £6,000 in 1726 yielded a handsome rental income until it was sold in 1762. In 1734, the hospital's finances were again transformed with the death of Magdalen, wife of Paul Dufour, a founding director who had been treasurer since 1719. His wife's fortune, from a previous marriage, was bequeathed to him with reversion to the French Hospital at his death. In 1739, he made his inheritance over to the hospital, swelling its coffers by £15,400.[2]

The timing of the Dufour donation was providential. From Christmas Day 1739 to mid-February 1740 England and the rest of Europe suffered the severest winter in living memory and the frozen rivers and water supply and bitter cold visited great suffering on the London poor. An Extraordinary Court, with a new governor, Pierre Cabibel, the deputy-governor Henri Guinand, the treasurer Pierre Gaussen, the long-serving secretary Philippe Champion de Crespigny (fig. 26) and twenty-eight directors took far-reaching decisions. This Court initially awarded £1,000 grants to the Westminster and Soho poor relief committees and £300 was donated to La Soupe in Spitalfields and La Marmite in Westminster. Alms were distributed to more than eighty married couples who received eight to ten shillings per month. This form of relief was extended until 1759.[3]

In addition to the flow of donations and bequests, special charities based on bequests from Esther Coqueau (1745), Étienne [Stephen] Mounier (1770) and Lieutenant-Colonel Isaac Bérenger de Boislin (1753) have assisted many hundreds of widows, apprentices, poor French Protestant refugees and others. The hospital benefited from a successful appeal in 1763 to meet the cost of rebuilding the bakehouse wing, which raised £1,600, almost all of it from the Huguenot community.[4]

An unlikely donation from a refugee in earlier days was a necklace of forty-seven orient pearls, given to the treasurer by Mademoiselle de la Croix, the daughter and executrix of Madame Magdalen de Saint-Leger, (*née* Muyssons), widow of Théodore Le Coq de Saint-Leger. Théodore had been one of the elders of the Huguenot temple of Charenton outside Paris.[5] They were sold to an unnamed purchaser by one of the nobleman directors, David Montolieu, baron de Saint-Hippolyte. Money came in too from the inmates, most of it in the early years from the sponsoring of their places by well-wishers. Maitland recorded in 1739 that 74 of the 220 inmates were paid for at the rate of £9 per annum.[6] A few had their own income which they paid to the hospital in return for superior conditions of life.

Jacques Duplessis and Henry Delouche shared a first-floor room,[7] next to the steward's, from 1729 until Duplessis died in 1743. Duplessis had been a 'gentleman private' in the First Troop of the Horse Guards and had his military pension transferred from the Royal Hospital, Chelsea. De Louche received regular sums from the account of Pierre Perchard – an old employer perhaps. Both left considerable sums to the hospital, in Duplessis's case to the great dismay of his nephew, also Jacques, whose training and ordination in Leiden he had paid for and who had come to the hospital as its chaplain in 1742. The nephew's expectations from

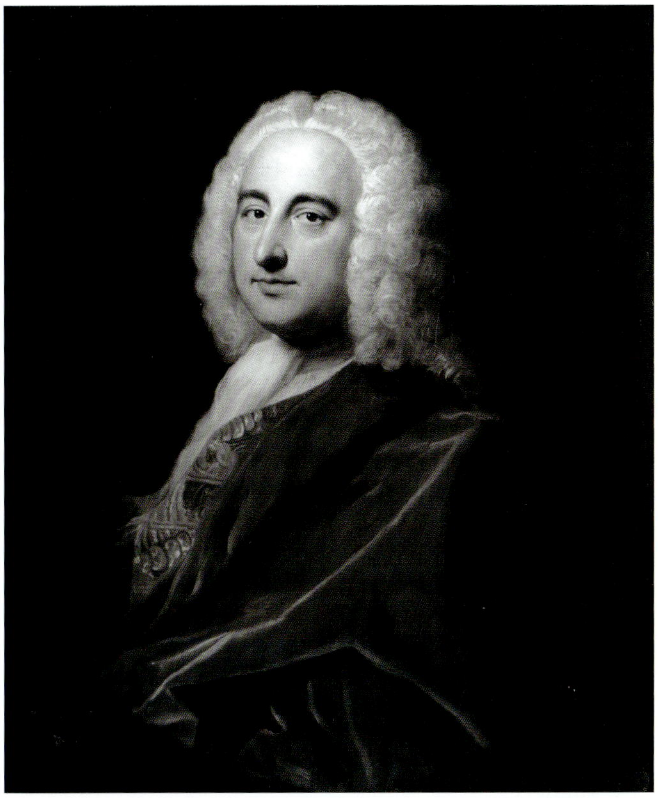

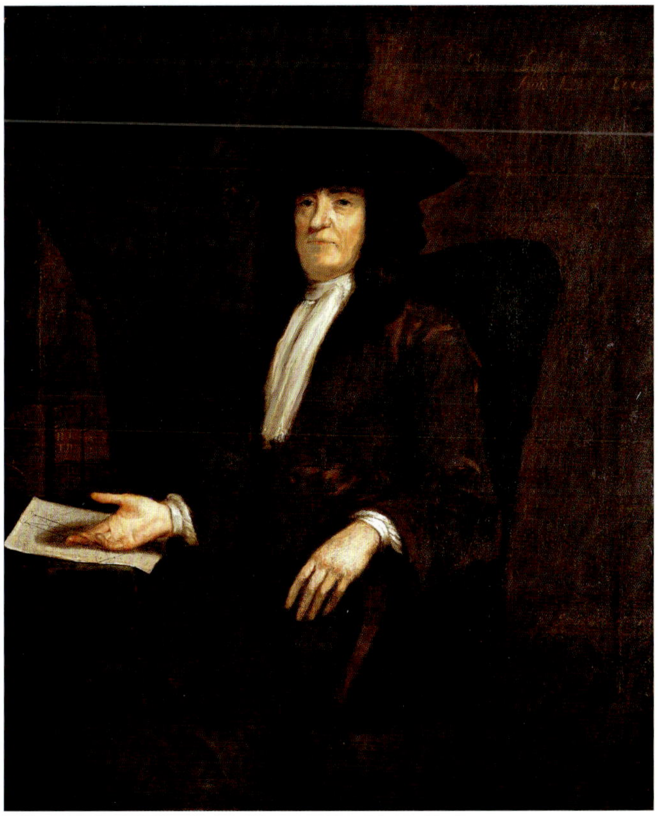

his uncle had come to nought, though, and the hospital benefited instead. Furthermore, the chaplain's £100 annual remuneration was not increased. The Revd Jacques married well – to Mary Ann Milxan, and among their three daughters' godparents at their christenings at the Chapel Royal, St James's, were Lady Elizabeth Hankey and Pierre Gaussen, a director of the French Hospital (and in 1756 deputy-governor).[8] The Duplessis story, in the hospital's archives, ends with a letter written by Richard Cox from North Audley Street asking the directors for financial help for Anne Duplessis, on behalf of the governor, Lord Ligonier.[9]

In 1735, Barthélemy Fresse made a gift of £65 in three per cent annuities, for which he was given a place in the hospital.[10] Generous benefactors could obtain places for their applicants, seemingly without extra payment. In the 1720s Madame d'Hervart, widow of the second governor, could nominate six, Paul Dufour, four, and Madame de Saint-Hippolyte, on behalf of Jacques Baudouin, two.

Initially much of the administrative work was shared between the steward, Philippe Ménard and Philippe Champion de Crespigny, the latter two between them serving as secretaries from 1718 to 1765. Later on it was performed by the clerk. From 1740 there was also a book-keeper. Matters affecting the directors and major financial issues were minuted in the diaries. They also record the gift by the governor, Lord Ligonier, of his equestrian portrait in 1752 (fig. 28) and the acquisition in the same year of an eight-day long-case clock by Charles Cabrier, Master of the

Fig. 26 (*left, top*) Philippe Champion de Crespigny (1704–1765), oil on canvas, British School. *Kelmarsh Trust*

Philippe's grandfather, Claude Champion, sieur de Crespigny, fled to England with his wife the comtesse de Vierville and their eight children and became a colonel under Marlborough. One of their sons, Peter, was a founding director of the French Hospital in 1718. Their grandson, Philippe, who lived in Champion Lodge, Camberwell, became a director in 1734 at the age of 30 and secretary in 1737. His brother Claude (1706–1782), who became a director in 1760, worked all his life in the office of the South Sea Company, starting shortly after the bubble burst in 1720.

Fig. 27 (*left, bottom*) Pierre Daudé (1653–1733), oil on canvas, Joseph Highmore, signed 'Jos Highmore, pint.' and dated, 1733

Pierre Daudé is shown three-quarter length seated in a high-backed chair, wearing a brown coat with white stock and a tricorn hat, his right hand is resting on a mathematical manuscript. Daudé came from Maruejols, and was educated at Saumur and Geneva. He came to England in 1680 and later became a tutor in the Trevor family.

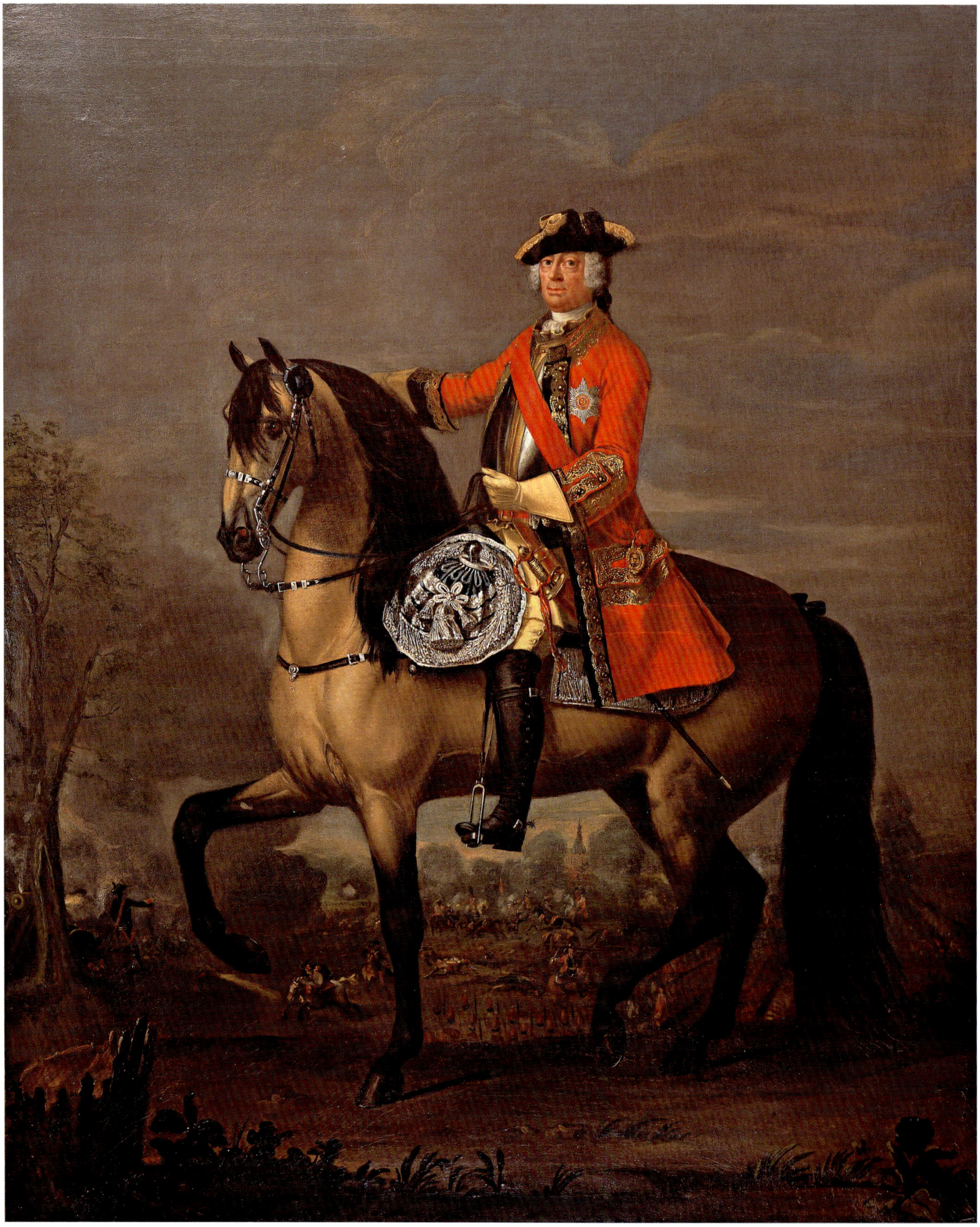

Fig. 28 Field-Marshal Sir Jean-Louis Ligonier, KCB (1680–1770), oil on canvas, Bartholomew Dandridge, c. 1745, in original contemporary frame

Governor of the French Hospital from 1748 to 1770, Ligonier was Commander-in-Chief of the British Army. Wearing the Star and Jewel of the Order of the Bath, he is portrayed against a backdrop of French blue coats and the red coats of the British Grenadiers illustrating the military campaign against the French between 1738 and 1747.

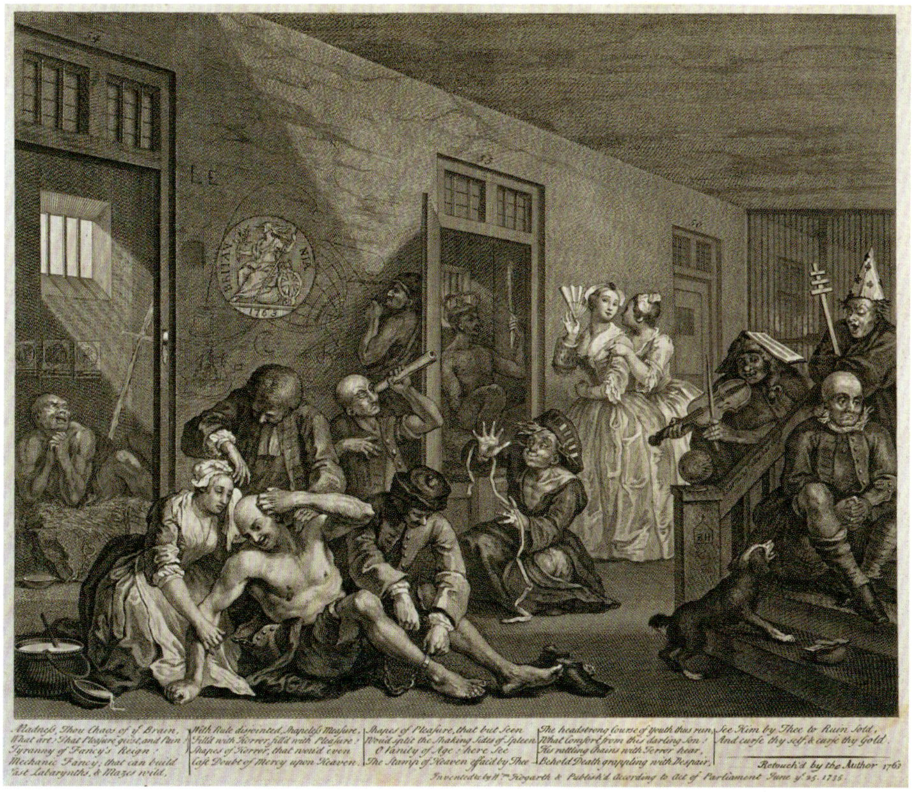

Fig. 30 *The Rake's Progress, Scene 8: The Rake in Bedlam*, engraving, William Hogarth, 1735. *Victoria and Albert Museum*

Tom Rakewell is shown in the foreground stripped naked. In the background, one inmate is wearing a crown and another is reclining on a bed of straw in spiritual ecstasy, whilst a light shines through the window onto a crucifix. A well-dressed lady and her maid are being entertained by the antics of the inmates. Visiting Bedlam was still considered one of the sights of London at that time.

Clockmakers' Company in 1756, which is recorded in the 1766 inventory as furnishing the directors' Court Room (fig. 29).

William Maitland's description shows how the French Hospital was setting an example to the many other institutions offering care that were then coming into being:

> The Hospital at present contains 220 poor and helpless men and women who … are plentifully supplied … with all the necessaries of life … The charity also extends to lunatics for whom accommodation in a large infirmary is provided. On the foundation there are always a chaplain, physician, surgeon and other proper officers who carefully attend to the pensioners and administer to their several necessities.[11]

The provision of special care for mental health was unusual but not unheard of at that time. An interesting comparison is provided by the Bethel Hospital in Norwich founded in 1713 by Mary Chapman, the daughter of

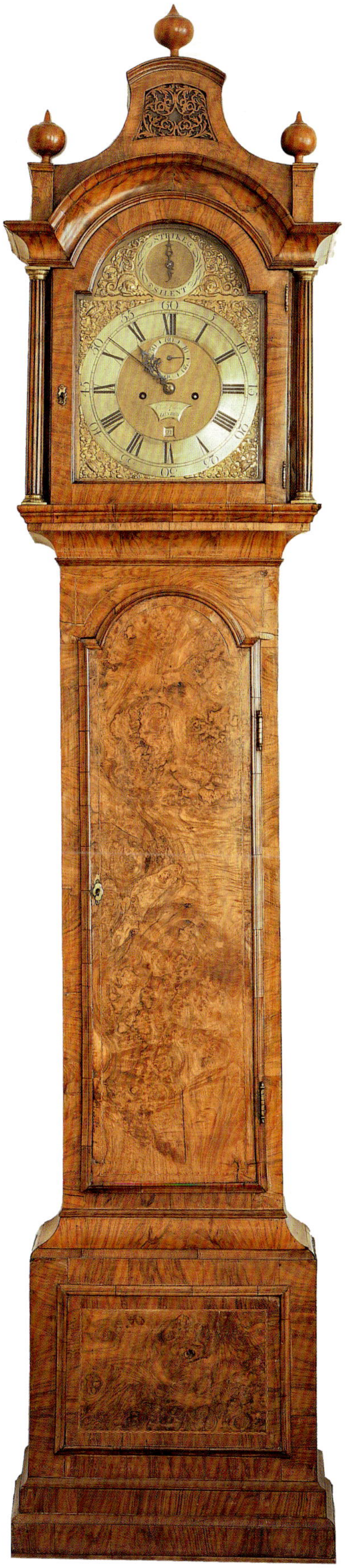

Fig. 29 (*left*)
Eight-day long-case clock by Charles Cabrier, walnut case, London, c. 1752

Apprenticed through the London Clockmakers' Company in 1719, Charles Cabrier was made free in 1726 and served as Master of the Company from 1757 to 1772.

John Mann, a well-connected Norwich Whig. At this foundation, the 'True Protestant Religion' played a central role with biblical texts hanging in each of the rooms. It catered for the 'Poor inhabitants from Norwich' providing 'care, maintenance and relief of them for clothes, food and physic and all other necessaries'. Given the strong Huguenot links with Norwich, where the Huguenot congregation had met since the mid-sixteenth century, it is possible that the Huguenot communities in London were aware of this pioneering regional charity. Their aim was to provide a 'place of confinement which would facilitate recovery'.[12]

In their humane treatment of lunacy, both the Bethel, Norwich, and La Providence, London, provide a stark contrast with Bedlam Hospital, St George's Fields, London, founded in 1675, which continued to serve as a source of entertainment for Londoners, who paid to watch the lunatic behaviour of the hapless inmates.[13] The scene is captured by Hogarth in *The Rake's Progress* (fig. 30). St Luke's Hospital in Moorfields, founded in 1751, provided an alternative to Bedlam for distraught Londoners. Provision for the mentally ill followed in the provinces: at the Manchester Royal Infirmary opening in the 1750s; at Newcastle in 1765, at the York Asylum opening in 1777 and at other hospitals in Leicester and Liverpool in 1794 and 1797 respectively.[14]

Of the physicians and surgeons serving as consultants to La Providence one stands out. He was Jean-Baptiste

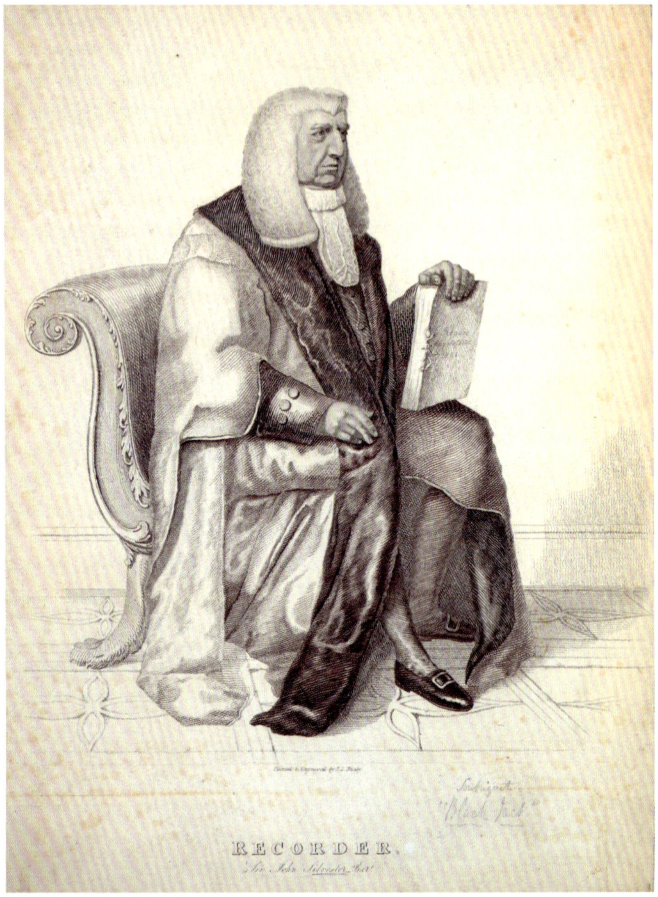

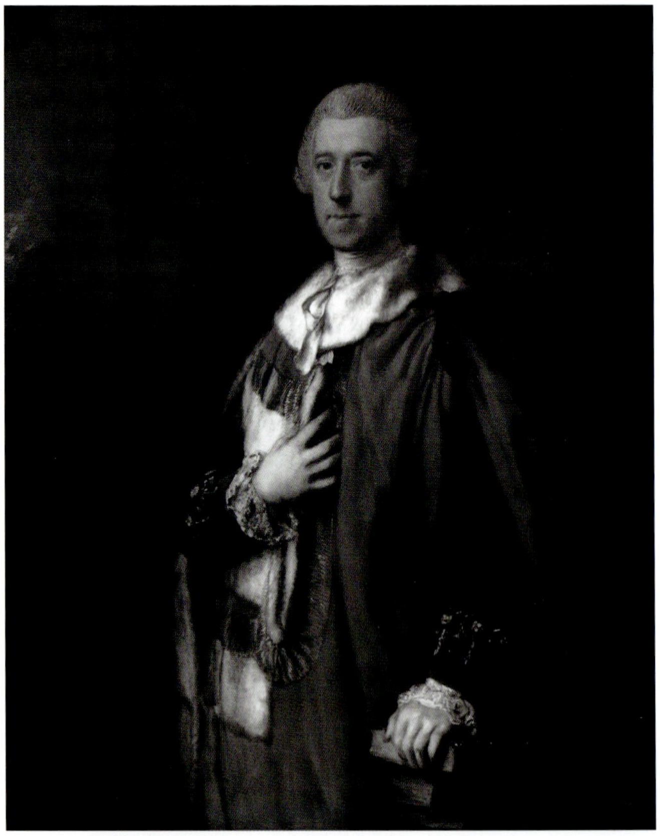

Fig. 31 *(right, top)* Sir John Silvester (1745–1822), engraving, T.L. Busby, 1824

Sir John Silvester served as Common Sergeant for the Corporation of London in 1790 and as Recorder of the City of London. Elected a Fellow of the Royal Society in 1780, a Fellow of the Society of Antiquaries in 1804 and awarded a DCL from Oxford University, he was made a baronet on 24 December 1814. His book-plate (see end-papers and pp. 109, 110) copies that used by his father, Sir John-Baptist Silvester (1714–1789), who served as physician to the French Hospital from 1742 to 1774. He was knighted in 1774.

Fig. 32 *(right, bottom)* William Bouverie, 1st Earl of Radnor (1724–1776), oil on canvas, Thomas Gainsborough, dated 1770. *Private collection*

William, 1st Earl of Radnor, became MP for Salisbury in 1747. He collected paintings and commissioned furniture from leading cabinet-makers. He was elected president of the Salisbury Infirmary. His great-great-great-grandfather, Laurens Desbouveries (1536–1610), son of a small landowner near Lille, came to England in 1568, settling first in Sandwich and then in Canterbury. The Earls of Radnor have continued to serve as governors of the French Hospital since 1770.

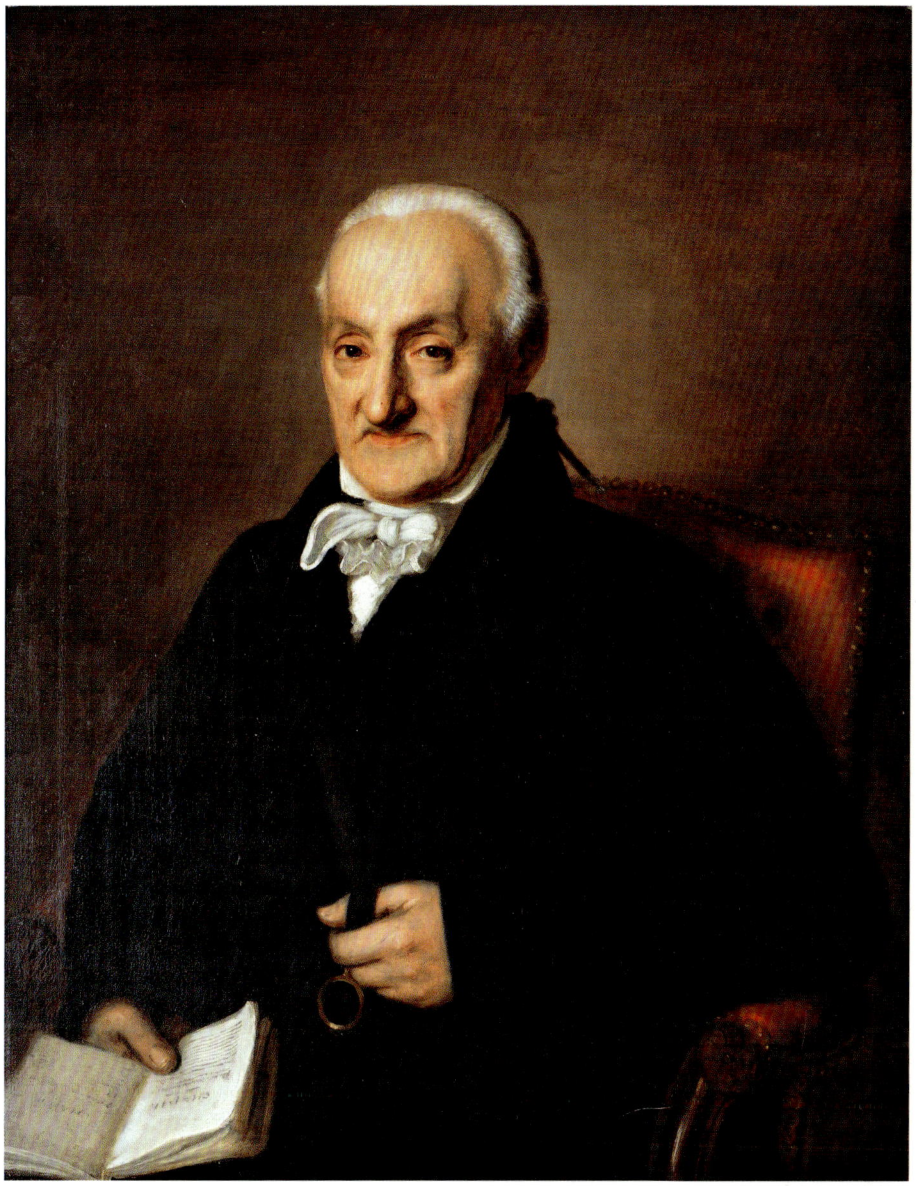

Fig. 33 David Duval (1751–1836), oil on canvas, artist unknown, c. 1830
Elected a director of the French Hospital in 1786, Duval was deputy-governor from 1813 until 1836. He is seated in formal attire in a late 18th-century armchair still in the French Hospital.

Zacharie Silvestre, who came from a family of distinguished physicians. His uncle was Pierre Silvestre, a refugee from Bordeaux, who came to England as physician to William of Orange, serving as an army doctor in Ireland and the Low Countries.[15] Jean-Baptiste became physician to both the London and French Hospitals. He was knighted by George III in 1774 and, as Sir John-Baptist Silvester, Kt, MD, FRS, LRCP, retired to Bath, where he died in 1789. His son, Sir John Silvester, Bt, Hon. DCL (Oxon.), Recorder of the City of London (fig. 31), became a director of the French Hospital in 1811.

Two of Jean-Baptiste Silvestre's letters to the directors survive. In the letter dated 1755 he reported that he had found, after examination, that Mathieu Baour, a refugee in his thirties from the Haut Languedoc, was deranged; and in the other, of 1762, he certified that Elizabeth Kendall (*née* Dambesieux), aged 22, and Anne Peltier of Spitalfields had 'recovered their senses and [could] be discharged'.[16] Medical officers were provided with their own consulting room. In 1739 the painter Lewis Giles was paid by agreement with Mr Du Bisson 'for guilding in the Chirurgiens cupboard' – the press that had been provided the previous year by Daniel Marsillat, carpenter – and for '14 drawers, scrowled, silverd and lackred'.[17]

While physicians and surgeons came and went as consultants, the stewards, chaplains, surveyors and bookkeepers were on the hospital staff. The board of management comprised the governor, who was elected for three years, the deputy-governor, the treasurer and the secretary, who were elected annually, and the directors, who were and still are, elected for life. After the brief governorships of Galway, Hervart, Robethon and Viçouse, all of them men of national stature, came four governors elected from the court of directors, Pujolas, the surgeon

Paul Buissiere, Cabibel and Gaultier. In 1748 there was a return to a major public figure, Field-Marshal Earl Ligonier, commander-in-chief of the British Army for much of his governorship (1748–70). Under Lord Chatham, Ligonier led his adopted country to victory against France in the Seven Years' War. He was followed by a descendant of the first flood of refugees from Spanish Flanders, William Bouverie, 1st Earl of Radnor (fig. 32), heir to Longford Castle and other estates, governor of the Levant Company and, according to his obituary (1776), 'an active and benevolent member of society, an affectionate and judicious parent, and a loyal and independent Peer of the Realm'.[18] His eight successors to the earldom have, three times with an interregnum, served as governors until today.

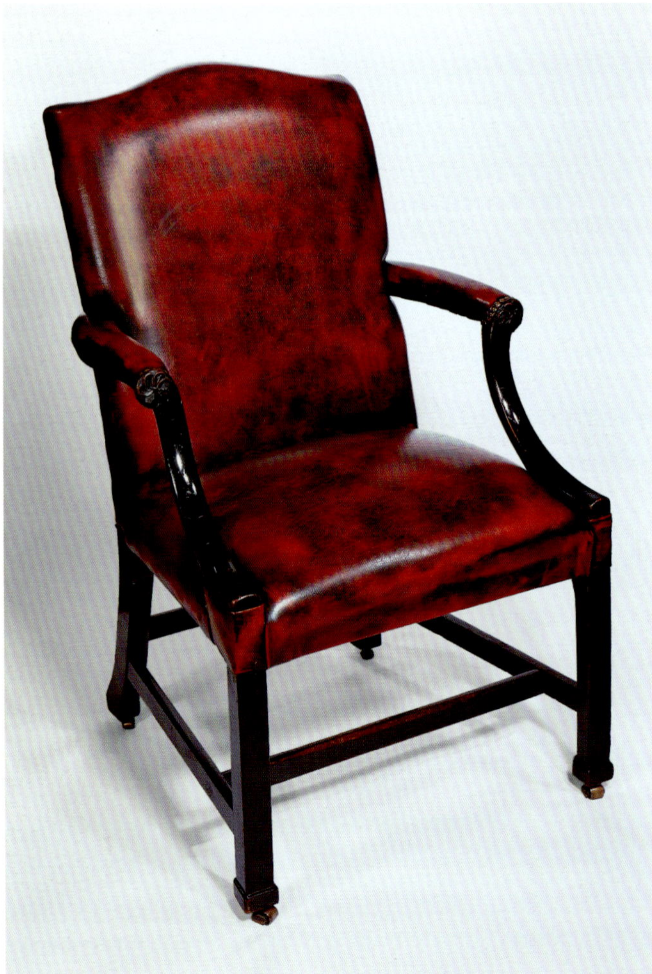

Fig. 34 Library chair, mahogany, c. 1765

The chair with its serpentine padded back and scrolled arm supports is carved with rosettes at the ends of the arms discernible in the portrait of the deputy-governor David Duval (fig. 33). The chair has been reupholstered in red leather with brass nail-head borders in keeping with its original appearance.

The only comparable dynasty among the officers is that of the Duvals as deputy-governors, which began in 1813 with David Duval (figs. 33–4), a director since 1786, the third Duval to be elected. Six Duvals have succeeded him, the current deputy-governor being Peter James Duval, elected in 1981.

One of the most active directors was Jean-Henri Guinand (fig. 16). Arriving from Geneva in 1713, he became an active member of the Huguenot committee and was a founding director and the deputy-governor of the French Hospital. He found time also to be deacon of the French Protestant Church of London, Threadneedle Street, co-secretary of the General Assembly of the French Protestant Churches of London in 1721 and, in 1728, founder of the French Almshouses in Black Eagle Street, Spitalfields, for forty-five needy church members. According to Maitland, Guinand, an 'eminent French merchant of Little St Helen's', collected £1,248 7s 6d for the French Almshouses, 'in a large pewter dish in his possession'.[19] Guinand's ancestors are recorded in Besançon in 1519. His descendants appear on the Huguenot pedigree of Their Royal Highnesses Princes William and Henry

Fig. 35 *(right, top)* *La Malheureuse Famille Calas*, engraving, C. de Carmontelle, 1765

The engraving shows the Calas family, with the exception of their father, the linen merchant, Jean Calas, in the Conciergerie, Paris, receiving the final judgement from the Maîtres de Requêts, the French High Court, on the death of the eldest son, Marc-Antoine, a frustrated scholar of 28, who was not called to the bar because he was a Protestant. Marc-Antoine committed suicide on 13 October 1761, but to protect the family's reputation, his father claimed that he had been murdered.

Jean Calas was accused of his son's murder and appeared in court in November 1761. In March, 1762, he was condemned to death on the wheel. The public mood of intense anti-Protestantism in Toulouse had convinced the judges of Calas's guilt. Jean Calas refused to abjure his faith despite being tortured. His courage redeemed the family honour and paved the way for defenders of the Calas family.

The youngest member of the family, Donat, fled to Geneva, where his presence inspired Voltaire to take up the cause. In March 1765, after the case against Jean Calas had been heard in the highest court of France, all concerned were acquitted. Copies of this engraving were sold in London and on the continent to raise funds for the Calas family. Dr Maty (see fig. 103), physician to the French Hospital, was amongst those who supported the cause in London. Jean Calas's mother Anne-Rose was born in Spitalfields the grand-daughter of Peter Cabibel, a member of a refugee family from Languedoc and a founding director of the French Hospital, deputy-governor from 1720 and governor until his death in 1745. He also served as treasurer of the Spitalfields 'Soupe' in the early 1700s.

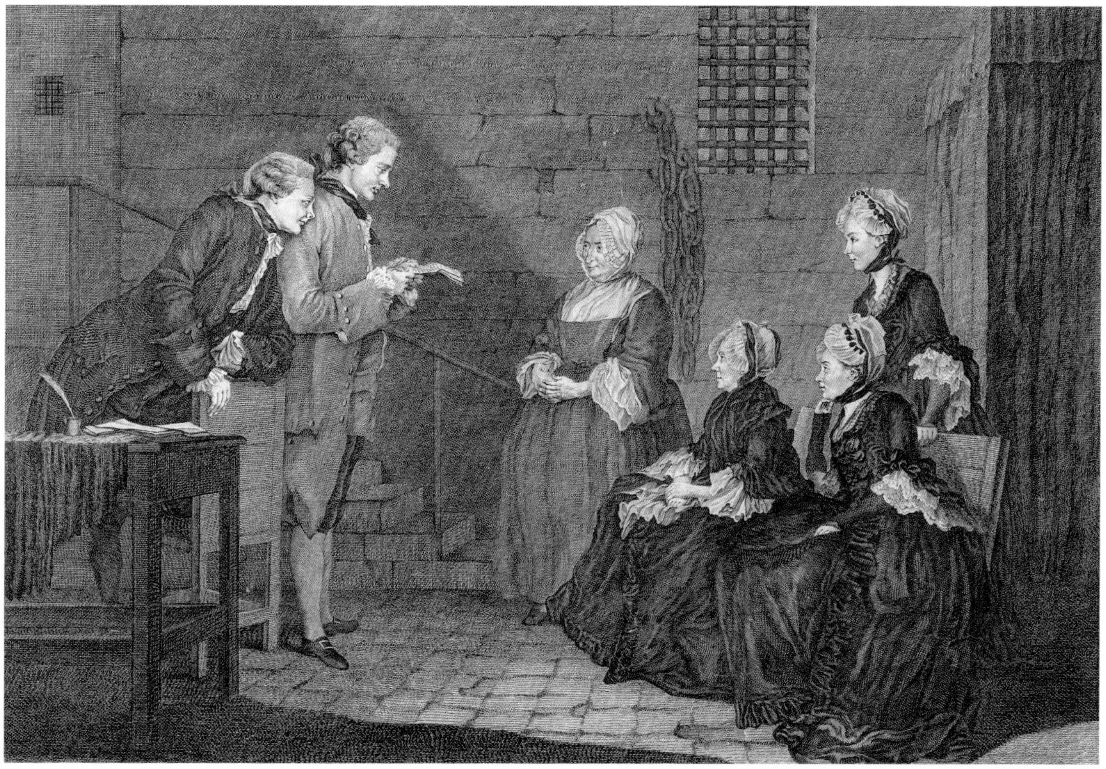

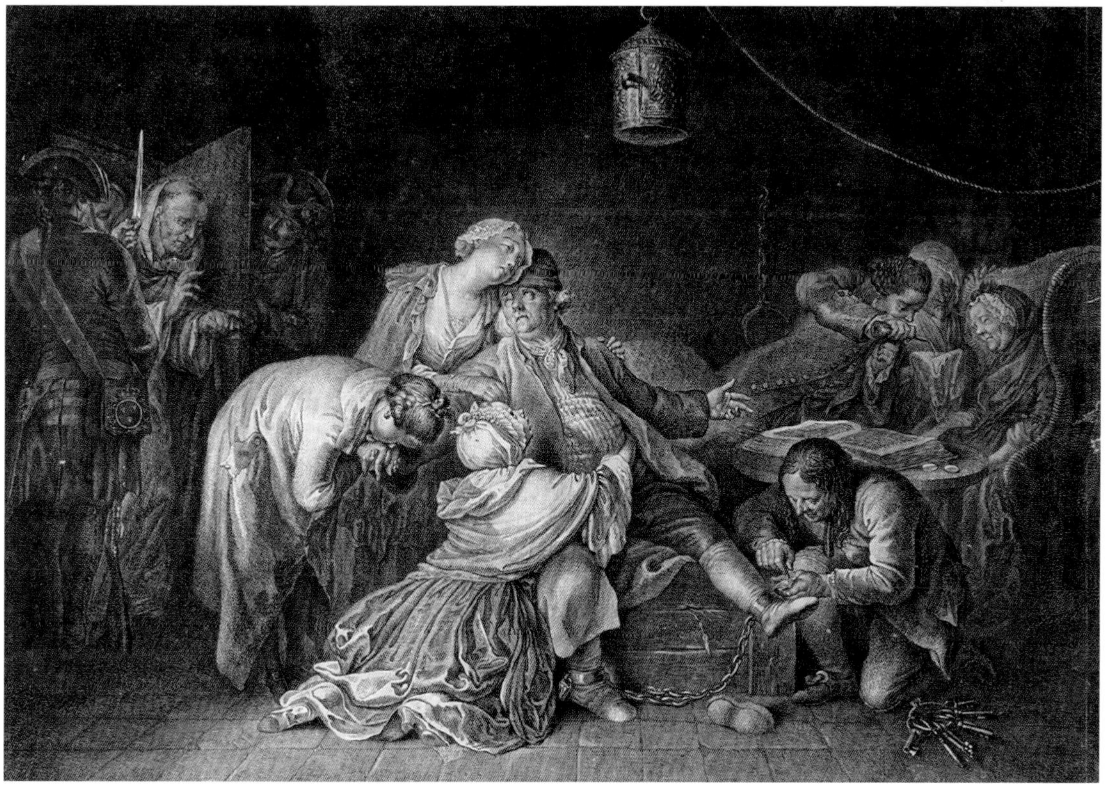

Fig. 36 *Les Adieux de Calas à sa famille*, engraving, signed: 'inv. peint & Gravé par D. Chodowiecki à Berlin', c. 1765
Anne-Rose Cabibel is shown kissing her husband's hand whilst his two daughters Rosine and Nanette embrace him on either side of their mother. Already tortured, Jean Calas is shown in prison, his manacles being released so that he can be led off to his final public torture and death in the Place St Georges, Toulouse, where his limbs were broken, and his body placed on the wheel. The scene is fictitious since Calas never saw his family again after his arrest. Subsequently, Voltaire persuaded Anne-Rose Calas to come to Paris, where she was received at the Royal Court and arranged for the two daughters to be released from the convents in which they had been confined. Voltaire championed the cause in his *Histoire d'Elizabeth Canning, et de Jean Calas*, published in London in 1762 by Jean Nourse, which did much to further the cause of tolerance.

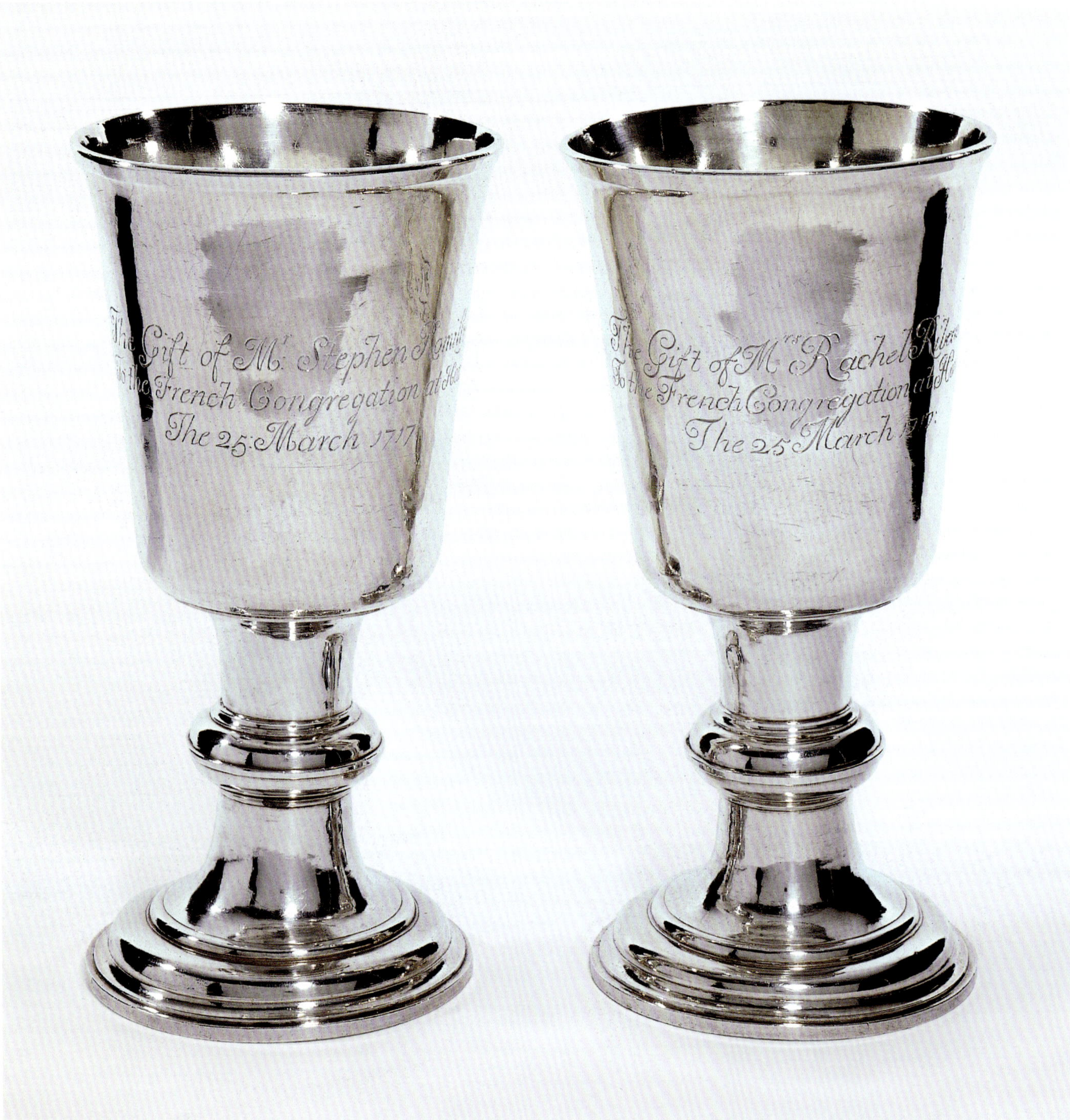

(fig. 105), since Guinand's grand-daughter Susanna Charlotte Guinand was the grandmother of the 1st Baron Fermoy, from whom the princes' mother descended.

The hospital flourished in the 1760s and 1770s. It was full to capacity. By 1763 the grounds were extended to four and a half acres, buildings were added, gardens well established and the orchards were productive. Legacies continued to fill the coffers and a high proportion of residents were paid for by sponsors. In 1774 to establish the corporation's leasehold rights, fifty-eight peppercorns were handed over to the Ironmongers' Company, the unpaid rental since 1716

Fig. 37 Communion cups, silver (Britannia standard), maker's mark of Robert Hill, London, 1716/17

Given by Rachel Ribeaut and Stephen Romilly to the French congregation at Hoxton, 25 March 1717, the cups were given to the hospital after the church closed in 1790. Romilly, the grandfather of the celebrated lawyer, ran a bleaching business at Hoxton. Ribeaut received external assistance from the French Hospital from April 1743 to July 1749.

(fig. 5). Future plans could now be made for generating income from four and a half acres of central London. A comparison of Rocque's (1746) and Horwood's (1792–9) London maps shows how bricks and mortar, in the form of terraced housing, were creeping ever closer to La Providence. Both maps still labelled Bath Street as Pest House Row.

International bequests reflected widespread sympathy for the refugees and their descendants. In 1740, Estienne Ronjat of Vevey, Switzerland, had enriched the corporation with a share of his deceased estate totalling £6,473.[20] Bequests continued into the 1770s, with £1,000 left by both the duchesse de La Force and Stephen [Estienne] Mounier, a director since 1750. Mounier added a long annuity of £20 to 'place out four poor boys as apprentices'.[21] Renewed sympathy for the ongoing plight of the Protestants in France was aroused by the fate of the Toulouse merchant Jean Calas, executed on the accusation of the murder of his son. The youth had in fact committed suicide, frustrated by not being able to pursue his chosen profession (figs. 35–6). One of the most surprising donations, in 1787, was sixty-three bottles of champagne sent to the hospital by the Chevalier d'Oraison as a gift from the young widow Marie Thérèse Louise of Savoy-Carignan, Princesse de Lamballe, the closest friend of Queen Marie-Antoinette and superintendent of the royal household in France.[22] The champagne was accepted, sold and brought each inmate a present of one shilling, with a small sum left over that was added to the funds.

The numbers of inmates indicate that persecution was still a vivid memory. Even in France of the 1720s there was still persecution: the duc de Bourbon, regent for the young Louis XV, had attempted to crush the surviving 'church of the desert', its secret pastors and worshippers. However, in 1787 Louis XVI convened a meeting of Notables which produced the Edict of Toleration, reversing the Revocation of the Edict of Nantes of 1685. In broader terms it reflected a decline in the intense Catholic-Protestant bitterness of earlier years. Yet the Gordon Riots in 1780 showed that anti-Catholic sentiment was still close to the surface in London.

In London, unemployment in the silk industry soared – Jacquard looms, importation of cheap silk and cheaper (Irish) labour led to severe unrest and, though the Spitalfields Act of 1773 brought peace, acute poverty was common. The weavers could do even less than before to support the aged, the *aliénés* and the sick amongst their community. But the more prosperous Huguenot families that had moved further out of London became integrated into Anglican churches. In 1790, following the closure of the Hoxton Huguenot church in 1785, Pierre Fargues gave the French Hospital two silver communion cups (fig. 37) and a silver paten, a welcome addition to the hitherto pewter-only chapel plate.[23] The last minister of the Hoxton Church, the Revd Pierre Lescure, had previously served the French church in Leicester Fields, which closed in 1778. This had occupied the Orange Street chapel, now behind the National Gallery, until its merger with the Le Carré church in Berwick Street (fig. 38). Lescure became chaplain to the French Hospital in 1790. Pierre Fargues's donation marks an early stage of the hospital's history as a treasury

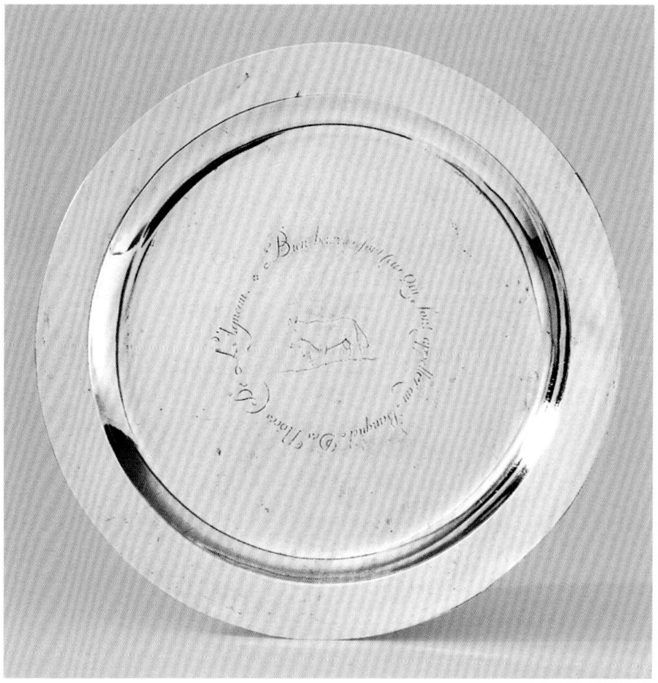

Fig. 38 Alms-dish, silver (unmarked), attributed to Jonah Clifton, London, c. 1720

The dish was bought by subscription by the congregation of the conformist church of Le Carré in 1720. This church had been established in Soho Square in 1689, although in 1694 it moved to Berwick Street, where its flock continued to meet until 1769. It then moved to Little Dean Street and closed in 1849. Its name derives from its original location in Soho Square.

One of the last members of the congregation, A.H. Rivaz, gave the church's silver service to St John the Evangelist, Limehouse, a church selected by the Bishop of London. Consigned for sale at Sotheby's in 1930, some French Hospital directors negotiated with the ecclesiastical authorities to purchase this most typical Huguenot piece. The service of nine items included two 'bassins' made in 1719 and 1720 by Jonah Clifton. A 'souscoupe' was withheld.

for artefacts, records, and later, books, of the Huguenot past, although in this case the gift was intended for regular use in the service of communion.

In the last decade of the eighteenth century political upheavals in France placed the former plight of Huguenot refugee settlers in London in the shade. Other priorities dominated those with charitable intentions. A new generation of officers and directors faced serious challenges to ensure that the French Hospital flourished in the nineteenth century.

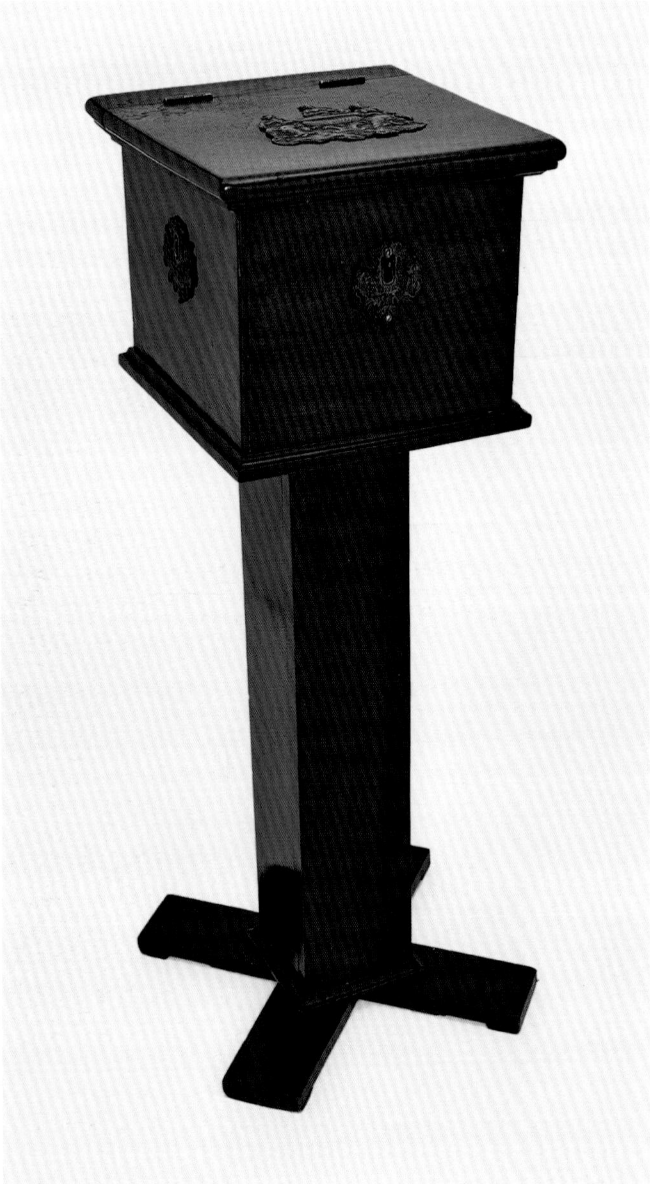

Fig. 39 Alms-box, mahogany, mid-Georgian, on later stand
The three key escutcheons are in gilt metal, cast and chased with rococo motifs and figures; the money slot is mounted with the three theological virtues, Faith, Hope and Charity.

1 PRO. PROB 11/579 (10 May 1921).
2 HL H.L1 Dufour Charity. See Gray, p. 81.
3 Gray, *ibid.*, pp. 3–4.
4 HL H.F2.9; Gray, p. 62.
5 Théodore de Saint-Leger's will mentions 'argenterie, perles, diamants, tapisseries, carosse et chevaux'.
6 Maitland, p. 1303.
7 The contents of their room are listed in the 1742 inventory, see p. 112.
8 *Registres des Eglises de La Chapelle Royale de Saint James et … 1700–56* (*HSQS*, XXVIII, 1924), p. 8.
9 HL H.H1.10. Richard Cox, first paymaster to Ligonier's regiment, then to the British army, became the Cox of Cox and King's, bankers.
10 HL H.E4.1.
11 Maitland, p. 1303.
12 M. Winston, 'The Bethel of Norwich: An Eighteenth-Century Hospital for Lunatics', *Medical History*, 1994, 38, pp. 27–51.
13 W. Parry Jones, *The Trade in Lunacy: a Study of Private Madhouses in England in the Eighteenth and Nineteenth Centuries*, London (1972).
14 Roy Porter, *Mind-forg'd manacles: a history of madness in England from the Restoration to the Regency*, London (1990); Richard Hunter and Ida McAlpine, *Three Hundred Years of Psychiatry 1535–1860* (1963).
15 Pierre Silvestre was later Inspector of Architecture and Gardens to the Duke of Montagu at Boughton, and literary executor to the Catholic exile Charles de Saint-Evremond. He served as physician to Ralph, Duke of Montagu.
16 HL H.D13.3.
17 HL H.B11.3.
18 Jacob Radnor, *A Huguenot Family*, Winchester (2001), p. 53.
19 Maitland, p. 1304.
20 HL H.E2.31.
21 HL H.L4.1. PRO.PROB.11/1013 (20 March 1775). The fund, augmented by later bequests, continues to this day to make an annual grant to assist a young person in craft or other work or training.
22 A.H. Browning, Presidential Address, Huguenot Society AGM, 1933, *PHS*, XV, 1 (1934), p. 11. See also F. Montefiore, *The Princesse de Lamballe* (1896).
23 Jones, p. 13, plate VII.

5

Waning fortunes in Finsbury

By 1800 the French Hospital was under pressure to justify its continuing existence and was facing financial problems. Bequests were diminishing in size and number, and running costs had risen steeply since the outbreak of war with France. In 1793 the deficit of over £350 had to be met by selling stock.

Political events in France brought demands for charitable support for French Catholic refugees. Between 1792 and 1802 over 12,000 French Catholic priests came to Britain. By the end of the Napoleonic wars, other smaller hospitals had been established in Mile End, London, including the Beth Holim for Spanish and Portuguese Jews and another for German and Dutch Jews. Huguenot descendants working in the highly successful luxury trades of the West End of London were already well integrated. They had belonged to French churches which conformed to the Anglican liturgy, but by the end of the eighteenth century the French churches had mostly closed and they

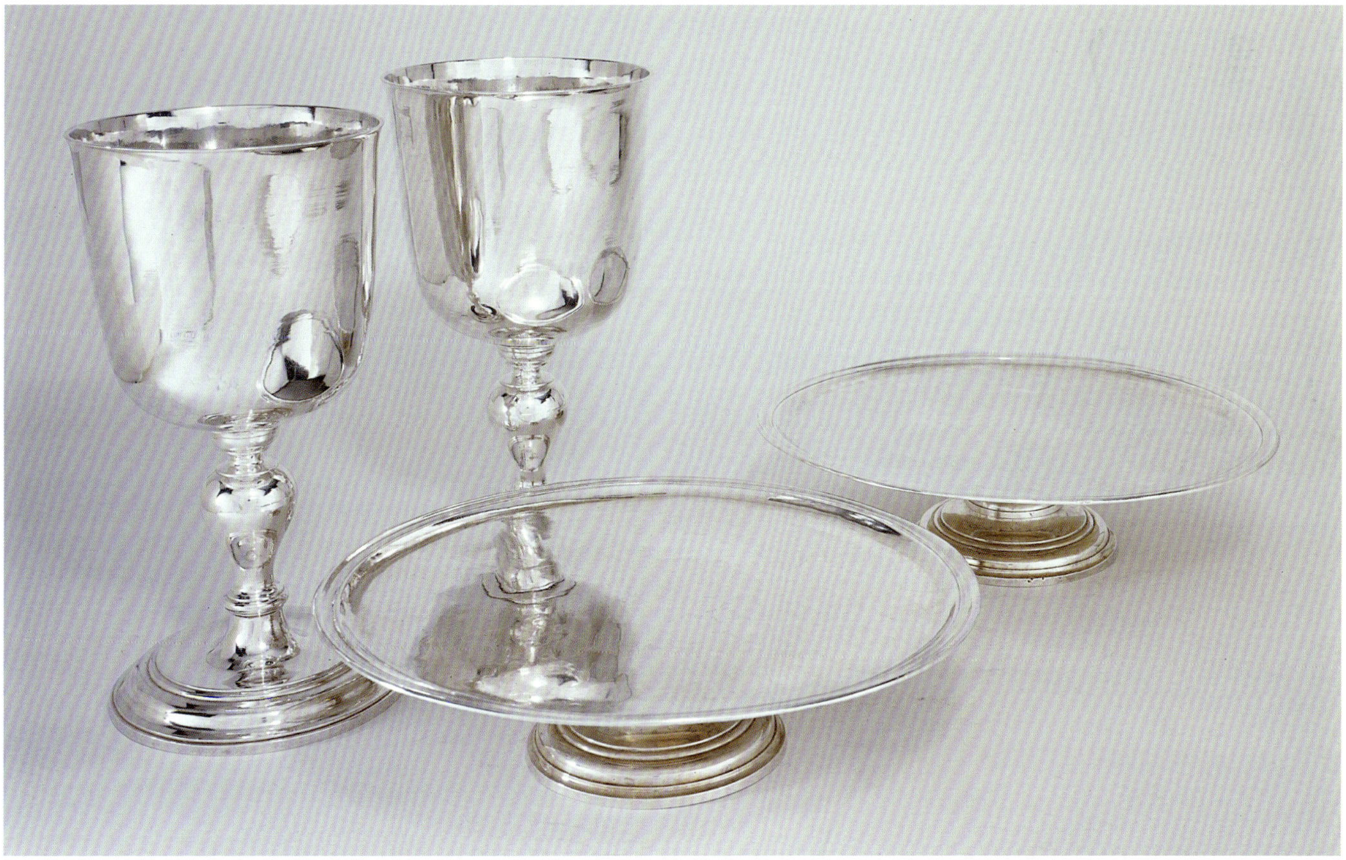

Fig. 40 Communion plate for the Savoy Chapel, 1717/18

A pair of communion cups, silver (Britannia standard), London, maker's mark of Lewis Cuny, 1717/18, and a pair of patens, silver (Britannia standard), London, maker's mark of Lewis Cuny, 1717/18

The cups are identical in form to the 1631 set of cups made for the Walloon congregation that met in the crypt of Canterbury Cathedral. In 1717–18, Jacob Margas supplied a set of four similar communion cups for the French Church in Threadneedle Street. The form of the paten is similar to an earlier example supplied by Cuny for Wishford Magna Church, Wiltshire.

The communion plate was used by the conformist congregation at the French Church of the Savoy until 1737 when it merged with its annexe the Church of Les Grecs in Hog Lane. In 1845 a new church was built in Shaftesbury Avenue. Lewis Cuny worked in Panton Street, Soho. It was presumably his widow 'La Veuve Cuny' who recommended Jacques Ray for admission to the French Hospital in 1737 (fig. 13).

were attending local Anglican churches. However, those families who had settled in the East End and strove to make their living through the fluctuating silk trades often still had recourse to the Huguenot charities established three generations earlier, including Huguenot friendly societies and the French Hospital.

The last of the mental patients was admitted to La Providence in 1785 and by 1791 the wing or Petites Maisons of the hospital for the mentally ill was empty and quickly adapted for other use. Those suffering in this way could now be placed elsewhere: at Bethlem or Guy's Hospital or, since 1786, at the specialist St Luke's, which occupied a fine new building a few hundred yards from the French Hospital, just north of Old Street.

The treasurer, Jean-Daniel Lucadou, appointed in 1794, had persuaded the Court by 1796 to limit the number of inmates to 140. Five years later there were only 100, less than half the number that had been cared for when Lucadou first became a director in 1769. The directors considered that their duty lay in caring for 'those among us who are in distress', as the Court Prayer entreated. They felt that this was more important than busying themselves 'too much with the perpetuity of an establishment whose nature it is to die out of itself in time'.[1]

With the continuing successful integration of the Huguenots in London, several Huguenot charitable organ-

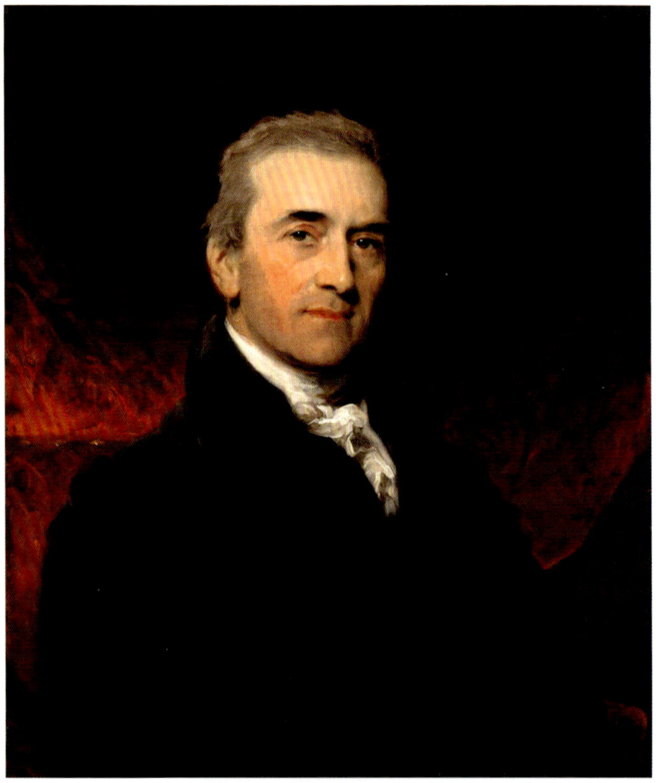

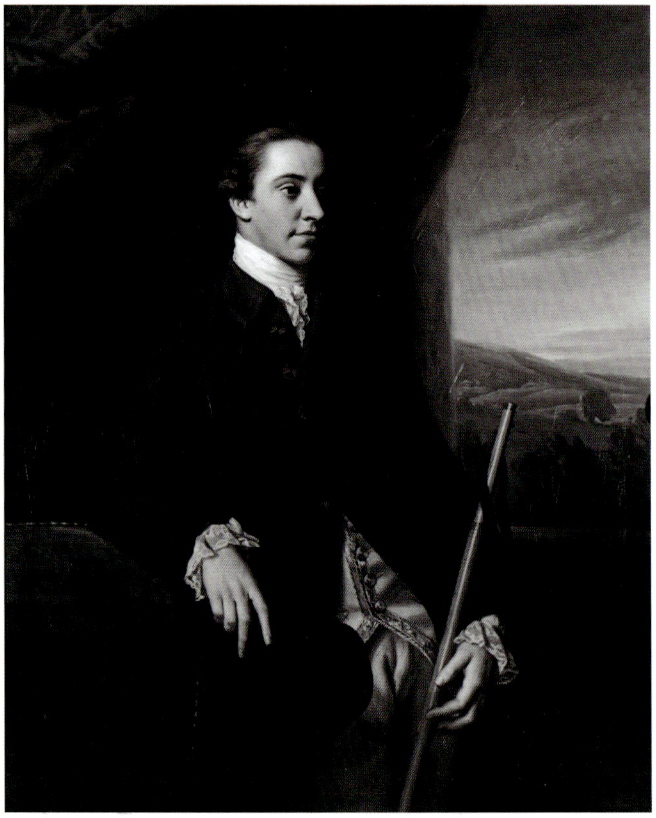

Fig. 41 (*right, top*) Sir Samuel Romilly, KC, MP (1757–1818), oil on canvas, Sir Thomas Lawrence. *National Portrait Gallery*

Romilly was a law reformer who became Solicitor General in 1806. He was the youngest son of Peter Romilly, a jeweller of Frith Street, Soho, and his wife Margaret Garnault, and was the grandson of Samuel Romilly, who presented one of the silver communion cups to the French Church at Hoxton in 1717 (fig. 37). The family had originally come from Montpellier. Sir Samuel Romilly was elected a director of the French Hospital in 1786. By 1802 he was one of the recognized leaders of the Chancery Bar. He was elected Member of Parliament for Queenborough. A man of mercy, reason and eloquence, he tackled with vigour the tendency of contemporary English criminal law to resort to the death penalty for trifling offences.

The Romilly family arms are displayed at Rochester. The Romilly book-plate (end-papers and p. 110) belonged to Sir Samuel's father, the jeweller Peter Romilly (1712–1784), who 'delighted in his library' at his home in Frith Street, Soho.

Fig. 42 (*right, bottom*) Jacob Pleydell-Bouverie, 2nd Earl of Radnor (1749–1828), oil on canvas, Nathanial Dance. *Private collection*

A great Francophile, the 2nd Earl of Radnor often stayed in Paris and in Caen. At home he employed the architect James Wyatt to extend Longford Castle and helped organize the Wiltshire Militia. He entertained the Prince Regent at Longford.

izations found that they had reached the end of their useful life. The corporation of the French Hospital assumed responsibility for administering their residue funds. Capital worth £1,600 in 1791 was held on behalf of the Société de Nismes, one of the friendly societies pioneered by the Huguenot refugees in England, and three places were allocated in the hospital for use by their members. The hospital bakery still supplied bread for the Spitalfields 'Soupe', renamed 'Le Pain' when bread became the main ration. In 1827, the French Hospital assumed responsibility for its capital amounting to £1,700, at which time there were 46 'Bread House Pensioners'.[2] The last payment was made on behalf of that charity in 1877.[3] Since 1841, the French Church (formerly St Mary the Less) in Norwich, has annually paid the residue of its apprenticeship funds to the French Hospital. In the twentieth century the Huguenot church of the Savoy made over its charitable funds to the French Hospital.

In a bid to put the corporation's finances on an even keel, the treasurer Lucadou made personal loans to the hospital. Although these were repaid by the sale of stock worth £1,000 in 1795, he organized a public appeal in 1803, with a printed handbill in French and English.[4] This was a failure. Targeted mainly at the Huguenot community in England it raised only £306, almost all of it from the governor and directors.[5]

Part of the building including the Petites Maisons wing was rented out in 1801. Yet the 'cash flow' problem persisted and land was sold to meet an annual overspend running to

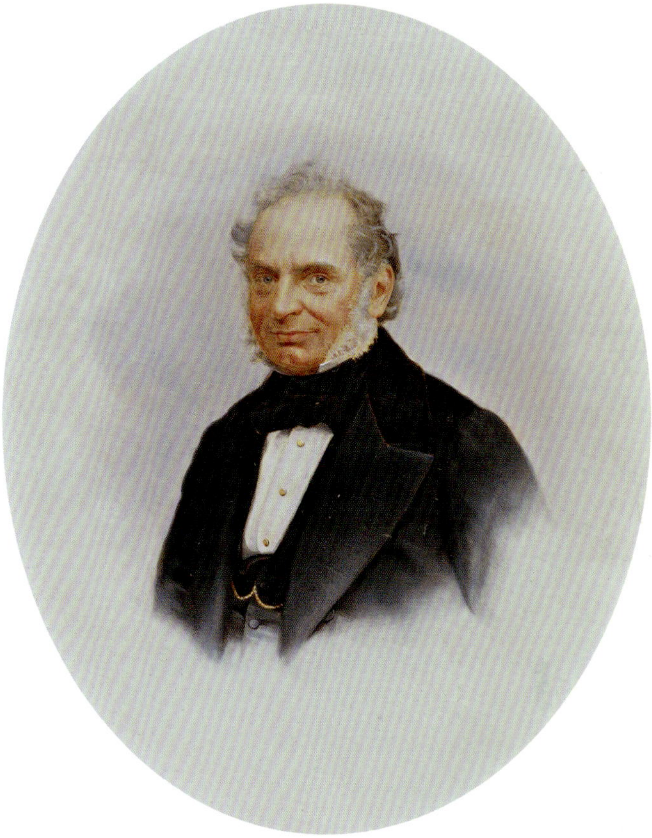

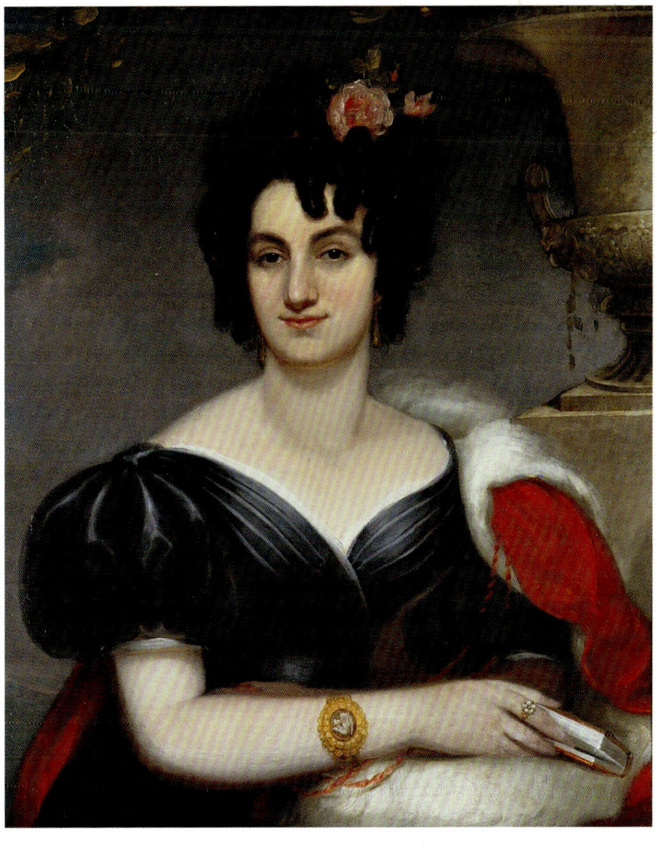

Fig. 43 (*right, top*) Richard Grellier (1801–1863), oil on card, unknown artist, c. 1855

Richard Grellier was the son of Peter Paul Grellier (1773–1828), who became a director in 1820. His grandfather was Leonard Turquand, also a director from 1770. This network of Huguenot families included the Aubertin family. Elected director in 1837, Richard continued the family tradition and served as surveyor to the French Hospital for twenty-five years. He wed (Mary) Louisa André in 1856. Her portrait (fig. 44) also hangs in the dining-room at Rochester. Christopher Grellier, a member of the family is currently a director, having previously continued the family's tradition of surveying for twenty-five years. His wife has served until recently as a trustee of the Idlewild Trust since its foundation by Peter Minet (fig. 107).

Fig. 44 (*right, bottom*) Mrs Louisa Grellier, *née* André (c. 1811–1879), oil on canvas, circle of George Henry Harlow, 1830s, in contemporary frame

Mary Louisa was the daughter of Jaques-Pierre André, who became a director of the French Hospital in 1814. She married Richard Grellier, the secretary, in 1856.

some £7,000. The sale of the building materials salvaged from the demolition of two empty wings brought in some cash.

In 1807, Sir Samuel Romilly (fig. 41), a director since 1786,[6] who became MP and Solicitor General in 1806, assisted the governor, Jacob Pleydell-Bouverie, 2nd Earl of Radnor (fig. 42), in bringing a bill through Parliament enabling the governor and directors to grant building leases. The ensuing Act of 1808 led to the granting, from 1810, of twenty-nine leases, all of about sixty years' duration. Tall tenements and rows of terraced housing on land leased by the hospital soon surrounded the high walls of La Providence and the green fields beside the footway to Islington became Galway, Gastigny and Radnor Streets.

As early as 1801 the court of directors had discussed the possibility of moving to a smaller building elsewhere to cater more economically for the dwindling numbers of inmates. In 1815 there were thirty, forty-four in 1827, but

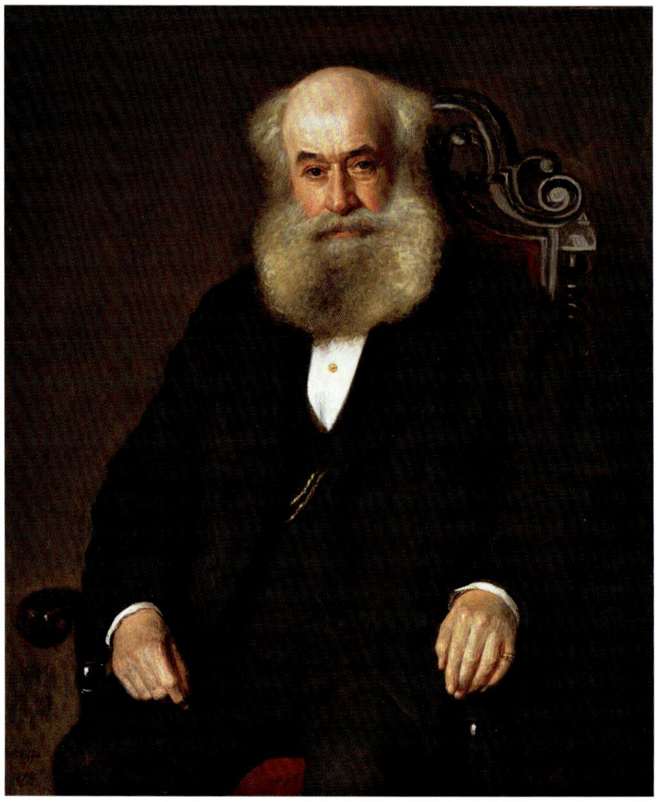

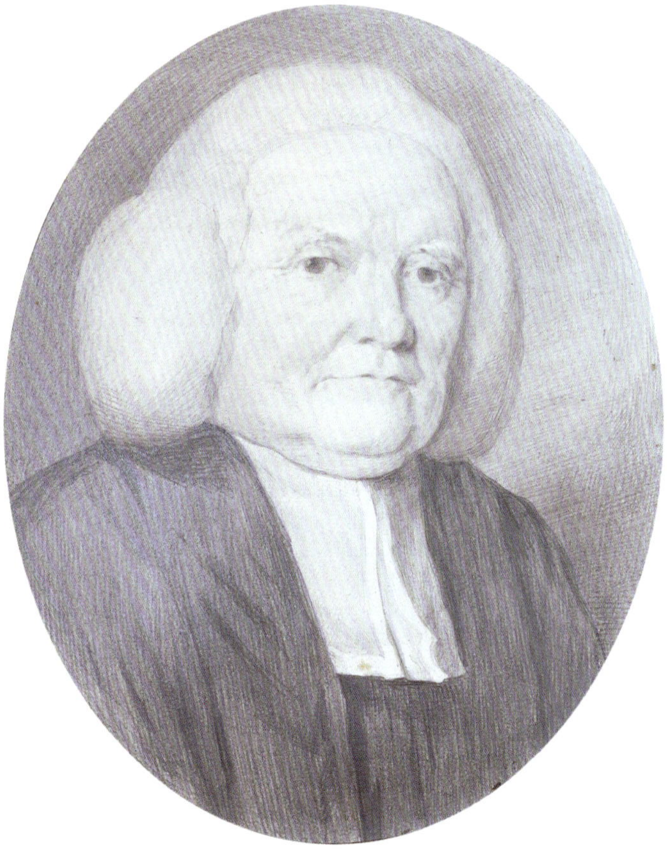

Fig. 45 (*right, top*) Richard Hervé Giraud (1800–1886), oil on canvas, signed W. Fyfe, 1874

Giraud is seated in a Jacobean chair. Elected a director in 1829, he served as secretary from 1836, treasurer from 1854, and deputy-governor in 1876. He was descended from the Revd Thomas Hervé, the minister of Les Grecs, the Huguenot church in Hog Lane. He was a cousin-once-removed of Arthur Giraud Browning (fig. 59), who presented this portrait to the French Hospital. A founder member of the Huguenot Society in 1885, he was also the first Master of the Huguenot Masonic Lodge founded in 1884.

Fig. 46 (*right, bottom*) The Revd Thomas Hervé, drawing, A.B. Connor, Wandsworth, 1904

This drawing of the minister of the Chapel Royal and of Les Grecs was copied from a miniature. A label on the back, signed 'A.G.B. [Arthur Giraud Browning] October 1904', includes the following commentary: 'Born in 1684/1688, Thomas Hervé was in early life a Capuchin Friar at La Rochelle. He was most zealous and active in persecuting the Protestants but from reading some of their books which he seized he became convinced of the truths they contained. After surmounting many difficulties he escaped to Holland. Later he came to London and from about 1727 to 1731 he was a member of the French Church in Hog Lane. In Hogarth's print of Noon (published 1738) the minister depicted standing at the door of that church as the congregation is leaving is said to be Mr Hervé. In 1758 he was appointed minister of the French Chapel Royal, St. James's and about the same time he was acting as French tutor to the Royal Princesses. Mr. Hervé married Elizabeth Gagnon (b. 1699 d. at Faversham 1765) by whom he had an only daughter Jane Elizabeth. He died at Faversham 1769/70. Jane Elizabeth Hervé b. in London 1733 married in 1758 the Revd Francis Frederick Giraud then Vicar of Westwell but afterwards of Preston near Faversham. She died in 1816 leaving issue six sons and two daughters v Giraud pedigree.'

the lean times lingered on through the 1830s and 1840s. In 1837, the surveyors Savage and Grellier (figs. 43–4) conducted a thorough scrutiny of the buildings and produced an estimate of £1,470 for repairs – the broken brickwork and stairways, dry rot and general decay demanded urgent action.[7] A new building was proposed the following year but the necessary funds and a strong conviction of the need to move were lacking.

At that time attendance by some directors fell and on occasion there was 'no quorum' so that decisions had to be deferred, but other directors worked energetically for the hospital. David Duval (fig. 33) served as a director for fifty years from his election in 1786 and was deputy-governor from 1813. Richard Hervé Giraud was appointed as a director in 1829 (fig. 45) retiring as deputy-governor in 1887. One of his forbears on his father's side had been sponsored for the Anglican ministry by Lord Galway, and one of his mother's ancestors was Thomas Hervé (fig. 46), the pastor of the Huguenot church in Soho known as Les Grecs, immortalized by Hogarth in *Noon*. Both Duval and Hervé would have known Joseph Claude Meffre, who became chaplain to the hospital in 1826. A former Catholic priest who had fled revolutionary France, he had joined the Church of England in 1798 (fig. 47). He was the last native French-speaking chaplain, serving the hospital until his death in 1846.

From 1836 the minutes, directors' first names and the Corporation's business were written in English for the first time.[8]

In one issue of the weekly *Household Words*, Dickens described a visit to the hospital in which he found that:

> [It] has lost much of its distinctive national character. Sixty years ago a visitor might have heard the inmates chattering away in antiquated French. They speak English now, probably some of them do not know a word of French, because the majority of their ancestors in four generations had been English.

He thought it 'a little amusing mark of deference to the land of their founders' that 'a Mrs Stephen (who was admitted after 1820) became Madame St Etienne as soon as she entered the French Hospital'.[9] When in 1841 an important step was taken to streamline applications, the forms known as 'Petitions' (fig. 48) were printed in English.

In 1851 the Revd Charles Weiss, historian of the *grand refuge*, recorded that in the early 1800s, 'the descendants of the exiles, whose interests were completely identified with those of the English, would no longer avow their origin', partly due to 'the fierce wars of the Republic which lasted till the end of the Empire, which had revived the old hatred between France and England ... the French colony in London no longer existed ...'[10]

From the mid-nineteenth century, most of the families whose elderly members were admitted to the French Hospital had previously been connected to the silk trade. The overwhelming majority came from the East End, especially Spitalfields, Bethnal Green and Mile End.[11] By then, as Charles Weiss noted, 'The Spitalfields workmen themselves seem to have little recollection of their foreign origin. Nevertheless, in their old age, they frequently claim the right of ending their days in the French Hospital, which they call their Providence'.[12]

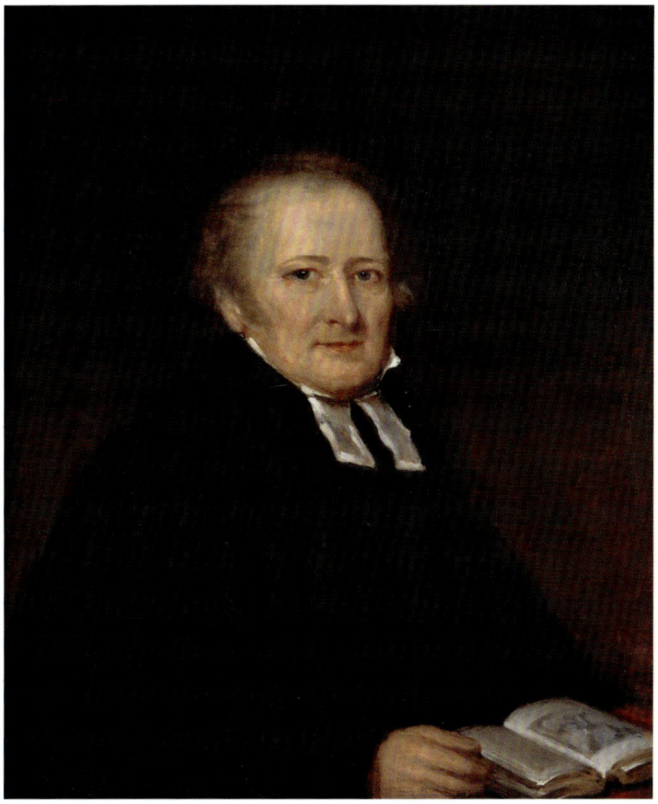

Fig. 47 The Revd Joseph Claude Meffre (1766–1845), oil on canvas, artist unknown, 1830s

A Catholic priest from the diocese of Toulon, Meffre fled from the aftermath of the French Revolution in 1794. He was involved in a public scandal in Salisbury and by 1798 had formally recanted his Catholicism in Winchester Cathedral. He published an Apologia for his religious position, which was printed in the *Winchester Repository*. Meffre joined the Church of England and declared that it was in conformity with 'the doctrine of the true Catholic Church'. From 1826 to 1847 he served as the last of the French Hospital's French-speaking chaplains.

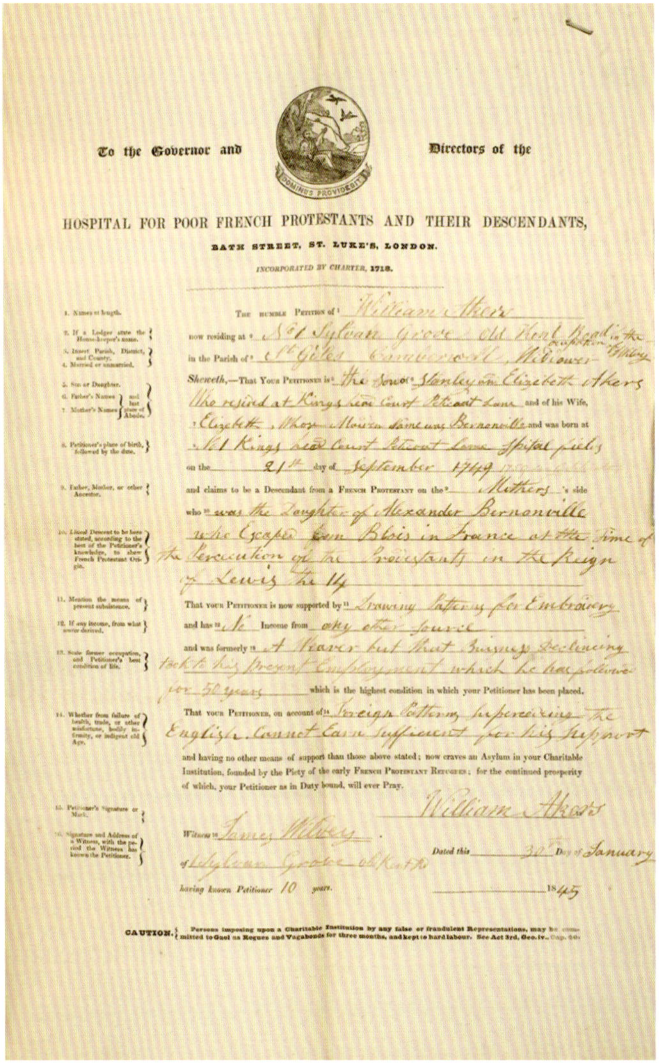

To the Governor and Directors of the

DOMINUS PROVIDEBIT

HOSPITAL FOR POOR FRENCH PROTESTANTS AND THEIR DESCENDANTS,

BATH STREET, ST. LUKE'S, LONDON.

INCORPORATED BY CHARTER, 1718.

1. Names at length. — The humble Petition of William Akers

2. If a Lodger state the House-keeper's name. — now residing at No 1 Sylvan Grove Old Kent Road in the

3. Insert Parish, District, and County. 4. Married or unmarried. — in the Parish of St Giles Camberwell Widower

5. Son or Daughter. 6. Father's Names and last place of Abode. 7. Mother's Names and last place of Abode. — Sheweth,—That Your Petitioner is the Son of Stanley and Elizabeth Akers Who resided at Kings Head Court Petticoat Lane and of his Wife, Elizabeth, Whose Maiden Name was Bernonville and was born at

8. Petitioner's place of birth, followed by the date. — No 1 Kings Head Court Petticoat Lane Spitalfields on the 21st day of September 1749

9. Father, Mother, or other Ancestor. — and claims to be a Descendant from a French Protestant on the Mothers's side

10. Lineal Descent to be here stated, according to the best of the Petitioner's knowledge, to shew French Protestant Origin. — who was the Daughter of Alexander Bernonville who Escaped from Blois in France at the time of the Persecution of the Protestants in the Reign of Lewis the 14

11. Mention the means of present subsistence. — That your Petitioner is now supported by Drawing Patterns for Embroidery

12. If any income, from what source derived. — and has No Income from any other source

13. State former occupation, and Petitioner's best condition of life. — and was formerly A Weaver but that Business declining took to his present Employment which he has followed for 50 years which is the highest condition in which your Petitioner has been placed.

14. Whether from failure of health, trade, or other misfortune, bodily infirmity, or indigent old Age. — That your Petitioner, on account of Foreign Patterns superseding the English cannot Earn sufficient for his support

and having no other means of support than those above stated; now craves an Asylum in your Charitable Institution, founded by the Piety of the early French Protestant Refugees; for the continued prosperity of which, your Petitioner as in Duty bound, will ever Pray.

15. Petitioner's Signature or Mark. — William Akers

16. Signature and Address of a Witness, with the period the Witness has known the Petitioner. — Witness James Wilvery of Sylvan Grove Old Kent Rd having known Petitioner 10 years.

Dated this 30th Day of January 1845

CAUTION. Persons imposing upon a Charitable Institution by any false or fraudulent Representations, may be committed to Gaol as Rogues and Vagabonds for three months, and kept to hard labour. See Act 3rd, Geo. iv., Cap. 40.

Fig. 48 A Petition: a printed application form submitted in 1845. *Huguenot Library*

In 1841 printed application forms for admission to the French Hospital known as 'Petitions' were introduced. William Akers was the grandson of Alexander Bernonville 'who escaped from Blois in France at the time of the Persecution of the Protestants in the Reign of Louis XIV. He originally worked as a weaver, but "that business declining" took to his present employment of drawing patterns for embroidery which he had pursued for fifty years, but foreign patterns superseding the English, could no longer earn sufficient to support himself.' At the time of his application he lived at No. 1 Sylvan Grove, Old Kent Road. His parents had lived in 1 King's Head Court, Petticoat Lane, Spitalfields, where he was born in 1759. He died in 1852 and was buried in St Luke's, Old Street.

1 HL H A4.2 Court Minutes 1780–1816. See also Marmoy, 'French Hospital', p. 236.

2 HL H.1.4, Memorandum Book of Jean Hebert, Steward, pp. 17–18, 79–80.

3 C.F.A. Marmoy, 'La Soupe: La Maison de Charité de Spittlefields', *PHS*, XXIII, 3 (1979), pp. 134–7.

4 The handbill indicates that services were held in the chapel twice a week in French according to the Anglican liturgy. The minister was responsible for preaching, visiting and comforting the elderly, infirm and sick.

5 HL H.J38. Marmoy, 'French Hospital', p. 237.

6 HL H.A1.2; HL H.E9.6.

7 HL H.F1.5.

8 *Ibid.*, p. 240.

9 *Household Words*, 8 (1853). There is, regrettably, neither a Stephen nor a St Étienne to be found in Charles Marmoy's *List of Inmates*.

10 Weiss, pp. 280, 283–4. Weiss was president of the Société de l'Histoire du Protestantisme Français, Paris.

11 Robert Nash, in a personal communication, May 2008.

12 Weiss, pp. 280, 283–4.

6

The French Hospital in Hackney

The hospital in Finsbury was now very run down and in urgent need of restoration. There is no evidence that any building works were carried out after the 1837 survey. Even though the number of inmates had fallen and funding was very tight, the idea of making a new building began to take shape in the directors' minds. The choice was to attempt to restore the present property, part of which had already been leased out, to rebuild or else to find a new site and start afresh. The old building had been modified, two wings had been demolished, one leased out. Rebuilding the hospital on its Bath Street site did not seem a very attractive option since the area had become quite built up over the last fifty years. Furthermore, part of the site was still leased from the Ironmongers' Company and the future prospects of development seemed unsure. Some directors suggested that the best idea would be to seek a freehold site somewhere slightly further out of the City but still within easy reach of the East End, whence most of the inmates hailed. On 2 May 1857 an Extraordinary Court was convened and it was decided, by nine votes to six, to obtain a site for building a new hospital. The opinion of the current inmates, including 'those troublemakers in the disorderly ward', was canvassed and they voted in favour by forty-three votes to ten.[1] The search by the directors then began in earnest.

The Building Committee was set up the following month. Henry Elliot, the steward, kept a 'Journal of Visits to Various Locations to Ascertain an Eligible Site for Building a New Hospital'[2] and recorded visits to sites including Beckenham, Finchley, Highgate, Holloway, Putney, Snaresbrook and Wimbledon, all of them still rural or

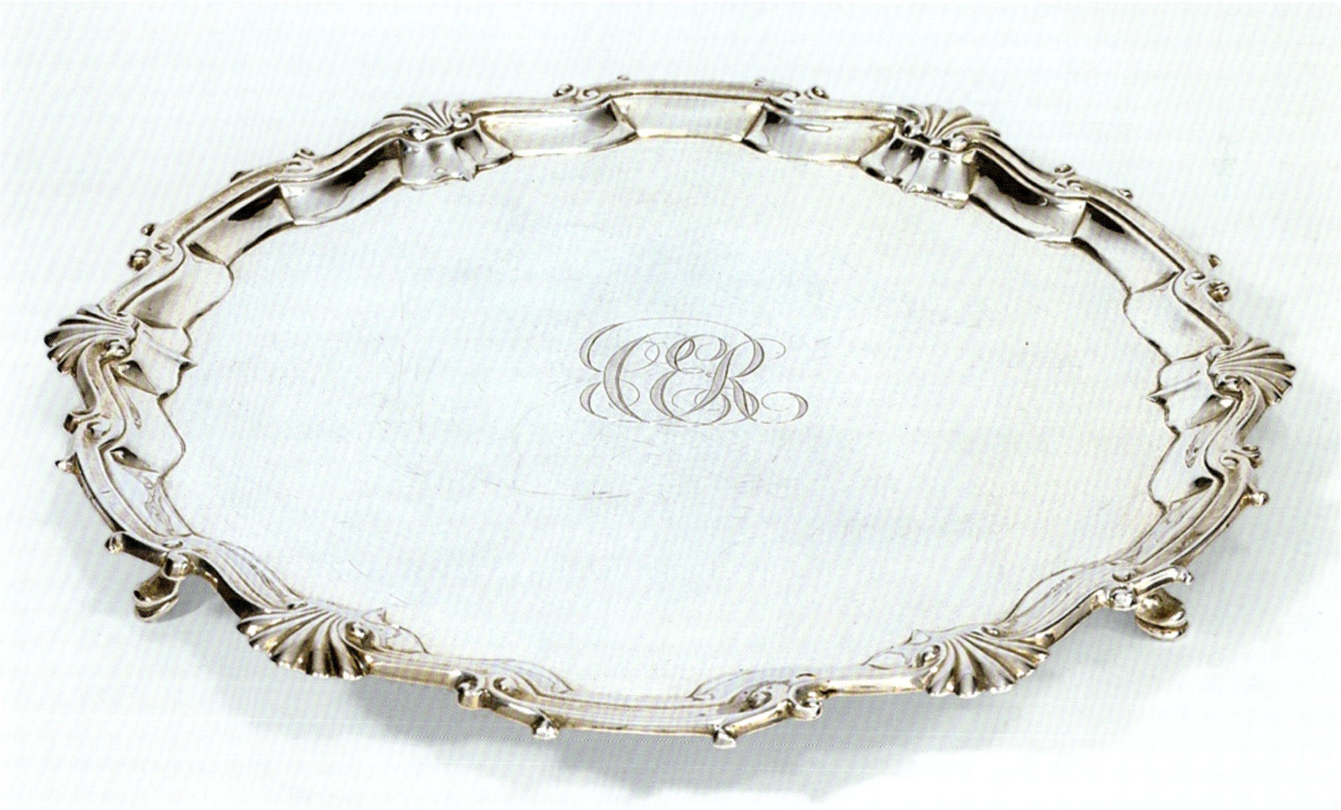

Fig. 49 Waiter, sterling silver, maker's mark of Edward Jay, London, 1791/2
Both this waiter and the salver in fig. 51 were given to the hospital by Francis Jolit.

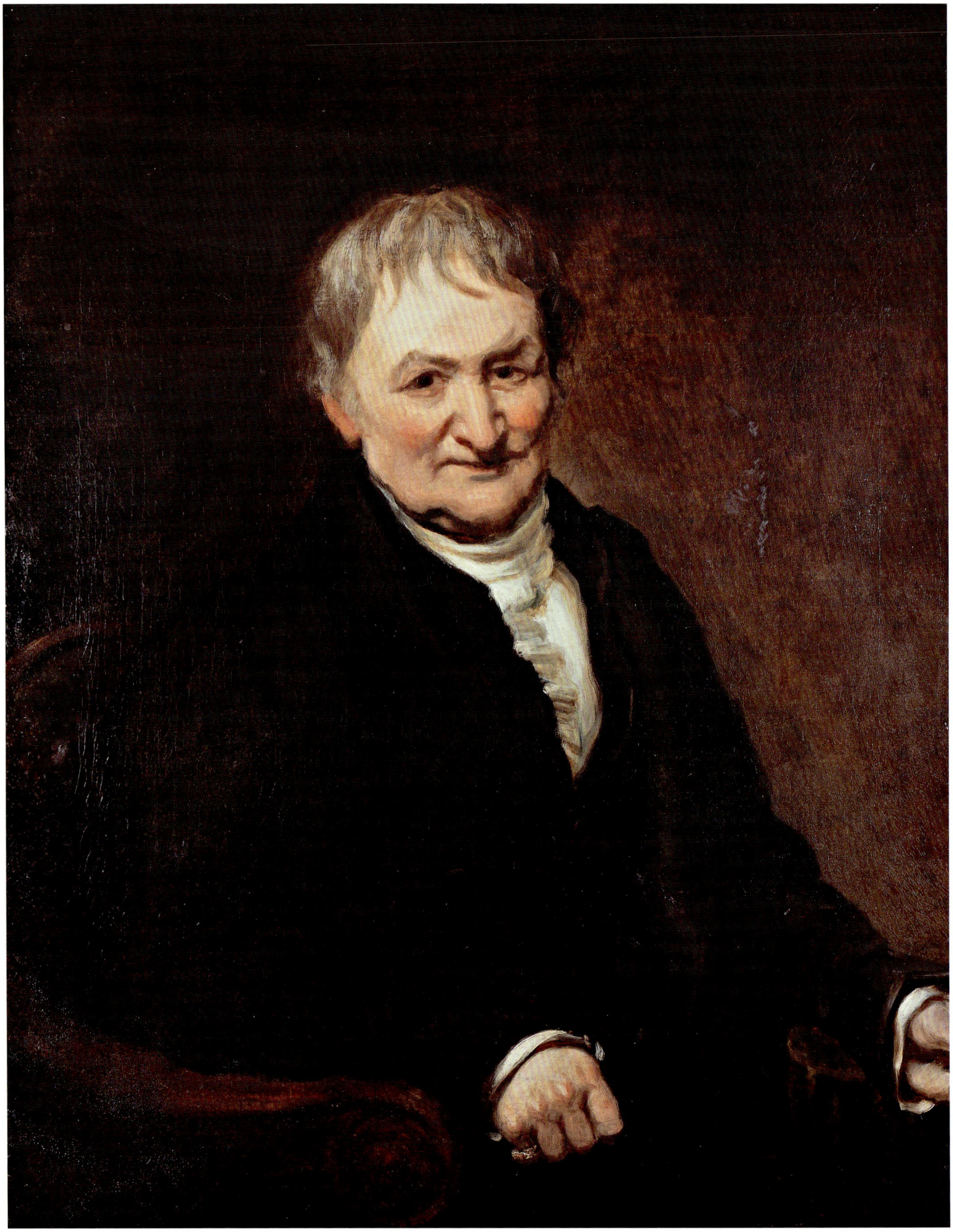

Fig. 50 Francis Jolit (c. 1754–1836), oil on canvas, John Opie, c. 1805

Director of the French Hospital from 1818, Jolit worked as an undertaker and is mentioned in the wills of many Huguenot descendants. His youngest son, Thomas Russell Jolit, was treasurer of the Charitable Society of Saintonge and Angoumois from 1838 to 1860.

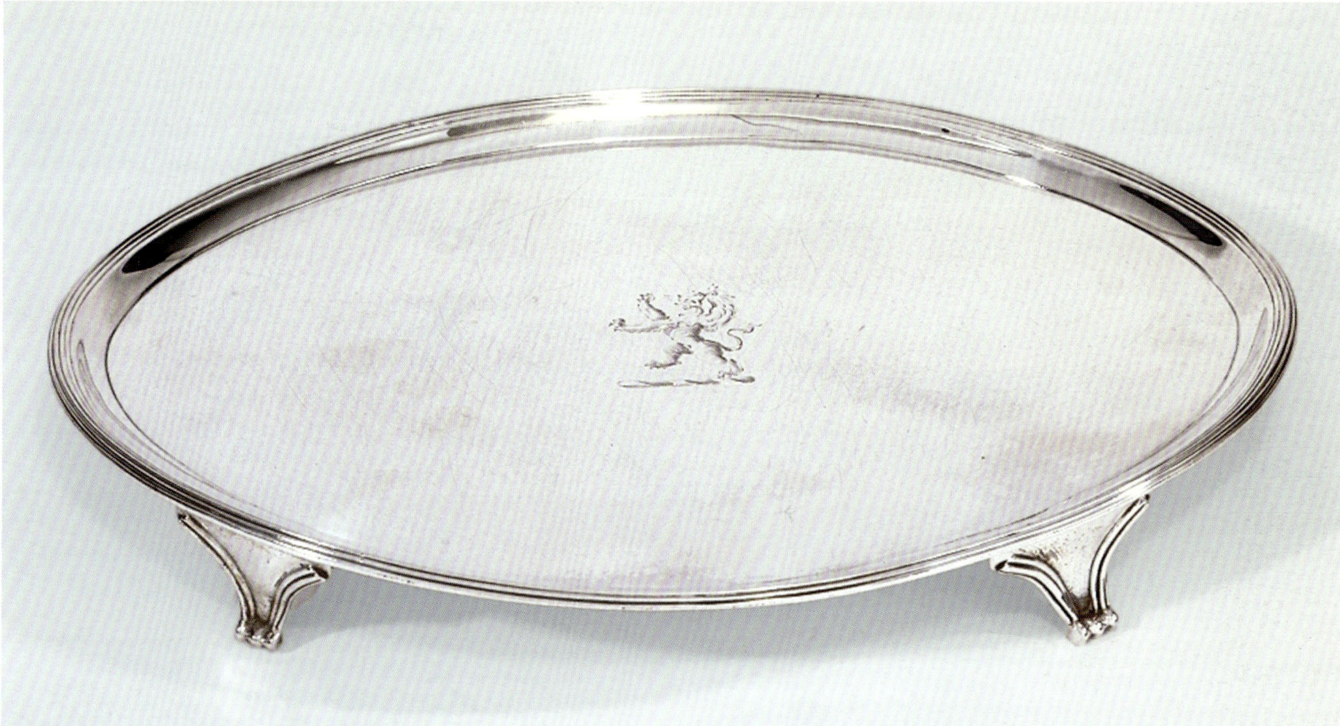

Fig. 51 Salver, sterling silver, maker's mark of William Peaston, London, 1754/5

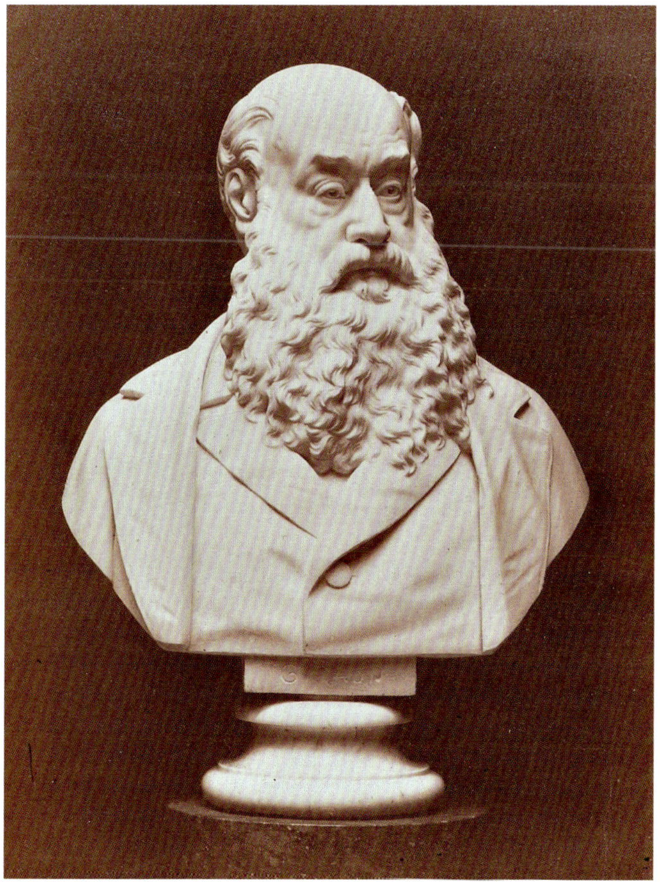

Fig. 52 Richard Hervé Giraud (1800–1886), photograph by H. Dixon of marble bust by J. Lawlor, 1882

Neither this marble bust of Giraud nor that commissioned by the directors of Robert Lewis Roumieu is any longer in the French Hospital collections.

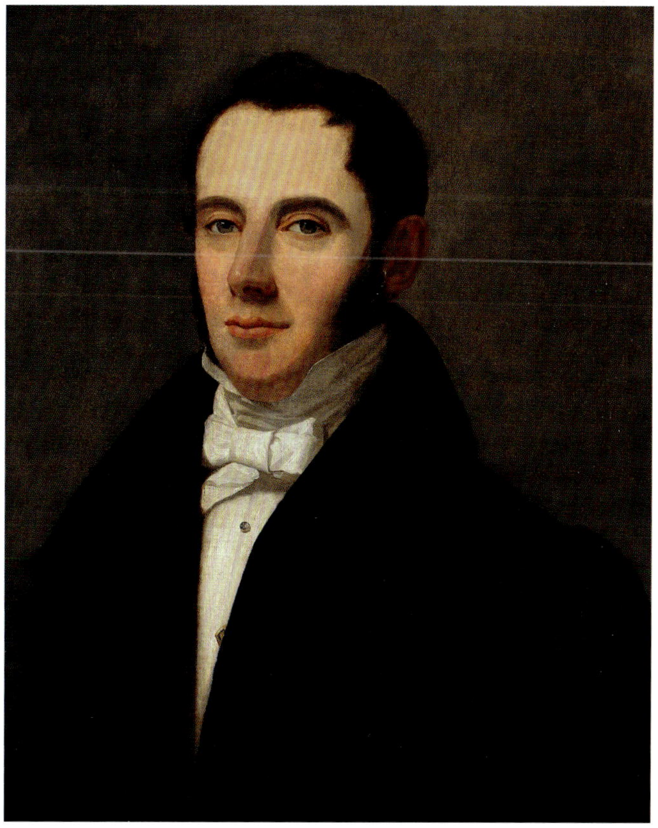

Fig. 53 Frederic Albert Winsor, oil on canvas, follower of Louis-Leopold Boilly, c. 1800, in an 1830s frame

Frederic Winsor was a director for nearly 40 years, becoming secretary in 1874. He was born Friedrich Albrecht Winzer, the son of a pioneer of the same name, who founded the Gas Light and Coke Company in 1812. His father was responsible for lighting Pall Mall in 1809–1810 during the Sessions of Parliament.

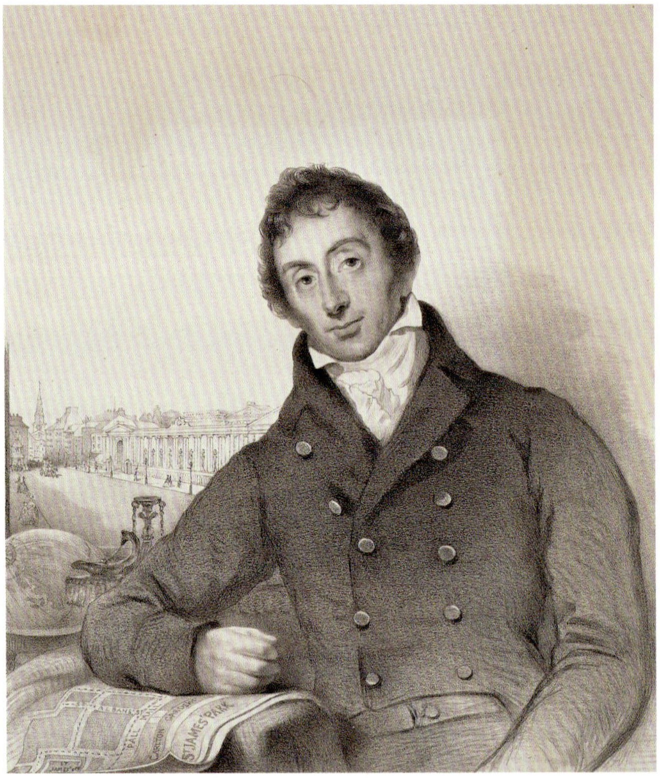

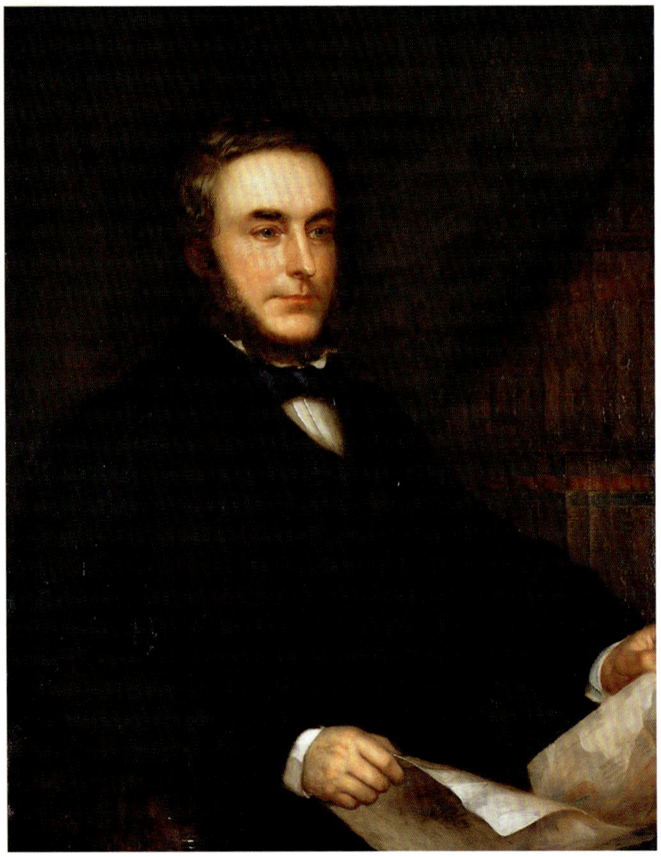

semi-rural. However, the committee was drawn to south Hackney, a 'perfectly healthful neighbourhood',[3] where a fine new park had been laid out and named after Queen Victoria and opened to the public by 1845. They had already begun using the new burial ground alongside, where in 1854 the widow Sarah Symons was the first inmate of the French Hospital to be interred. Her undertaker had been Francis Jolit (figs. 49–51). Her grandfather was the silk weaver Charles Gentil, from Bolbec, Normandy, who had died in the hospital in 1777.

In 1859 three directors were delegated to select a site on Victoria Park and negotiate its purchase. They were Richard Hervé Giraud (fig. 52), treasurer since 1854, William David Jourdain, a director since 1834, and Frederic Albert Winsor (fig. 53), elected in 1836, the barrister son of a German immigrant (fig. 54) who had pioneered gas lighting in England.

A three-and-a-half-acre site 'extensive and studded with a pleasing variety of fine old trees' was chosen, on Wick Lane.[4] A price of £1,600 per acre was agreed. The land had been owned by the Norris family and its forbears for two hundred years. The Norrises had Huguenot connections, notably with the early Walloon family of Du Quesne, a member of whom, now called Du Cane, was Henry Norris's agent for the property.[5] On 1 August 1862 plans of the proposed new building were presented by Robert Lewis Roumieu (fig. 55), a prominent London architect who, with his partner Alexander Gough, had worked on the restoration of St Pancras Old Church and the building of the Almeida Theatre. His French Hospital (fig. 56) was in the style, wrote the *Builder* (2 June 1866), of 'the French

Fig. 54 (*left, top*) Frederic Albert Winsor (1763–1836), lithograph, J. A. Vinter after Dupont

The sitter is shown half-length with a view of Pall Mall in the background.

Fig. 55 (*left, bottom*) Robert Lewis Roumieu (1814–1877), oil on canvas, signed, 'J. Desanois Eques p 186[?]'

Robert Lewis Roumieu, FRIBA, was a distinguished architect of Huguenot descent. Seven years after his election as director in 1856, he became honorary architect to the hospital and designed the new and imposing building in Victoria Park, Hackney. This opened in 1865 and was equipped with the most modern facilities of mid-Victorian England. It provided accommodation for 58 inmates as well as staff. Roumieu became treasurer of the hospital in 1876. On his death, the directors commissioned a memorial tablet for the chapel and a portrait bust which stood in the corridor of the hospital at Hackney.

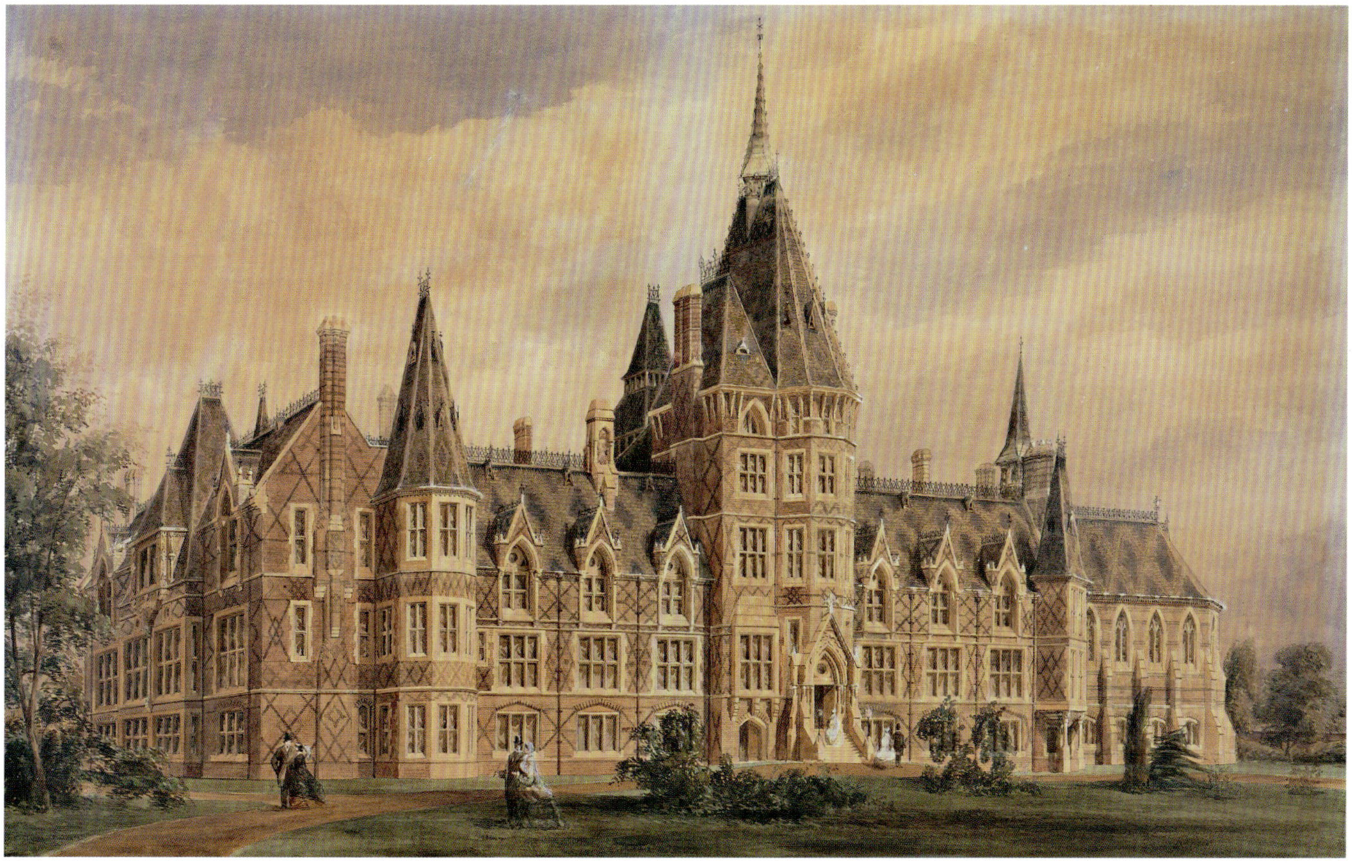

Fig. 56 *The French Hospital, Victoria Park, Hackney, from the south-west*, water-colour, attributed to R.L. Roumieu, c. 1876

Set in three and a half acres of grounds, the new buildings provided accommodation for forty women and twenty men, the steward and his wife and nurses and servants, as well as a chapel, library and spacious day-rooms. After World War II the building became St Victoire's School for Girls. In the 1970s the Cardinal Pole Roman Catholic School took over.

châteaux of the age of Francis I' and modelled on the Château de Chambord.

The new hospital building was greatly admired both for its magnificence and its utility. The *Builder* described the court room and chapel, men's and women's day-rooms, refectory, bed rooms and even the lavatories, reproducing the floor plan. The periodical opined that the sixty inmates were 'perfectly provided for' and declared it 'an ornamental feature of Victoria Park'. The cost of the building was put at £20,000 but Roumieu generously waived his fee. The financing of the operation, the sale of the leases and stock that had raised the money, was handled by another director, Francis de La Mare.

The *Illustrated London News* of 15 July 1868 was impressed by the Price's Patent 'hot water apparatus' for heating the rooms, the running hot and cold water and the dumb-waiter system for sending up dinners by lifts, and praised the hospital's suitability as a home for the inmates.

Robert Lewis Roumieu had known the hospital well. He had been a director since 1856 and his father John had been a director before him. His grandfather, Abraham Roumieu, was also an architect and his great-uncle, Adam Roumieu, succeeded as steward in 1742 and served until 1770. A.G. Browning later described the 'beautiful and commodious building which had sprung, as if by magic, from the fertile brain and generous heart of one of their own "body"'.[6] The directors commissioned a memorial bust of Roumieu and a tablet for the hospital corridor at Hackney.[7] The distinguished architect, Samuel Sanders Teulon, a director from 1862, also served on the Building Committee.[8]

Philip Smith Duval, deputy-governor (fig. 57), and Richard Hervé Giraud, as secretary and then treasurer, had overseen the rebuilding and the move. On completion, Duval presented a silver communion flagon (fig. 58) for use in the new chapel. Giraud, who succeeded Duval as deputy-

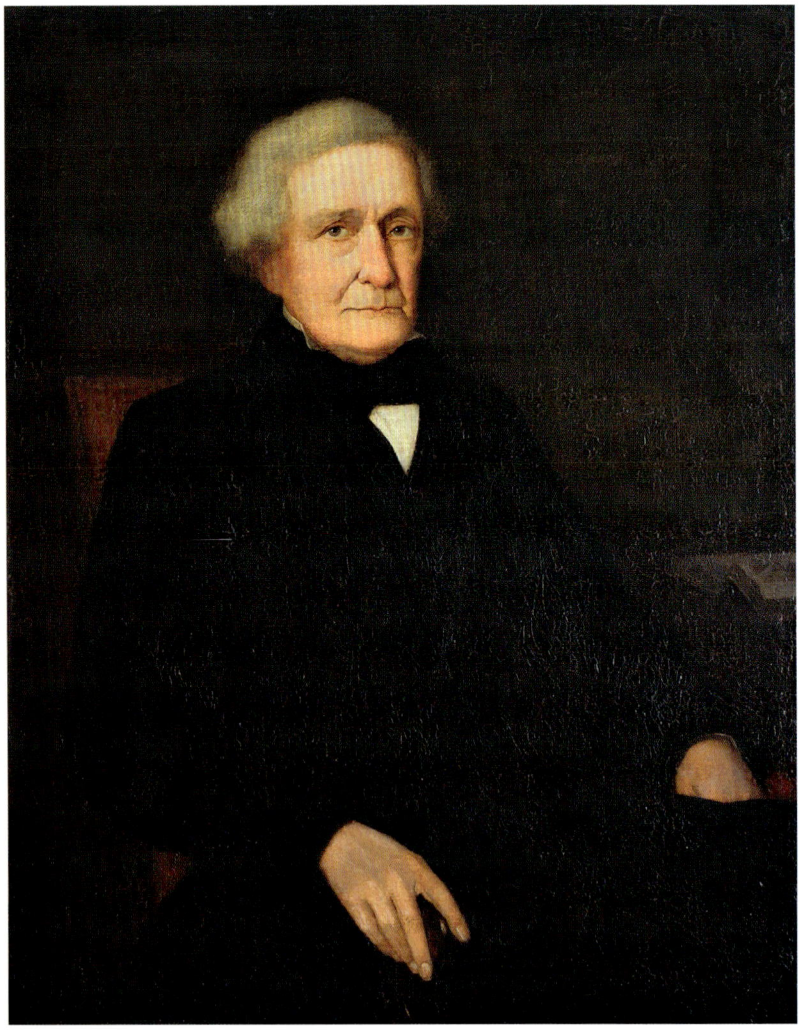

Fig. 57 (*left*) Philip Smith Duval (1837–1878), oil on canvas, artist unknown, English school, 1860–70

Philip Smith Duval became a director of the French Hospital in 1826 and deputy-governor in 1859. Philip was still serving as deputy-governor when the hospital celebrated its 150th anniversary in 1868.

Fig. 58 (*right*) Communion flagon, sterling silver, makers' mark of Edward and John Barnard, London, 1866/7

The silver flagon presented in 1867 by Philip Smith Duval, deputy-governor, for the use of the new French Hospital chapel at Victoria Park, Hackney, replaced the pewter 'pot' in use from at least 1742.

governor in 1876, dealt with the compulsory sale of the old Bath Street site and buildings to the London School Board in 1879. He had not been in favour of the move to Victoria Park, complaining of the long journey from central London, the shortage of cabs, and the sight, to the east, of 'several tall chimney shafts ... belonging to manufactories which do not consume their own smoke'.[9]

Despite the dwindling size of the Huguenot community in London, the new French Hospital could boast state-of-the-art equipment for the care of a mere sixty inmates. The Huguenot community could pride itself on successful integration into the fabric of English society. The Hackney hospital was a monument to that achievement and its French style appropriately symbolic. It was seen as a lasting testimony to the community's origins and history and its endurance. Besides serving the immediate needs of the sixty inmates it would provide physical and pastoral care for Huguenot descendants for a long time to come. It also laid the foundations for a remarkable revival of interest in Huguenot history and achievement that continues to this day.

1 HL H.F1.6.

2 HL H.F1.5.

3 HL H.F1.5, 'Journal of visits to various localities ... for building a new hospital', August–September 1857.

4 Agnew, 1886, p. 526.

5 Isobel Watson, *Gentlemen in the Building Line ... The Development of South Hackney* (1990), p. 88. Charles Norris, whose mother was a Grellier, and who served as a director of the French Hospital in 1865 and as a founding member of the Huguenot Society twenty years later, appears not to have been related.

6 A.G. Browning in R.S. Faber, *Bibliothèque de La Providence: Catalogue of the Library ...* (1901), p. vii.

7 Now at Rochester, It reads 'R.L. Roumieu Esq. FRIBA Elected Director 1856, Honorary Architect 1860 Treasurer 1876. Died on the 159th Anniversary of the Hospital 28th June 1877. In affectionate remembrance of his personal character and in recognition of the talent and care which he gratuitously devoted to the interests of the French Protestant Hospital, Particularly in the Design and Execution of this Building and in the management of the Hospital Estate. This Tablet is dedicated'.

8 His brother William Milford Teulon was also elected in 1863.

9 HL H. F1.6 Giraud to Grellier, 21 August 1861.

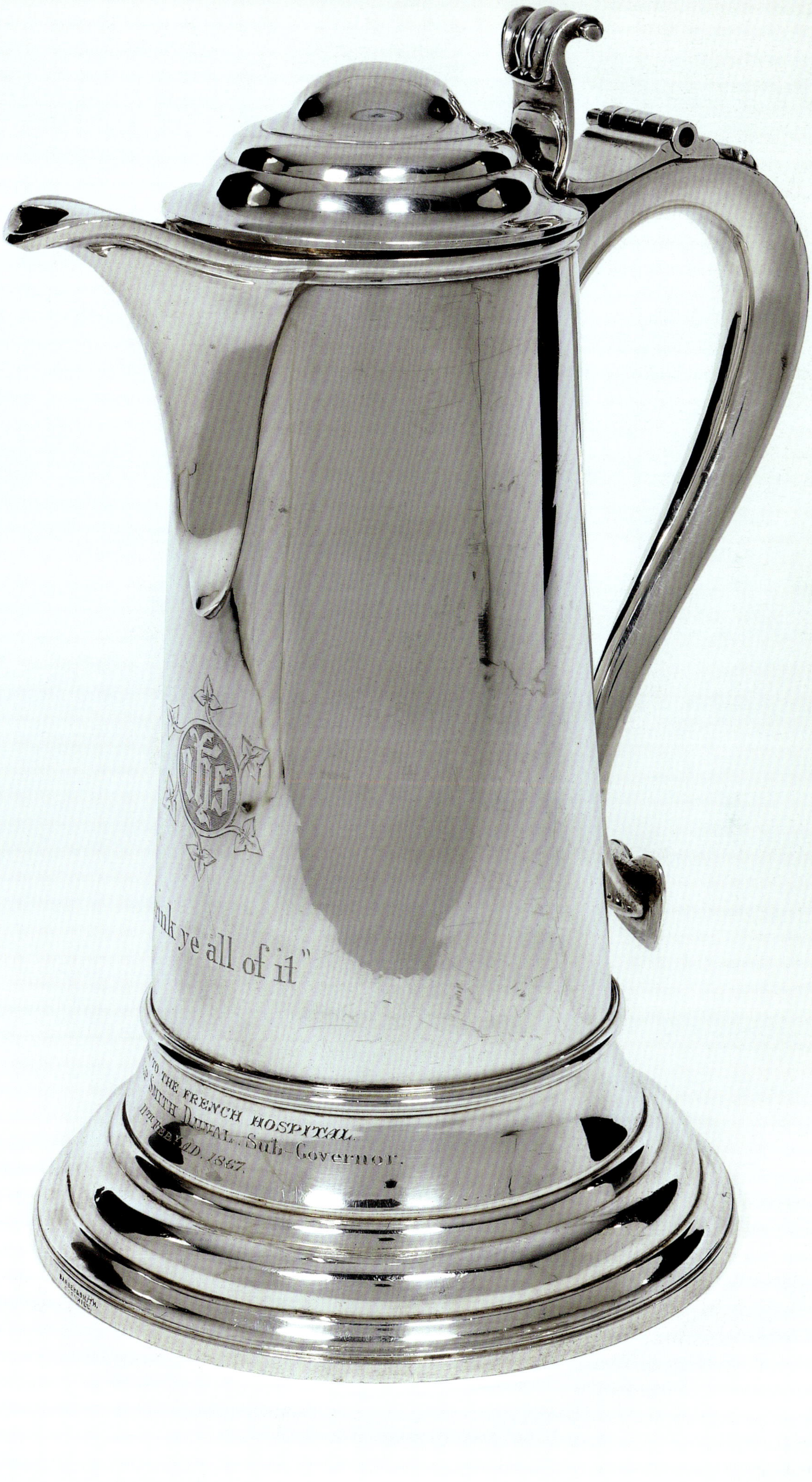
ye all of it"
TO THE FRENCH HOSPITAL
Sub-Governor.
1867.

7

Health and heritage: 'The chief Huguenot foundation in this country', 1867–1938

The idea of the French Hospital as a centre for memorabilia illustrating the history of the Huguenots had already taken shape in the minds of the directors in the early nineteenth century. The 1810 edition of the *Ordres et Réglements* noted that:

> [T]he descendants of the refugees ... [were] more happy, [and had] more confidence and comfort in a charitable establishment, founded for their particular benefit, under a body of Directors connected with them by common ties, in a society in which they [found] the same habits and the same remembrances, and in the frequent recurrence of religious aid, so particularly suited to their age and circumstances.

And the statute book concluded that the hospital should be maintained 'as a monument of the piety of their ancestors'. The new hospital at Hackney was the embodiment of this viewpoint, continuing to provide care for the aged and infirm among poor Huguenot descendants, and at the same time serving as a repository for artefacts, portraits, documents and books belonging to the Huguenot tradition.

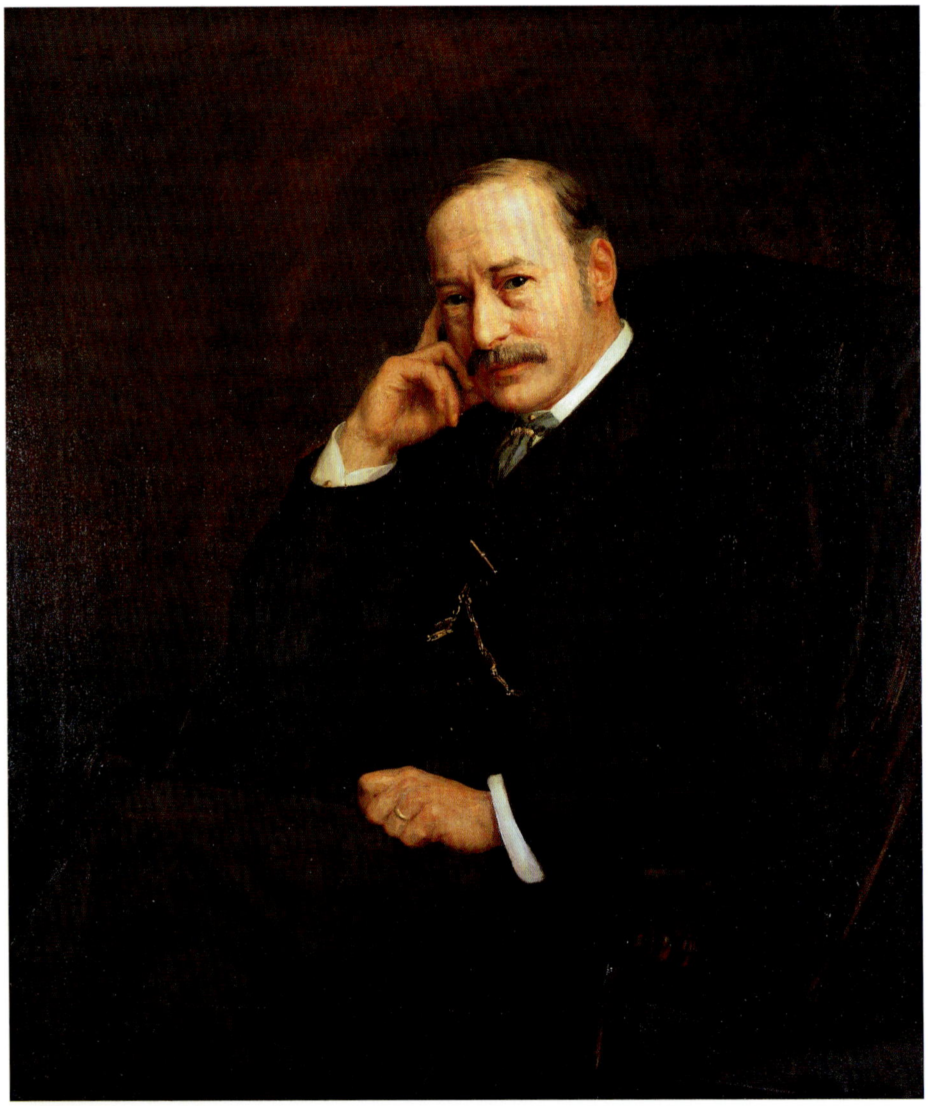

Fig. 59 Arthur Giraud Browning, FSA (1835–1907), oil on canvas, A. B. Connor, c. 1900, in original composition frame

Elected a director in 1873, Browning served as secretary in 1875 and deputy-governor in 1898. Browning was also a governor of the French Protestant School in Westminster, by then in Shaftesbury Avenue. The school children would visit the French Hospital in Victoria Park to sing psalms in French to the residents.

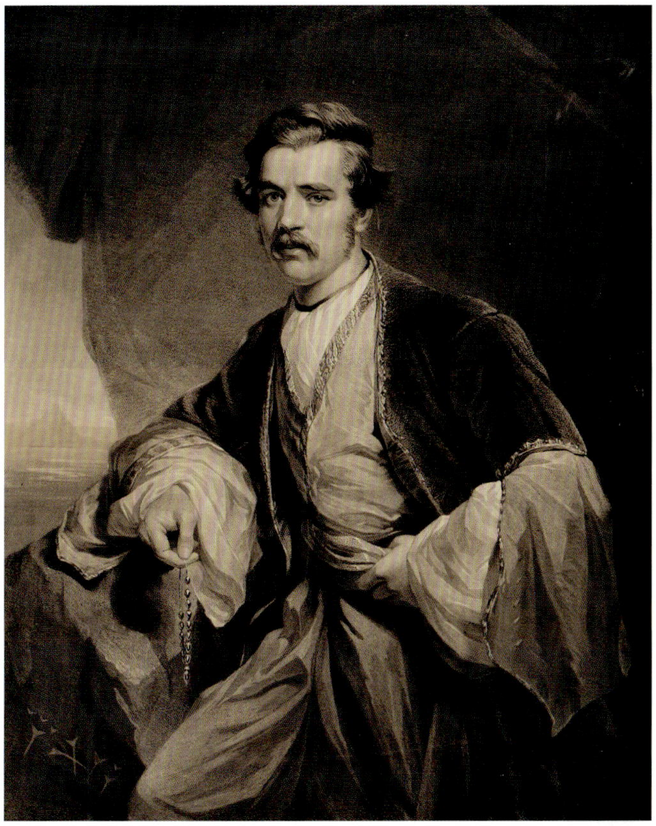

Arthur Giraud Browning (fig. 59),[1] a civil engineer, served as secretary from 1875. In 1876 he began by appealing to fellow directors to donate books about, and pictures of, the Huguenots and their history, or to contribute to a fund to make purchases, since the corporation's own funds were not to be so used.[2] These were still early days in the revival of interest in the Huguenots already popularized by Meyerbeer's opera *Les Huguenots* (1836) and Millais's painting *The Huguenot*, exhibited at the Royal Academy in 1852.

Browning arranged a dinner at the Criterion restaurant in Piccadilly on 21 May 1885, at which the diplomat and archaeologist Sir Henry Austen Layard ('Layard of Nineveh') took the chair (fig. 60). Browning proposed the formation of the Huguenot Society of London (fig. 61). He was seconded by Thomas Archer, one of the many directors present. The first object was 'the interchange and publication of knowledge' about Huguenot history, in France and in the diaspora, genealogy and heraldry, and the registers of the Huguenot churches in Great Britain. Publication of the registers was a major objective from the outset: this was a practical use of the new society, since the hospital's

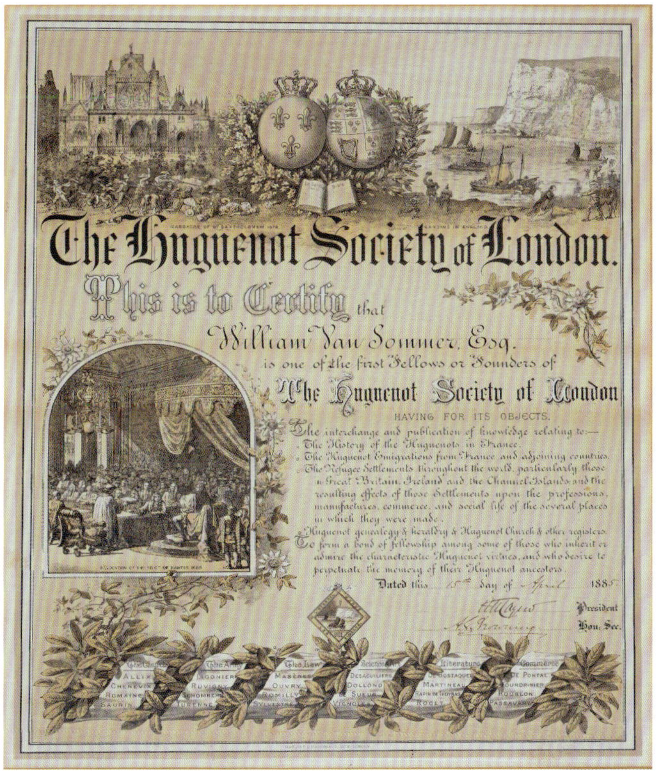

The Huguenot Society of London.
This is to Certify that
William Van Sommer, Esq.
is one of the first Fellows or Founders of
The Huguenot Society of London
HAVING FOR ITS OBJECTS.
The interchange and publication of knowledge relating to:—
The History of the Huguenots in France.
The Huguenot Emigrations from France and adjoining countries.
The Refugee Settlements throughout the world, particularly those in Great Britain, Ireland and the Channel Islands and the resulting effects of those Settlements upon the professions, manufactures, commerce, and social life of the several places in which they were made.
Huguenot genealogy & heraldry & Huguenot Church & other registers.
To form a bond of fellowship among some of those who inherit or admire the characteristic Huguenot virtues, and who desire to perpetuate the memory of their Huguenot ancestors.
Dated this 15th day of April 1885
President
Hon. Sec.

Fig. 60 (*left, top*) Sir Henry Austen Layard (1817–1894), lithograph, S.W. Reynolds, published by P. & D. Colnaghi, 1850

Layard is shown in exotic dress, his arm on a rock; with beads in his right hand. Born in Paris, Henry Austen is remembered today as an archaeologist for his excavation of Nineveh in the 1840s. Through his energy and brilliance, Layard enlarged the treasures of the British Museum and prepared publications of his discoveries. His *Nineveh and Its Remains* was published in London in 1853. It was largely thanks to his discoveries that the British Museum became the centre of cuneiform studies. One example is a tablet from the library of Ashurnasirpal, at Nimrud, which tells part of the epic of Gilgamesh and his search for immortality. Layard served as ambassador to the Sublime Porte. He also enjoyed a distinguished political career and served as a Member of Parliament and Under Secretary for Foreign Affairs. Proud of his Huguenot origins, Layard became a director of the French Hospital in 1884 and served as the first President of the Huguenot Society of London (fig. 61). He also served as a trustee of the National Gallery from 1892. His great-grandfather Daniel Peter Layard was physician to the Middlesex Hospital.

Fig. 61 (*left, bottom*) Certificate of the Huguenot Society of London, 1885

This belonged to William Van Sommer, whose forbears were artists and silk designers. See also Paul van Somer's engraving of Aufrère (fig. 112). The certificate lists the names of Huguenots who made distinguished contributions to the Church, the Army, the Law, Sciences, Literature and Commerce. The strongest claim of the officers of the French Hospital was their contribution to the Army with the names of two distinguished military figures, Ruvigny and Ligonier, who were early governors.

by-laws required that 'none but French Protestants or their descendants, being Protestants, shall be eligible as inmates of the Hospital' and the Huguenot church registers were indispensable if the directors were to satisfy themselves of the eligibility of applicants.

The society flourished and in time took over some of the social and scholarly functions Browning had felt the hospital should undertake. Yet for the commemoration of the bicentenary of the Revocation of the Edict of Nantes in October 1885, the hospital was still at the centre of activities.

In the 1892 'Blue Book' Browning wrote that 'the erection of the present stately building' served 'a twofold purpose ... to provide a peaceful asylum for some of the poor and aged descendants of the French Protestants, and ... to erect a standing memorial of the practical piety of

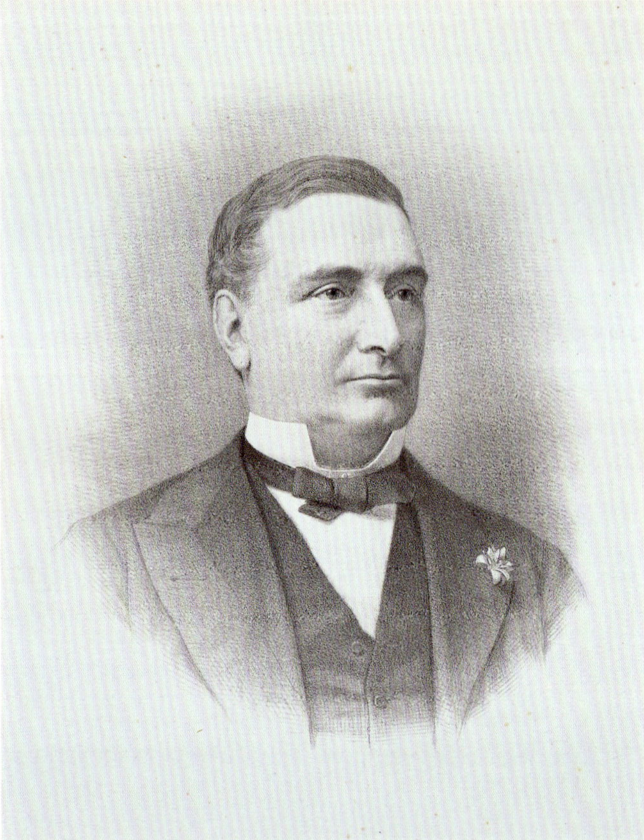

Fig. 62 (*right, top*) Sir Henry William Peek, Bt, MP (d. 1898), photogravure

Sir Henry Peek was a director from 1846 and served as deputy-governor from 1897 until his death in 1898. His mother was a Le Maitre and her family came originally from Dieppe. Sir Henry and his family founded the biscuit-making firm of Peek Brothers. He was Member of Parliament for Mid-Surrey from 1868 to 1884, and was a public benefactor instrumental in saving both Burnham Beeches and Epping Forest from development. He was a founder member of the Huguenot Society in 1885 and became one of the two first vice-presidents.

Sir Henry Peek was active in collecting portraits of earlier directors for the French Hospital and with A.H. Browning acquired the portraits of Sir John Ligonier and Lieutenant-General Louis de Jean at auction in 1898 (figs. 9, 11). After his death, his son commissioned the badges of the governor and deputy-governor of the French Hospital in his memory.

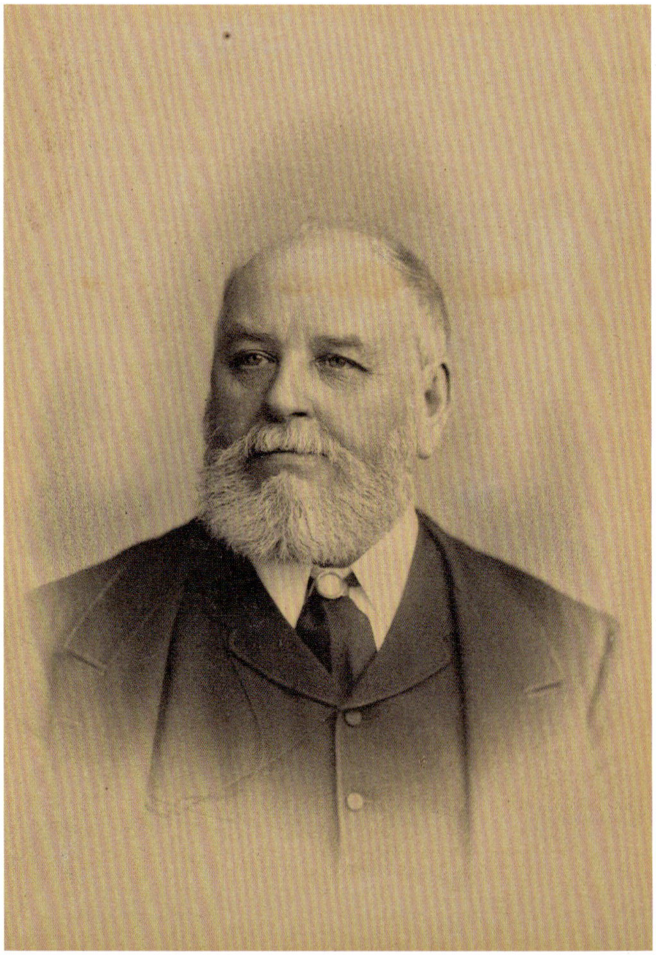

Fig. 63 (*right, bottom*) Charles John Shoppee (1823–1897), photograph, Fradelle & Young, The Photo-Mezzo-Tint Gallery, 246 Regent Street, London

Charles John Shoppee was an architect and surveyor who designed the new hall for the Barber Surgeons' Company in 1864. In 1877 he designed and commissioned a Master's Badge for that Company which was supplied by Lambert's. He built up an important architectural library and a museum of architectural woodwork and metalwork at his home in Mecklenburgh Square, London, WC1. Some of these objects were acquired by the Victoria and Albert Museum after his death. His great-great grandfather Jacques Chapuis was born in Condrieu, near Lyons and served as an officer in the French army. Taken prisoner at the Battle of Oudenarde, he was brought to England.

Shoppee was a founder member of the London and Middlesex Archaeological Society. He was a keen bibliophile who collected and designed book-plates and was a founder member of the Ex Libris Society in 1891.

Becoming a director of the French Hospital in 1867, he served as treasurer in 1877 and deputy-governor from 1887 to 1897. He was a founder member of the Huguenot Society in 1885.

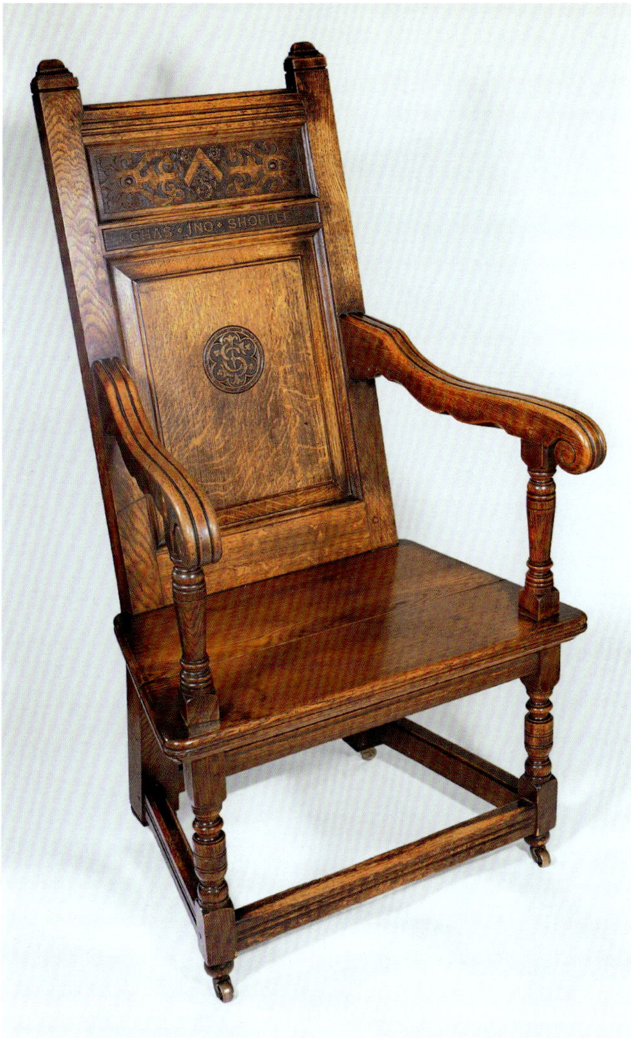

Fig. 64 Armchair, oak, 17th-century style

The panelled back of this armchair is carved with the name 'Chas Jno Shoppee' with CJS in monogram. Shoppee presented the chair for the use of the governor.

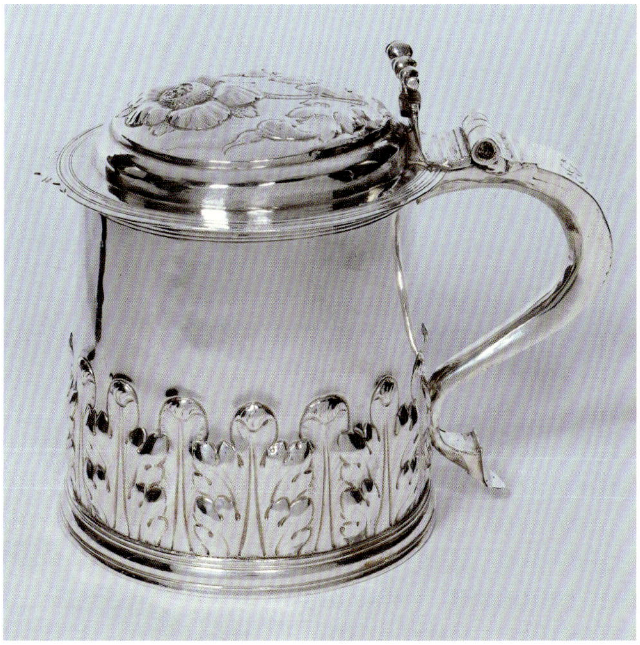

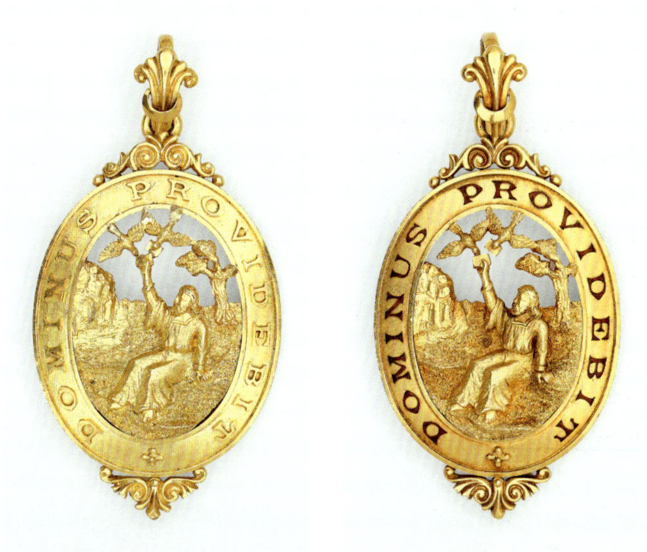

Fig. 66 Badges of the governor and the deputy-governor, gold and enamel, maker's mark of George Lambert, London, 1898

Both badges are chased with the scene of Elijah and the ravens, surrounded by the motto 'Dominus Providebit'. They were presented by Sir Cuthbert Edgar Peek, a director, in memory of Sir Henry William Peek, a director from 1846 to 1898 and deputy-governor from 1897 to 1898.

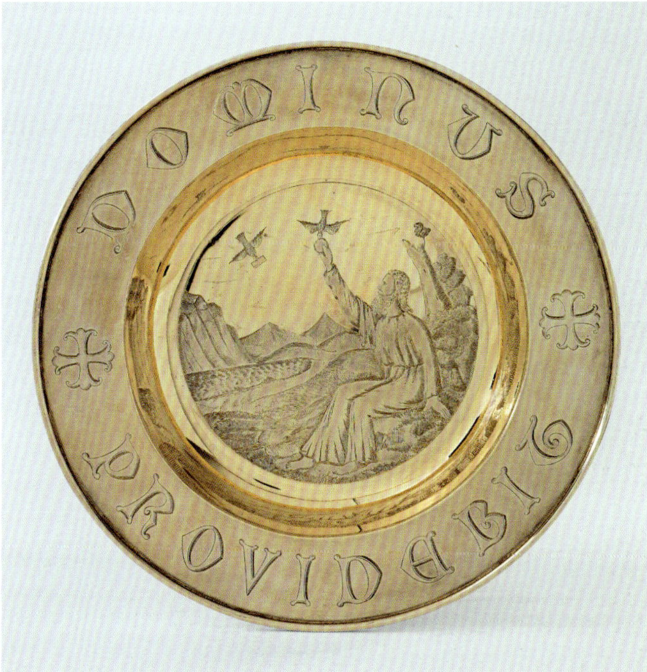

Fig. 67 Alms-dish, silver-gilt, maker's mark of George Lambert, stamped 'LAMBERT 12 COVENTRYST', London, 1897/8

In the 1890s the anniversary of the granting of the royal charter was celebrated on the fourth Wednesday in June, when a sermon was preached in the French Hospital chapel at Victoria Park. The alms-dish, given by the deputy-governor Sir Henry William Peek, was first used at the anniversary service in June 1898 and at regular Sunday services thereafter.

Fig. 65 (*left*) Tankard, sterling silver, maker's mark SL in monogram, London, 1685/6, presented to the French Hospital in 1893 by Sir Henry William Peek

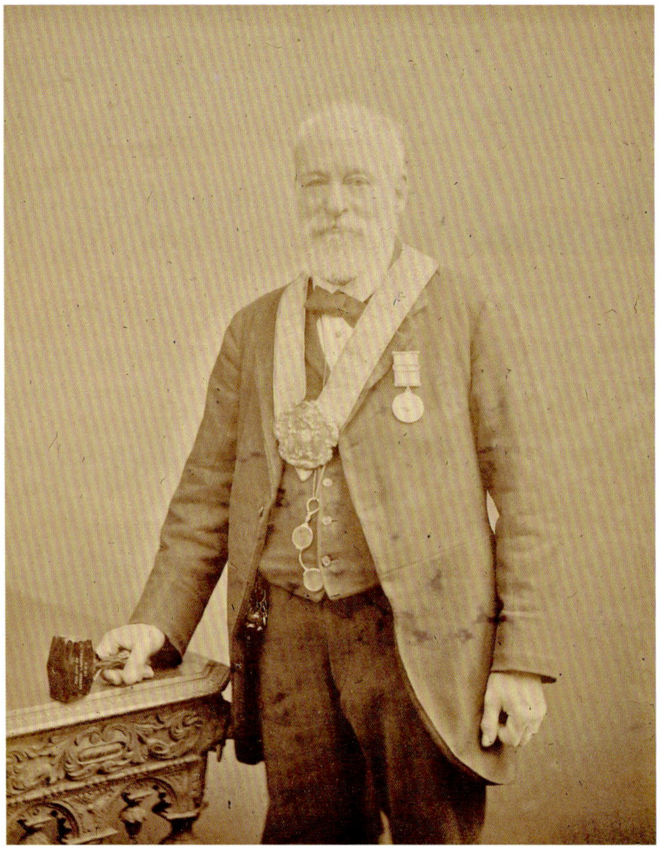

Fig. 68 George Lambert, photograph, Maull & Fox, 187a Piccadilly, London

In 1837 George Lambert was apprenticed through the Goldsmiths' Company. He later became a liveryman of the Horners', Glovers', Tinplate Workers', Gold and Silver Wyre Drawers', Gardeners' and Pattenmakers' Companies.

George Lambert ran a thriving goldsmith's and jeweller's business in Coventry Street, taking on twenty-two apprentices between 1868 and 1887. He became Prime Warden of the Goldsmiths' Company in 1887, Queen Victoria's golden jubilee year. He presented a number of gifts to the Company including an 18th-century cup and cover. A steeple cup, not unlike the example presented to the French Hospital, was commissioned from the London goldsmith Robert Stocker, although George Lambert himself contributed to its manufacture in 1886. On the cup were recorded the principal events of the Queen Victoria's fifty-year reign to date. He also gave the Company eighteen communion cups and patens ranging in date from 1561 to 1751 and thirteen silver-gilt apostle spoons with the same maker's mark BY and the date letter for 1626 which is said to be the most complete set in existence. He gave the Company fifteen other spoons ranging in date from 1661 to 1718 and eight tipstaves.

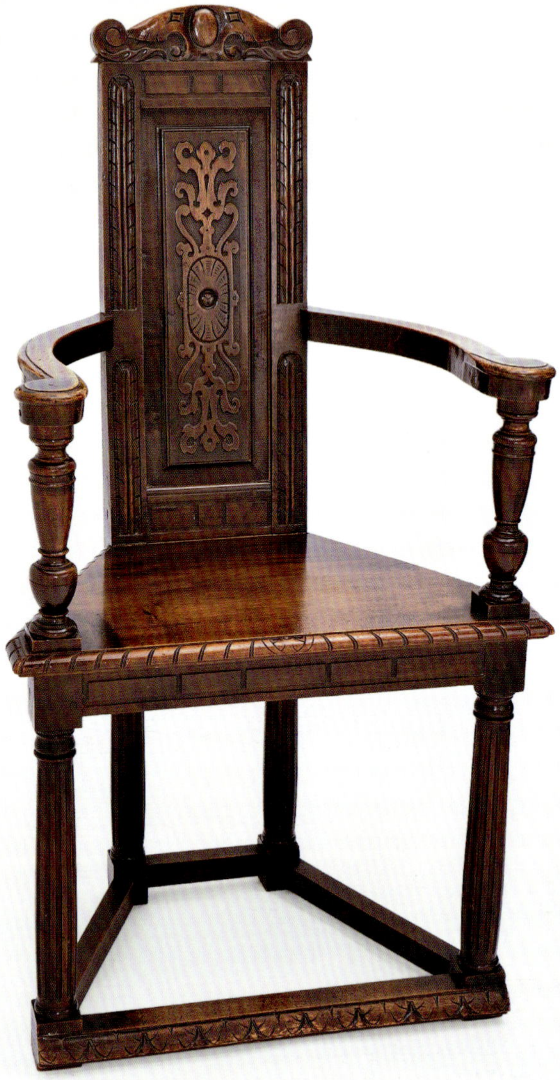

Fig. 69 (*right, top*) Calvin's chair (19th-century copy), oak

A 16th-century style carved oak *caquetoire*, copying Calvin's chair in the cathedral at Geneva.

the early French Refugees ...' He had been more specific about this second purpose when the year before he wrote that the directors 'rightly determined that this, the chief secular memorial of the Huguenot immigrants in this country, should be made to enshrine as far as possible the history and traditions of its Founders and to become the central *rendezvous* of all who by descent or by association are interested in ... the study of Huguenot history'.[3]

Two of Browning's closest confederates were Sir Henry Peek, Bt, MP (fig. 62)[4] and C. J. Shoppee [originally Chapuis] (figs. 63–4), who were deputy-governors in turn after Giraud. In 1885, Sir Henry Peek presented a tankard hall-marked in London in 1685 (fig. 65) to mark the bicentenary of the Revocation of the Edict of Nantes. Browning succeeded Shoppee as deputy-governor in 1898. In that year Sir Cuthbert Peek presented two gold badges of office for the governor and deputy-governor in memory of Sir Henry

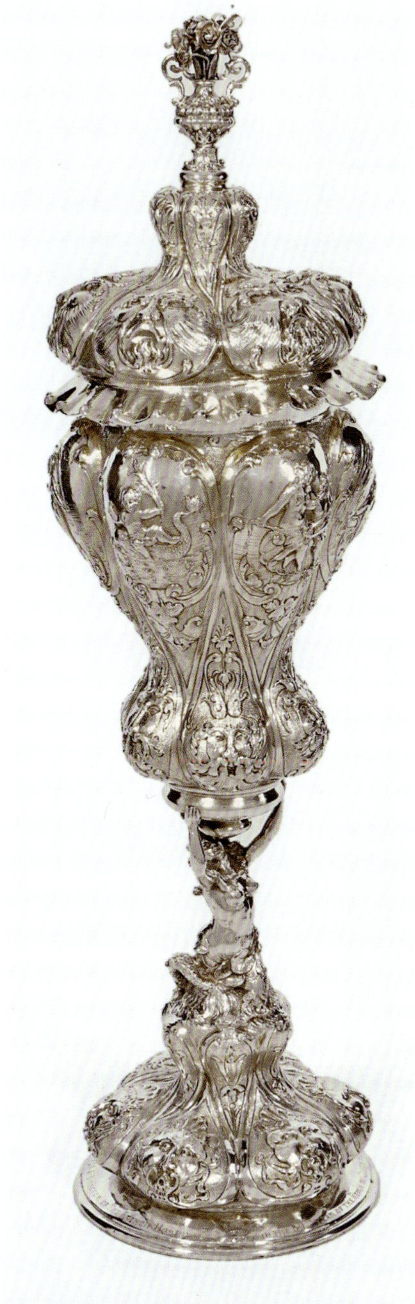

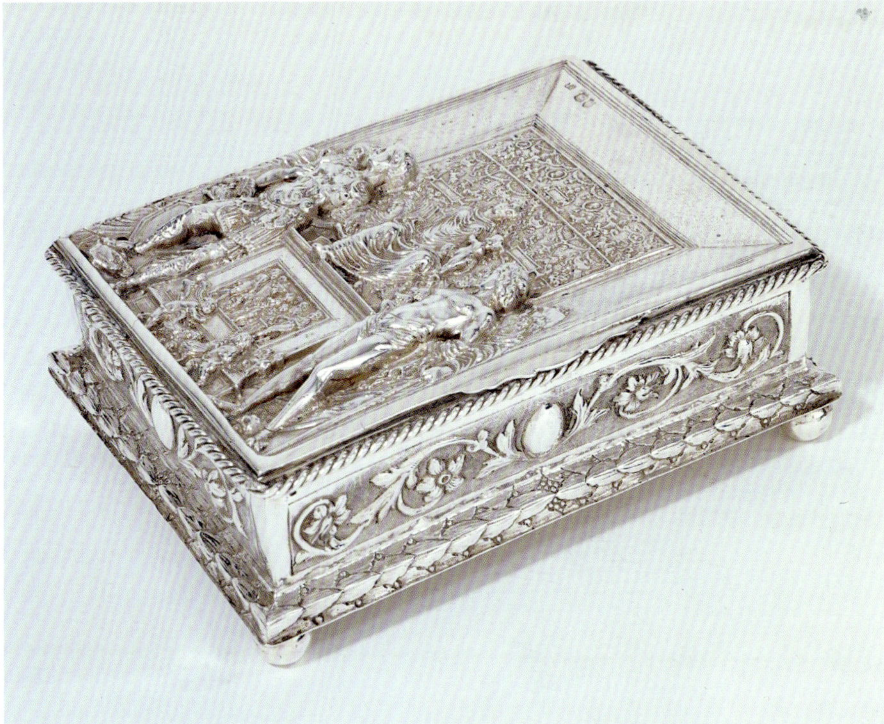

Fig. 71 Cigarette box, sterling silver, maker's mark JO, London, 1879/80

The lid of this cigarette box is cast from an Italian plaquette showing the Madonna and Child flanked by Saints George and David. The centre of the star on the inside of the lid is engraved with Elijah and the ravens.

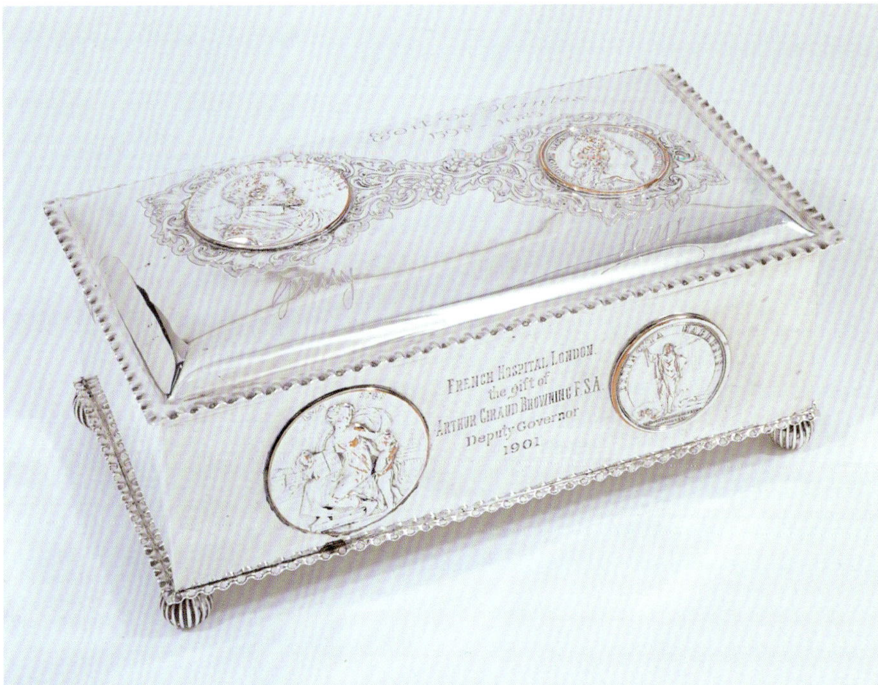
FRENCH HOSPITAL LONDON
the gift of
ARTHUR GIRAUD BROWNING F.S.A.
Deputy Governor
1901

Fig. 70 Standing cup and cover, sterling silver, German, 1895/6, imported by Berthold Müller

Of lobed form, the foot of the cup is chased with masks, the stem formed as a mermaid, the bowl chased with panels of tritons and sea-nymphs. The cover has a flower-vase finial.

Fig. 72 Cigar box, sterling silver and copper, maker's mark HB, London, 1901/2, with fluted ball feet, the lid and front inset with two silvered copper medallions, one representing Louis XIV of France.

Peek (fig. 66) and an alms-dish for the use of the chapel (fig. 67). These were made by the jewellery and goldsmith business belonging to fellow director George Lambert, who became Prime Warden of the Goldsmiths' Company in 1887 (fig. 68).

Browning presented a cigarette box and a cigar box (figs. 71–2) to the corporation in 1895. Also in that year he founded a trust for the purchase of books and manuscripts with a gift of £300 (figs. 73–4).[5] By 1801 there were between 2,000 and 3,000 volumes, mainly gifts from directors. A major contributor of documentation to the library was Henry Wagner (fig. 75). Having been appointed a director in 1867, he was inspired 'to turn his taste for genealogical research in the direction of Huguenot families.'[6] His own great collection of Huguenot wills, abstracts and pedigrees was later bequeathed to the French Hospital.[7] Wagner was also a keen collector of early Italian paintings which he gave to the National Gallery in the 1920s.

The Court meetings held quarterly were followed by dinners to which guests were invited, a succession of toasts made, in French, with the final one, as today, in English: 'To the safety and prosperity of old England', and a loving-cup ceremony, devised in about 1884, performed. The cups used later for this were almost certainly the pair presented by George Lambert in 1892 with covers added through the gift of Arthur Giraud Browning in 1907 (figs. 79–80). Brought in to the assembled company by the steward, the secretary announced that the cups contained:

> The choicest WINE of France commemorating our Huguenot Ancestors, FORTIFIED with SPIRIT, the SPIRIT of admiration for their faith and courage, and SWEETENED by SYMPATHY with the poor and aged among their Descendants. The Deputy Governor responded with a toast to the memory of the Huguenot founders of the hospital and to guests.[8]

Those present may also have been entertained with a four-part song, 'The Huguenot Refugee', set to music by Windham Ryves, the words written by Dr Samuel Byles (d. 1856), the medical officer at the hospital for thirty years. The chorus was suitably patriotic:

> Hey! For our land, our English land,
> The land of the brave and free;
> Who with open arms in the olden time,
> Received the Refugee.[9]

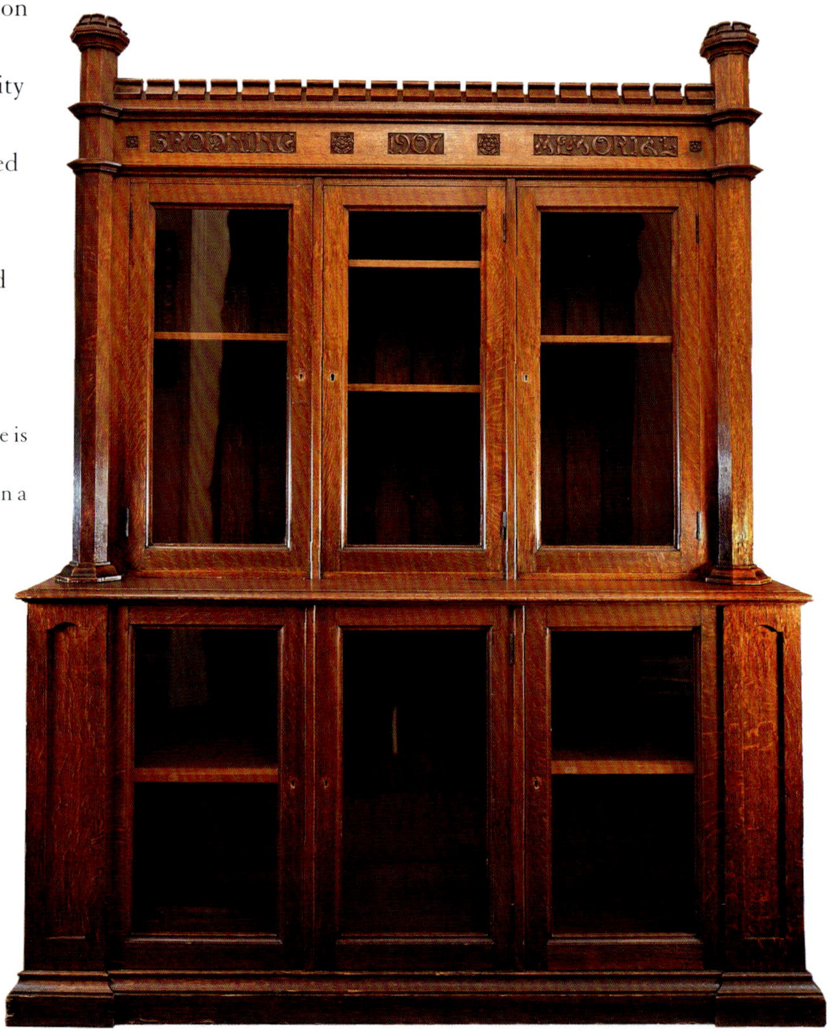

Fig. 73 (*right*) The Browning Memorial bookcase, oak, 1907

The upper part of this Gothic-style oak library bookcase is surmounted by a crenellated and turreted cornice with three glazed panelled doors between parallel pilasters on a moulded plinth. The Huguenot Library holds a manuscript catalogue of the books and manuscripts purchased through the French Hospital Library Trust Fund subscribed in memory of Arthur Giraud Browning along with a copy of the Trust Deed, 1895. A printed catalogue of the library was compiled by Reginald Stanley Faber with an introduction by Arthur Giraud Browning. The most frequent donors of books were Sir Henry Layard, Messrs Teulon, Charles John Shoppee, Henry Wagner, Cronin and William Morris Beaufort. The latest accession was the collection of books formed by the Huguenot Society of London which in 1900 was transferred to the Corporation of the French Hospital under conditions which secured the right to use the united collection at all reasonable times. Donations of historical works of the 17th and 18th centuries, which have now become 'excessively scarce', were encouraged.

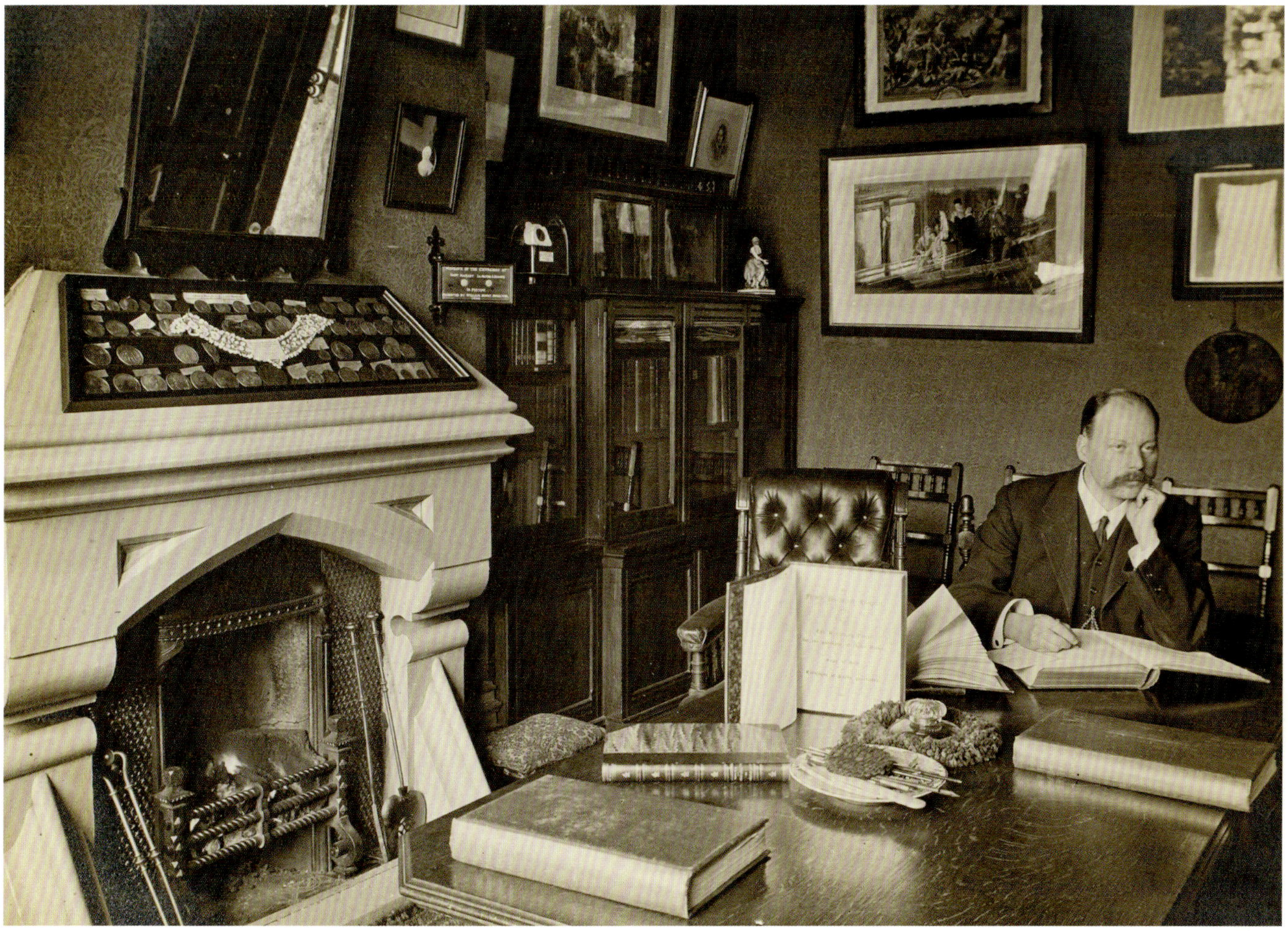

Fig. 74 The Library, The French Hospital, Victoria Park, Hackney, photograph, 1907. *Huguenot Library*

By 1900 the library contained nearly 4,000 volumes, a collection of engravings and was open to interested readers by appointment. Below the 1733 looking-glass (fig. 25) on the left is a display of medals built into the mantelpiece and next to it a frame containing two communion tokens or *méreaux* from two churches in Poitou. Contributions of appropriate books or engravings were often made by the directors.

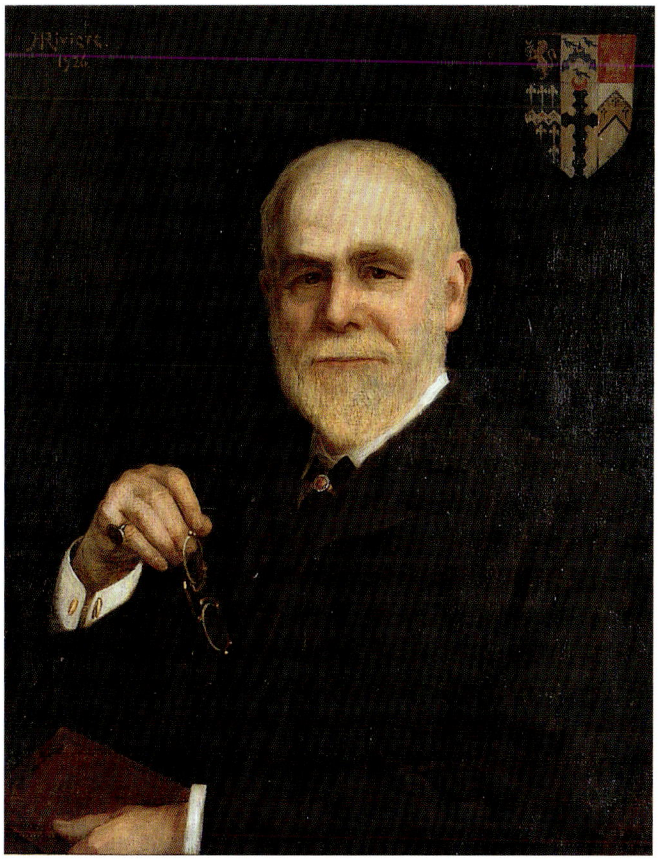

Fig. 75 Henry Wagner (1840–1926), oil on canvas, Hugh Goldwyn Riviere, signed 'H Riviere, 1926', in a copy of an 18th-century frame

Henry Wagner came from a wealthy Brighton family originally from Silesia, but they claimed Huguenot descent through the Wagner immigrant's marriage to a Teulon of Valleraugue in Languedoc, as the armorial shield in this memorial portrait demonstrates. Henry Wagner developed a passionate interest in genealogy, which was inherited by his cousin Sir Anthony Wagner, Garter King of Arms, who became a director in 1929.

Wagner was elected a Fellow of the Society of Antiquaries in 1875. He had started to collect paintings as an undergraduate at Merton College, Oxford, but his premises in Half Moon Street, Piccadilly, were later so crammed full of paintings that they were even screwed onto the doors. In 1921 he moved back to Brighton. He gave a painting by Lorenzo Monaco to London's National Gallery in 1912 and further gifts followed in 1918–19 and in 1921. In 1924 the National Gallery chose twelve more of his early Italian paintings. He left the hospital invaluable research papers – Huguenot will extracts and over 900 pedigree files – now in the Huguenot Library.

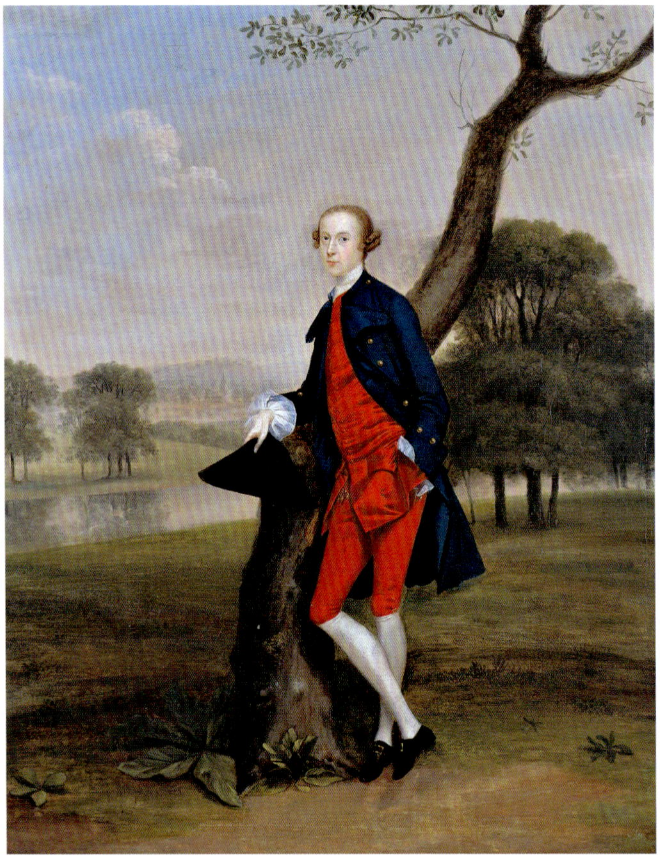

Fig. 76 Uuidentified man, formerly called 'Gainsborough Dupont' (1754–1797), oil on canvas, Arthur Devis

This painting was acquired as a portrait of Gainsborough Dupont, who was elected a director of the French Hospital on 9 April 1794, just three years before his death. He was the nephew of the artist Thomas Gainsborough and worked in his studio and was buried with his uncle at Kew.

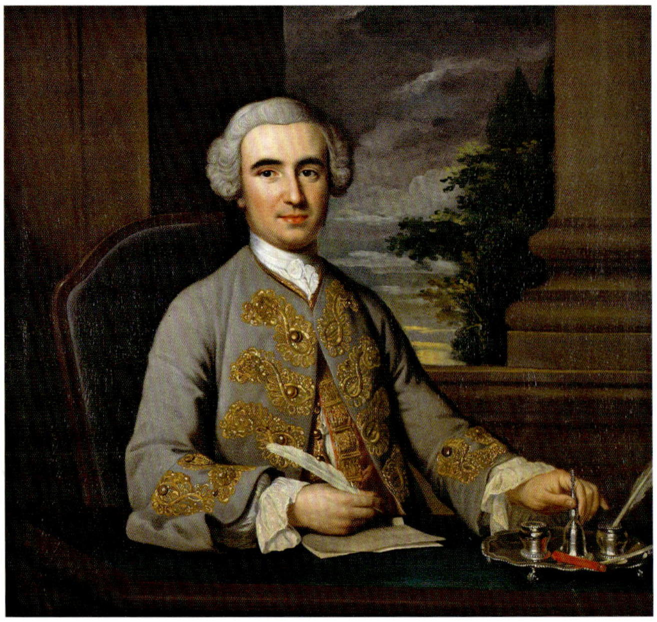

Fig. 77 (*right, top*) Peter Le Heup (1699–1777), oil on canvas, John Giles Eckhardt, 1747, in a 1770s frame

Half length, in a gold embroidered grey coat and red waistcoat, white frilled stock and lace cuffs, Le Heup is seated at a table with a silver inkstand and sealing wax, his hand on the bell, a column and a landscape beyond.

Peter Le Heup was the son of Thomas Le Heup one of the thirty-seven original directors of the French Hospital. Peter Le Heup was a banker, marrying in 1722 Clara, the daughter of William Lowndes of Winslow, Buckinghamshire, Secretary to the Treasury. They lived in Albemarle Street, in the parish of St George's, Hanover Square. Another member of the family Michel Le Heup was made a director in 1741. A Marie Le Heup was resident in the French Hospital in 1739 when her husband Edward Le Heup wrote to the directors in July begging them to prevent his wife from leaving the hospital as her demented state made his life intolerable. In 1739 one of the witnesses was another Edward Le Heup, a weaver of the parish of Christ Church, Spitalfields. Edward Le Heup sponsored his wife's readmission in 1751 (Gray, p. 66). The Le Heup family were connected with the family of the baron de Saint-Hippolyte.

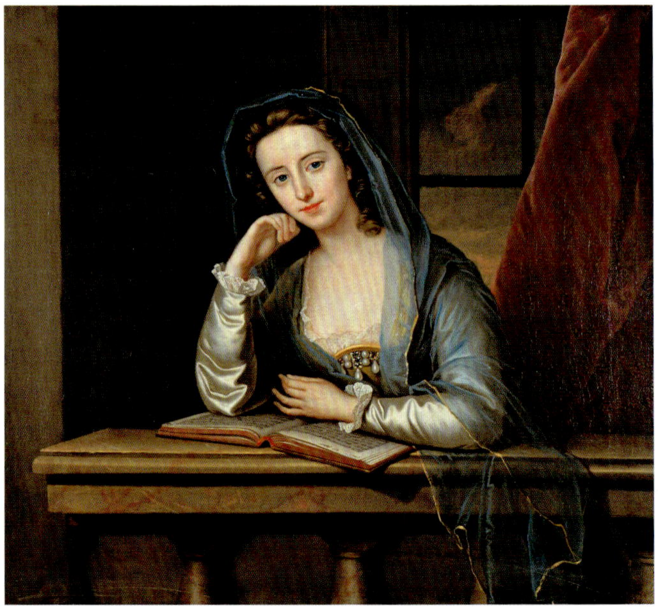

Fig. 78 Clara Le Heup (d. 1773), oil on canvas, John Giles Eckhardt, 1747

Clara, the wife of Peter Le Heup is portrayed half-length in a white satin décolleté dress and blue gauze scarf, standing by a window, her arms leaning on a book. Henry Wagner first saw the portraits of Peter and Clara Le Heup and Louis Montolieu (fig. 10) at Beauport, Battle, Sussex, the home of Sir Archibald Lamb in the 1850s; Lamb was the great-grandson of Marie Molinier, baronne Montolieu de Saint-Hippolyte (1684–1777).

Figs. 79–80 (*right and overleaf*) Loving cups and covers, silver-gilt, maker's mark of George Lambert, London; the cups, 1892/3, the covers, 1907/8

Inset with medals including those of Louis XIV and William and Mary, the cups were presented by George Lambert and 'Three Friends' in 1892 and the covers by Arthur Giraud Browning in 1907 to mark the tenth anniversary of his election as deputy-governor. The 'Ceremony of the Loving Cup' had been adopted in about 1884. Both donors were Fellows of the Society of Antiquaries and keen to develop the French Hospital collections as a resource for the study of Huguenot history.

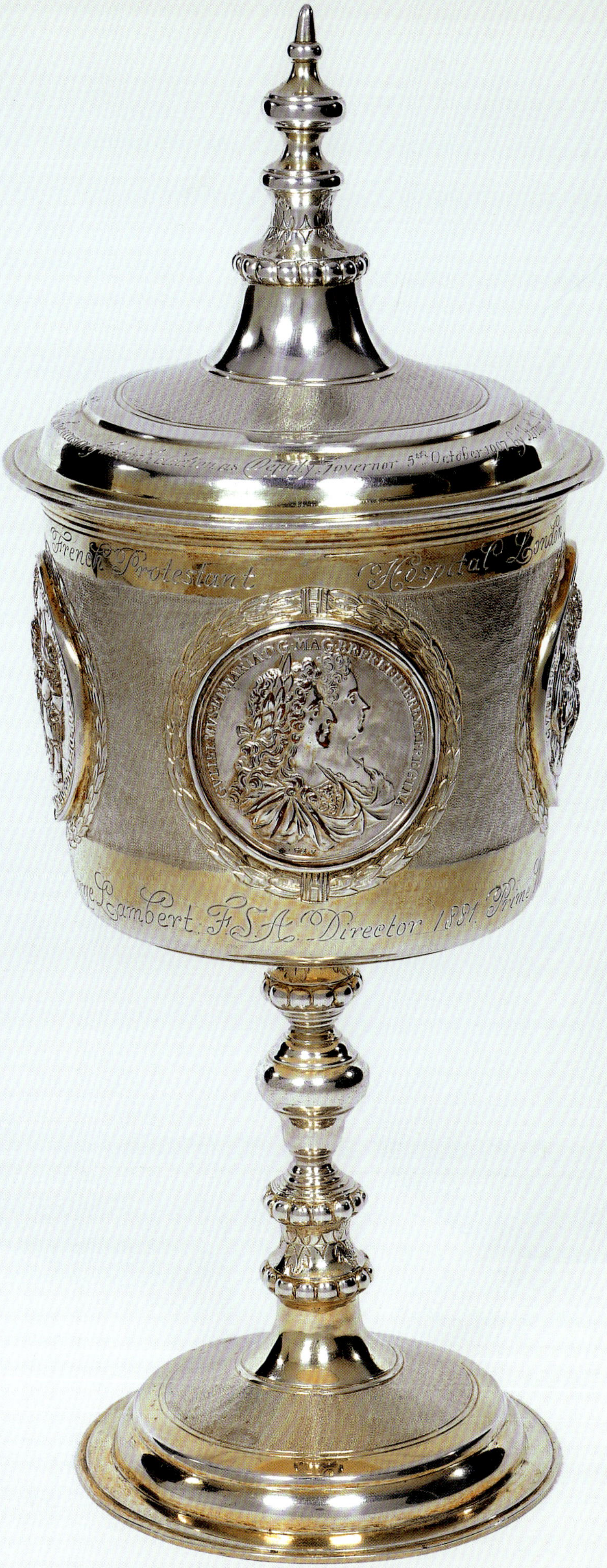
French Protestant Hospital
Lambert F.S.A. Director 1881

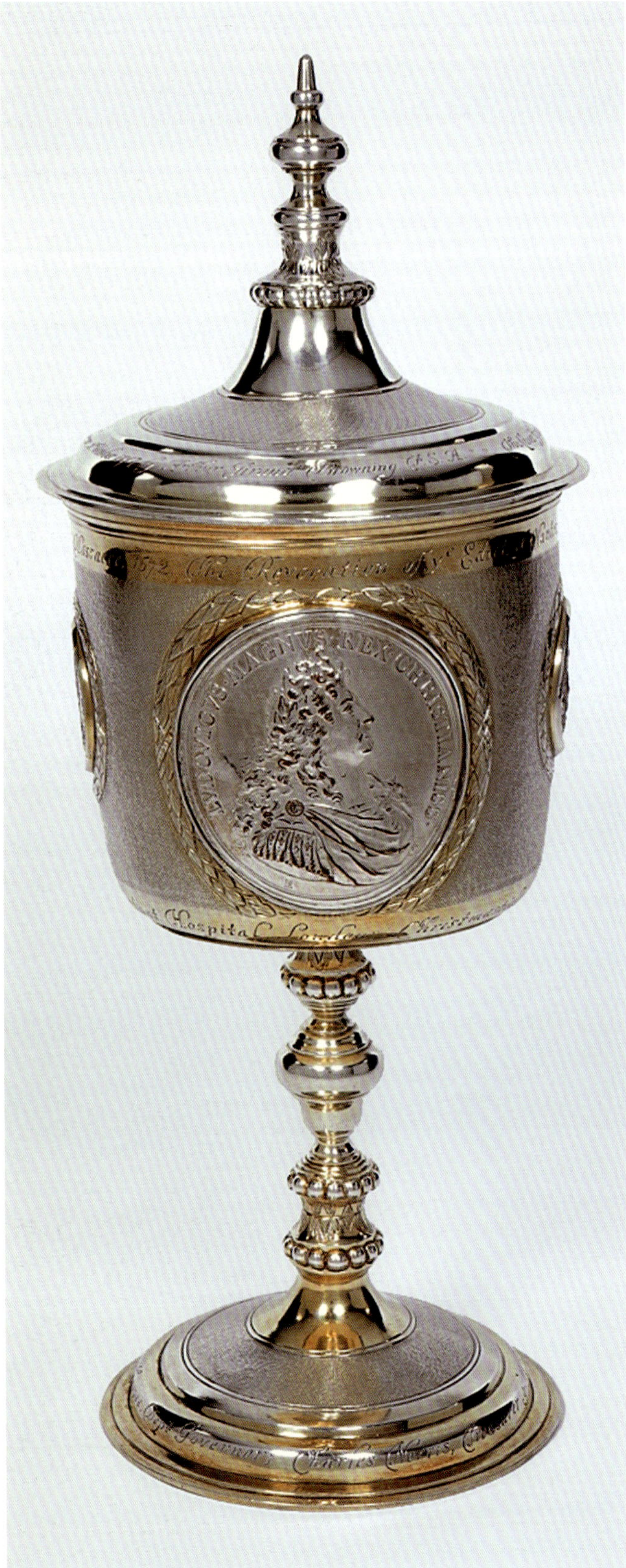

The anniversary of the granting of the royal charter was celebrated each June and 'a sermon preached at Divine Service'. During the feast which followed, the directors mingled with the inmates (figs. 81–2). This tradition lives on to this day and the welfare of the inmates still remains at the core of the directors' activities. Printed copies survive of 'The Inmate's Story', a tale by A.G. Browning, which he read 'at an entertainment given by some of the Directors and their friends to the inmates of the French Protestant Hospital, Victoria Park' on 23 May 1884. Concerts, recitations and cultural diversions of this kind were not to be found at the workhouse.[10]

Following their inspection in 1875, the Charity Commissioners observed:

> The Hospital, including the Chapel, is a handsome building, too handsome indeed for the purpose for which it was designed, viz. the board and lodging of aged weavers and weaveresses, ordinary labourers and domestic servants ... It appears to me that this Institution ... is eminently adapted to aged and decayed French Governesses who ... have been accustomed to more care, better accommodation and greater consideration than were ever dreamt of in the wretched hovels of Spitalfields.[11]

True, there were still weavers among the inmates, four of whom wove the splendid black silk dress presented to the old Queen for her Golden Jubilee in 1887. One of the four, James Dabbs, had entered the hospital at 74 in 1884. In his youth he had woven the silk for a white dress with an ivy pattern worked in silver for Princess Victoria.[12] His sister, Mrs Mary Bond, who had come to the hospital in 1879, presented the directors with a framed piece of her needlework 'in gratitude for the care and attention shown to her'.[13] She left her small estate to the hospital – £50 in the post-office and other items – at her death at 74 in 1884. James died in 1891 aged 81.

The hospital had its own loom in the men's day-room, while in the women's day-room residents were industriously employed in reading and needlework. The *Graphic* illustrated these scenes in an article in its 26 October 1885 issue (figs. 83–84).

Throughout the Edwardian era and into the 1920s the hospital ran smoothly (fig. 85). Joseph Irwin Marshall, who had been appointed clerk of the corporation in 1894 and doubled as steward from 1900 to 1930 'devoted himself to the welfare and happiness of the old people'. During the war years of 1914–18 and in the post-war period when

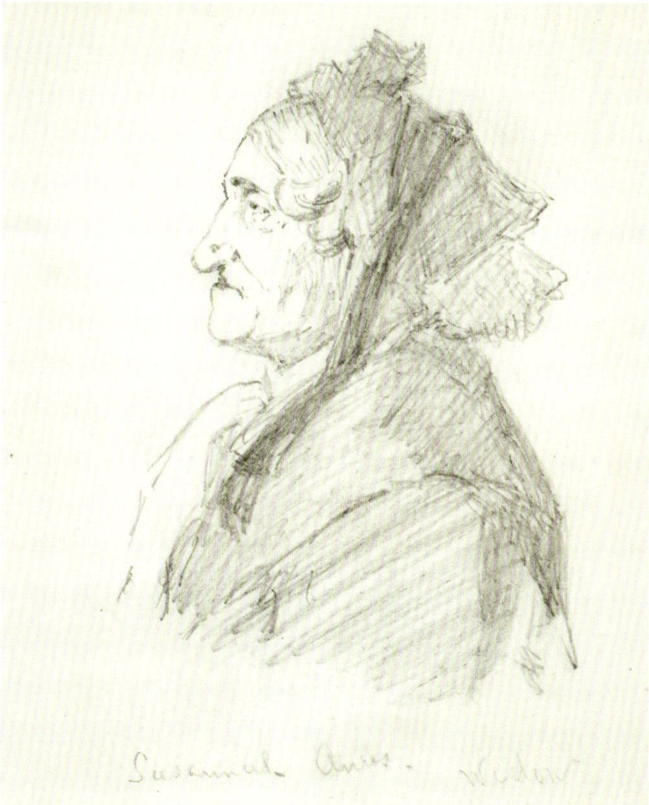

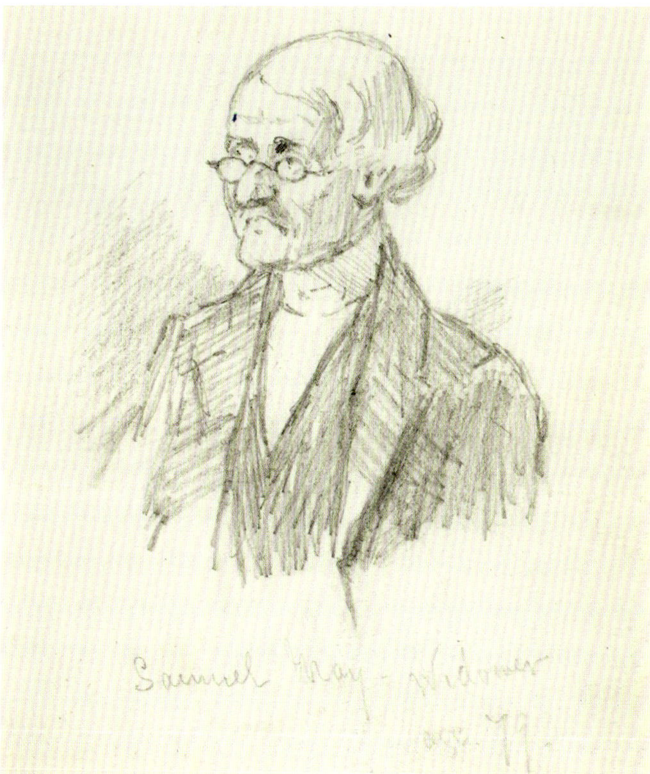

Figs. 81 and 82 Sketches of residents, pencil, 1881. *Huguenot Library*

Fig. 81 (*left*) Susannah Ames, widow

Fig. 82 (*left, bottom*) Samuel May, widower, aged 79

The daughter of William Chappell of 37 Wilmot Street, Bethnal Green, Susannah Ames (*née* Chappell) was admitted to the French Hospital in 1876. Her paternal grandmother Catherine Piquet was of Huguenot descent, the family coming from Lyons. Mrs Ames died in 1887. Samuel May was admitted to the hospital in 1878 with failing sight. Born in Bethnal Green, the son of William May and Sarah Manchée, he trained as a silk weaver, but also worked as a printer's messenger. His mother's great-grandmother had come from France as a refugee.

the income of the hospital was considerably reduced, Mr Marshall's 'skilful management prevented any appreciable hardships being felt by the old people under his charge'.[14] Seven of the youngest directors served in the First World War, among them were E.C. Ouvry and Thomas Aubertin, who later became deputy-governor.[15] In 1925, Richard Austen-Leigh, a director from 1919, caught the spirit of the post-war years in comic verse:[16]

> ... how each revolving moon
> The French Hospital Committee
> Spend a strenuous afternoon
> Dealing promptly with petitions,
> Reading this and that report,
> Taking note of new admissions –
> Being businesslike, in short.

After dinner they

> Pass the port and speed the sherry,
> Place them in the Chaplain's reach,
> Till the Chairman, waxing merry,
> Calls on Browning for a speech.

It was the Browning of this light-hearted verse, Arthur Hervé Browning, who in 1934 warned the Huguenot Society in a lecture on the history of the French Hospital that this happy existence was under threat.

1 He was the son of a first cousin of Richard Hervé Giraud.

2 A late 19th-century prospectus noted that 'A Library of works relating to the early history of the French Protestants, and to the Settlements of the Refugees in this country, is now in course of formation at the Hospital. It already contains nearly 4,000 volumes, many of them of great rarity and value, also some historical engravings, almost all of which have been presented by the Directors and their friends. The Library is freely open to those who take an interest in this special branch of history, and contributions of appropriate books or engravings will be very thankfully received.'

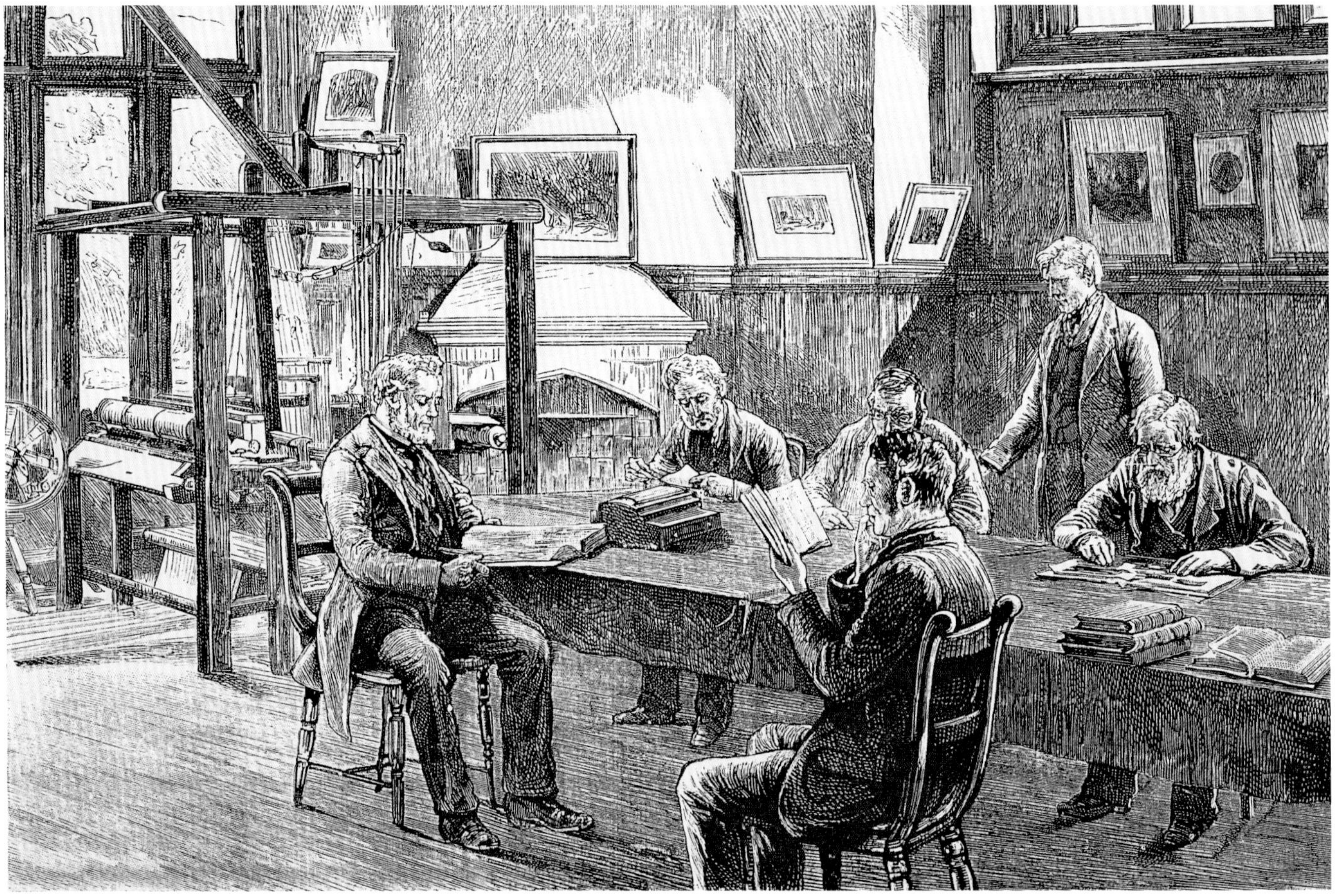

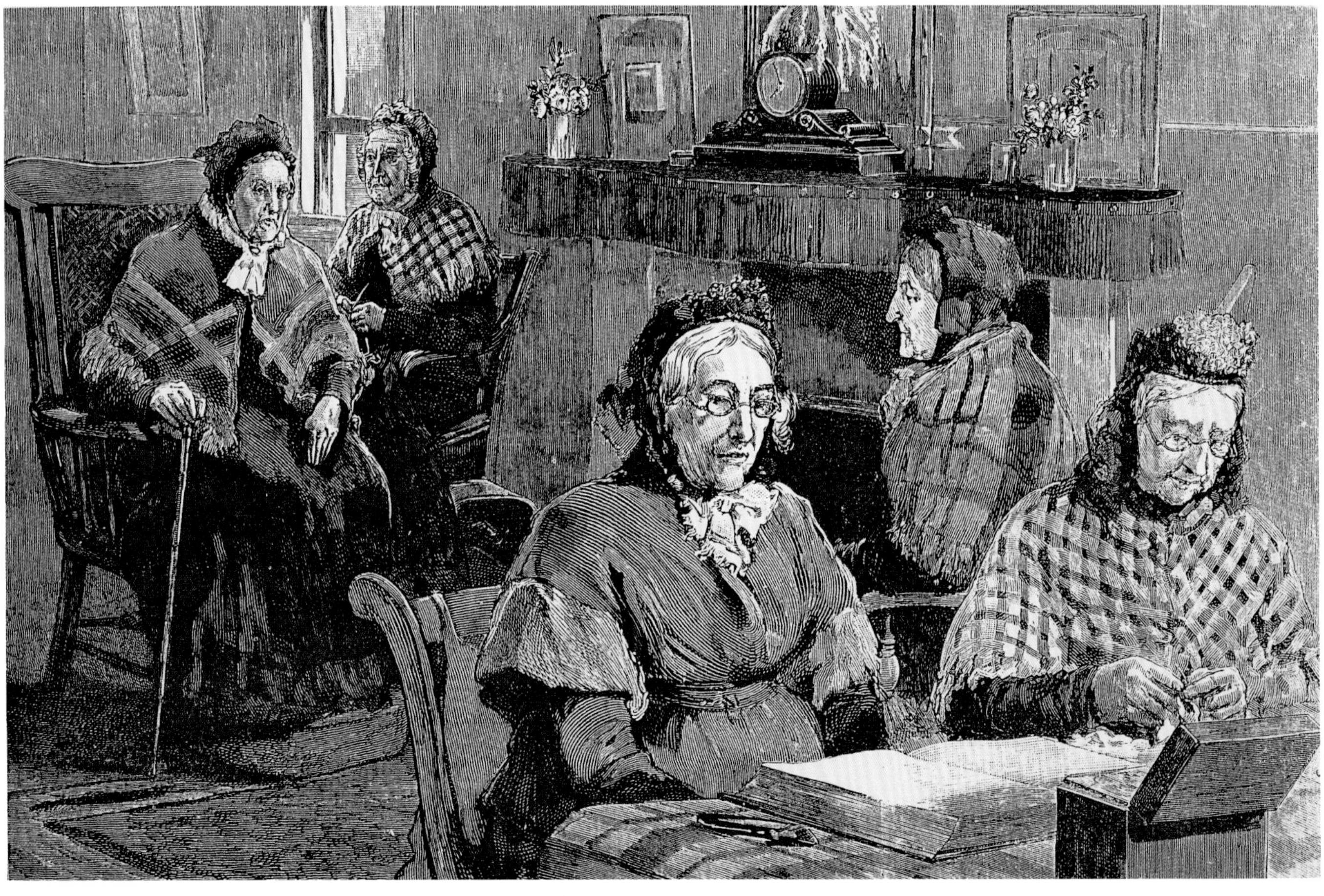

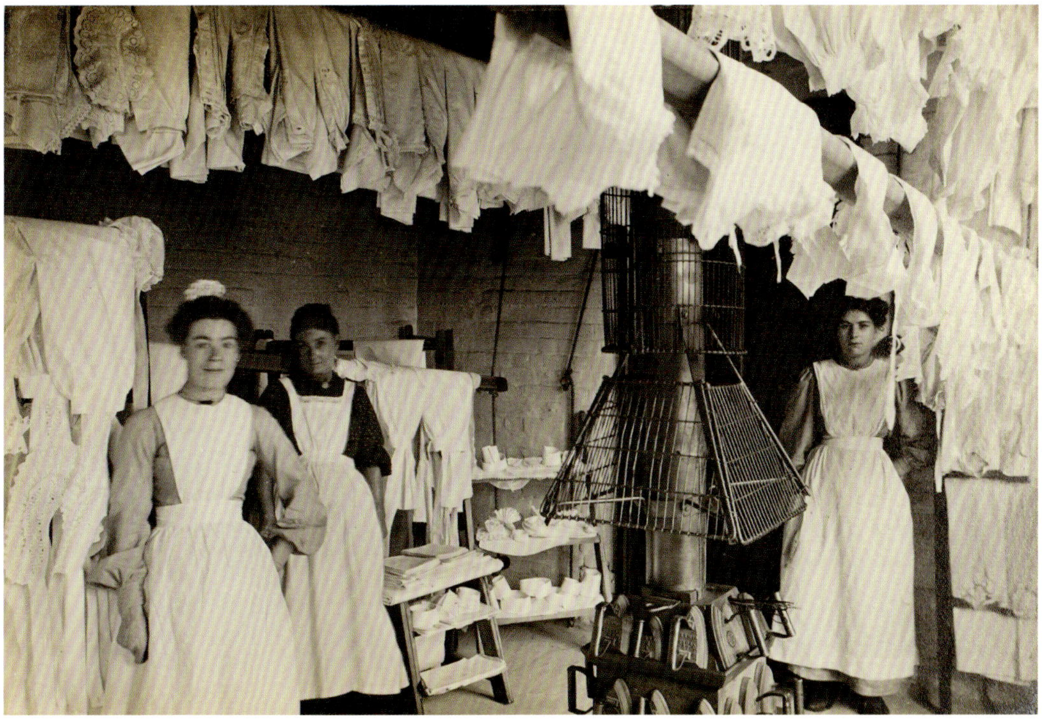

Fig. 85 The laundry, the French Hospital, Victoria Park, Hackney, photograph, 1907. *Huguenot Library.*

The basement laundry was staffed by three laundry maids responsible for bed and table linen and the inmates' clothing. Other staff including the chaplain and the medical officer attended the hospital daily and reported to the directors' committee at their monthly meetings. The steward remained in general charge of the hospital assisted by an efficient staff of nurses and servants, who had their own kitchen.

Figs. 83 and 84 Illustrations from the *Graphic*, 26 October 1885

Fig. 83 *(left, top)* Looms in use in the men's day-room, the French Hospital

Fig. 84 *(left)* The women's day-room, the French Hospital

The day-rooms were situated on the ground floor. During the morning the inmates would 'render what help they are able' towards the general economy. 'The old ladies do most of the needlework required in the provision and maintenance of their own dress and of the household linen etc and the men render a number of little services about the establishment.' According to an early 19th-century prospectus, the 'Women's Day Room contain[ed] a small Library of suitable works for the inmates' use.' In the men's day-room 'is a Billiard Table, presented by one of the Directors, and in both Day Rooms the tables are furnished with the *Sphere*, *Black and White*, *Strand Magazine*, *Quiver*, *Chambers' Journal* and other periodicals.'

'In sunny weather the more active of the old people may often be found enjoying a game of bowls on the lawn or giving their companions an airing in the bath chair, while, whatever the aspect of the sky overhead, the men's smoking room is pretty sure to be tenanted.'

The Browning memorial photograph album contains photographs of the men's and women's convalescent rooms and their communal bedrooms. Married couples and persons under fifty years of age were still not admitted.

3 *Charter and By-Laws* (1892), Preface, p. xxvi.

4 Sir Henry Peek was descended from the Le Maitre family on his mother's side.

5 The income was to be devoted to the purchase of books costing more than £3. The Huguenot Library has a manuscript catalogue of the items purchased through the French Hospital Library Trust Fund subscribed in memory of Arthur Giraud Browning with a copy of the Trust Deed, 1895.

6 Wagner's obituary in *The Times*, 27 April 1926 describes the French Hospital as 'the chief Huguenot foundation in this country'.

7 Wagner, *Wills.*

8 Transcribed from the printed 'Ceremony of the Loving Cup, The French Hospital, London', preserved as a loose sheet in the 1892 Blue Book in possession of the present deputy-governor, Peter Duval. It is inscribed on the verso: 'Invented circa 1884 by Mr. A.G. Browning when Secretary, but believed by those who hear it for the first time to be coeval with the Corporation.'

9 The song, of which the Huguenot Library retains a copy, was transcribed in full in Murdoch, p. 318.

10 HL H.J60.

11 Marmoy, 'French Hospital', pp. 246–7.

12 HL H.H2a3. Marmoy, *Inmates and Applicants*, vol. 1, Dabbs, James. Inmate. He also wove silk for dresses for the Duchess of Kent and Queen Adelaide.

13 HL H.A1.6. Marmoy, *Inmates and Applicants*, vol. 1, Bond, Mary (*née* Dabbs). Inmate.

14 A.H. Browning, *PHS*, XVII, 1 (1942), p. 90. Marshall was a former employee of Browning's.

15 *PHS*, XII, 4 (1921), pp. 281–320.

16 HL K.J61.

8

Under threat, enemy action and evacuation

After the First World War, the social climate had changed radically. There was a much greater awareness of social issues, brought further into the limelight by the Jarrow marchers and the General Strike. At a local level the London County Council (LCC) felt obliged to improve general living conditions in east London. Change came to Hackney as the LCC set about dealing with the grinding poverty of large swathes of London's population to the east and north.

At the Annual General Meeting of the Huguenot Society in May 1934, Arthur Hervé Browning, its president, let the fellows know what lay ahead for the French Hospital.[1]

> During the past six months the Directors of 'La Providence' have been, and still are, confronted with the grave possibility that their beautiful building and grounds in Victoria Park Road may be ruthlessly taken from them.
>
> Under their Slum Clearance Scheme the London County Council have set envious eyes on our little Naboth's vineyard[2] ... and in spite of our representations and repudiation of any desire to sell, have threatened to exercise their powers of compulsory purchase. ... The problem of providing not only a new home for our old people, but also for our invaluable collection of Huguenot relics, pictures, books, memorial windows, etc., is one that will not, and indeed cannot, be easily solved.

The story of Naboth the Jezreelite is told in the Old Testament. Naboth owned a vineyard near 'the palace of Ahab, the king of Samaria'. Ahab coveted it for a herb garden and offered Naboth 'a better vineyard', or its worth in money: 'And Naboth said to Ahab "The Lord forbid it me, that I should give the inheritance of my fathers unto thee".' All ends badly for Naboth, when Jezebel, Ahab's wife, sets up false witnesses against him and he is stoned to death, but Ahab is admonished by Elijah acting as God's spokesman, and Ahab and Jezebel are punished.

There is added poignancy in the metaphorical use by Browning of Naboth's vineyard for there is an earlier passage in the First Book of Kings in which Elijah is fed and watered by God's command. 'Get thee hence ... and hide thyself by the brook Cherith ... And it shall be that thou shalt drink of the brook; and I have commanded the ravens to feed thee there.' The image of Elijah and the ravens had been chosen over 200 years earlier by the founding directors as the seal of the hospital with the motto *'Dominus providebit'*.

The French Hospital's Court Minutes record the battle of wills that ensued during these troubled years. When the storm broke, Hugh Dumas, a county court judge, was deputy-governor of the hospital.

Prolonged negotiations had already begun in October 1933 when London County Council (LCC) made a written offer for £35,000 for the French Hospital buildings and grounds through a Notting Hill estate agent. Through the secretary, the directors replied that they had 'no intention of selling the Hospital'.[3] The LCC valuer, Frank Hunt, to whom the directors had been referred, told the directors that 'we were invited to inspect the property with a view to its being acquired by the Council' to provide housing for up to 3,000.[4] There was:

> An urgent necessity for providing rehousing accommodation in this part of London to deal with the numerous slum areas in the immediate vicinity ... here is a site of 3.2 acres with less than 100 people, mainly pensioners, residing thereon.

Then came the threat that the LCC would 'consider making a compulsory purchase if negotiations [were] ... abruptly terminated'.

The deputy-governor, Judge Dumas, and a number of directors met the LCC valuer and colleagues in July 1934. Dumas stressed the importance of the hospital to the inmates and their friends and families in Spitalfields and Bethnal Green, declaring that the hospital was:

> An outstanding memorial of the settlement of the Huguenots [who] had enriched the country in the arts, sciences and industries; it was a treasure house of memorials to past Huguenots ... its unique building was becoming more and more the centre of research [into] the Huguenots in England. The building and its surroundings were probably the most beautiful adornment to the Borough of Hackney.

If the proposal were carried forward, he asserted, they would have to 'resist it to the utmost'. The LCC retreated, and proposed to take 50,000 square feet to the west of the building for the erection of five-storey blocks of council flats. Frank Hunt wrote that the LCC 'would endeavour to preserve the setting of the Hospital so that memorial of the Huguenot Invasion might remain as at present'. The directors reluctantly agreed and haggling over the broad strip of well-planted land continued until September 1934 when a poorly attended committee meeting decided by seven votes to six not to authorize the sale of the smaller parcel of land but instead 'take the risk of compulsory purchase of the whole site by the LCC'.

Gallantly, however, the proposer, E.C. Fâche, seconded by Owen Fortrie Parker (of a sixteenth-century Walloon refugee family), accepted that the reversal had been agreed by too few directors and at a further meeting the directors voted by seventeen to four to accept the LCC's offer of £13,000 for the land to the west of the hospital. After a further year of argument over details – the fencing of the lodge, the height of the wall – the sale finally went through in October 1935.

The council flats were built and the hospital found itself overlooked, despite the high wall. In 1938, E.C. Ouvry, president of the Huguenot Society, a director of the hospital and its honorary solicitor, spoke as Browning had done four years earlier:[5]

> A considerable portion of the Hospital garden has now been taken away and large housing flats built, which dominate the Hospital and the grounds that have, so far, survived. Housing sites in the Hackney neighbourhood are scarce. The Hospital site is indeed a 'Naboth's vineyard'. It is not only a hospital, it is the Huguenot centre for learning. It is the Huguenot Museum.

He ended his presidential address:

> What is to happen if the re-housing claims of the East End masses become too strong to allow an ideal site, already partly acquired and partly built over, to escape the compulsory powers of a Socialist Council? If the time comes when the Hospital is compelled to close down on its present site, what is to be done?

Ouvry suggested as alternatives either 'a central institution ... as at present' or 'separate apartments round a court, allotted to the more active inmates', with 'a central building for the less able-bodied', the central building should be the 'recognized centre of all Huguenot institutions, library, museum and meeting place for all our charities and societies'. This, he suggested, would have to be in London.

Ouvry's alarm was soon dwarfed by a far greater menace. The day after Chamberlain's Munich Agreement with Hitler, the directors resolved on 1 October 1938:

> In view of the anxious experience of the prospect of war, to look into immediate steps to be taken by the Steward ... to protect the Hospital from the danger of Gas and Bombs.[6]

One thousand sandbags were obtained. In February 1939, the directors let the LCC know that one of the hospital's nearby properties, 87 Cazenove Road, could be used as a home for refugee children. In May, with war with Nazi Germany imminent, the need for 'air raid precautions' was discussed but it was decided that there was no need to evacuate the inmates and the collections. With the outbreak of war, an air-raid shelter was built for the inmates and staff. In October, with the war in its second month, the Royal Charter and some of the most valuable silver were sent for safekeeping to Longford Castle, Wiltshire, home of the governor, Lord Radnor. The *Grand Livre*, dating back to 1728, and other important documents were housed by the solicitor, E.C. Ouvry, in his home in Kent.

The hospital was soon to suffer from enemy attack, the fabric being damaged by Luftwaffe bombing in July 1940, as were its houses in Cazenove Road. In September the Blitz caused damage by 'shell splinters' and fires from an incendiary bomb, put out by the Hackney Fire Brigade. In October, a 'high explosive bomb' landed in the kitchen garden, the chapel windows were shattered including the memorial window dedicated to the memory of Arthur Giraud Browning in 1908[7] and brick- and stonework were damaged.

The destruction of some of the hospital's remaining properties in the parish of St Luke's, Finsbury, was far worse. Houses in neighbouring Galway Street, Bath Street and Gastigny Place were destroyed and claims made to the War Damage Commission.

As the Blitz went on—until May 1941 – inmates and staff in the Victoria Park Hospital were spending every night in the basement shelter, and life was 'becoming intolerable'. It was decided after the October air raid, to evacuate the inmates. 'Hosts' – mainly seaside landladies with no holidaymakers – were found at Littlehampton, through the efforts of the deputy-governor the Revd Dr S.P. Duval, Vicar of nearby Lyminster and Rural Dean of Arundel.

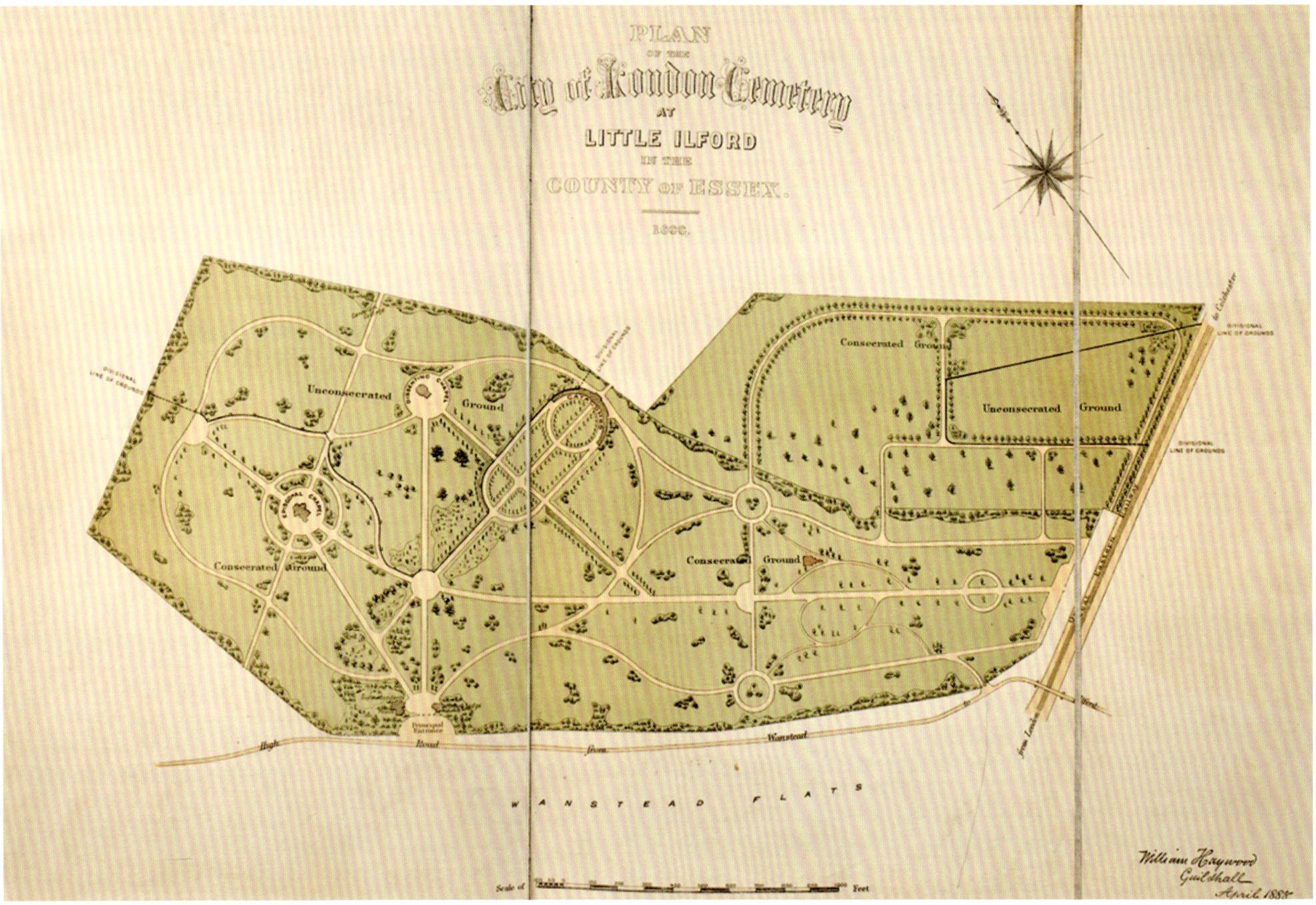

Fig. 86 *Plan of the City of London Cemetery at Little Ilford in the County of Essex*, water-colour, William Haywood Guilshall, 1888. *Huguenot Library*

The French Hospital Burial Ground was marked by a monument inset with the seal of the French Hospital and the inscription: 'Here rest many "Children of the Stranger" whose last days were spent at the Hospital or Hospice founded by French Protestant Refugees early in the XVIII Century for the reception and care of the poor and aged among their fellow exiles, and their descendants.'

This is followed by a quotation from Matthew 25: 31–2: 'When the Son of Man shall come in His Glory and all the Holy Angels with Him, then shall He sit upon the Throne of His Glory, and before Him shall be gathered all Nations.'

Others were housed in Broxbourne in Hertfordshire, where a director, Colonel Davy, kept in close touch.

The directors were much exercised over the care of the evacuated 'old people'. What to do about the old lady who tore up the postal orders she was sent? In 1943 new suits were sent to the male evacuees – at £4 each. Several inmates died in exile and were buried at the hospital's expense in the hospital's ground in the City of London cemetery (figs. 86–7). One was James Hurlin, aged 81, a former 'chair carver journeyman', who died at Littlehampton in 1942. He was a great-grandson of Daniel Marchand, a child refugee from Alençon who, a former silk weaver, had died in 1801, aged 84 in the old hospital at Finsbury. Hurlin had other relatives who had lived at La Providence: he belonged to one of the many family dynasties among the inmates.

The Fourmy family is another example. Anne Fromey [*sic*] entered the hospital in 1730 and the latest descendant of the Fourmy family to take up residence at La Providence died in 2001. Florence May Smart had entered the Rochester Hospital in the early 1970s. Her elder sister Grace had entered in 1969 and died there thirty years later, possibly the longest ever resident. Other members of this family are recorded there during the eighteenth and nineteenth centuries.[8]

The French Hospital at Victoria Park was requisitioned and opened as a day nursery for mothers doing war work, although the directors retained their Court Room and Library, the latter maintained by the librarian, Winifred

Turner, on her weekly visit.[9] The portraits, framed engravings and some valuable books went to Ystrad, near Llandovery, to the care of an elderly widow, Dame Margaret Pryse-Rice. The fencing and the old entrance gates of the Norris Estate were requisitioned for scrap but were saved after the clerk, J.I. Marshall, pointed out that they were of 'considerable antiquity'.[10]

The French Hospital still held property at the old Finsbury site, which was badly damaged by enemy action in November 1943. Then, on 19 February 1944, the adjacent Radnor Street School was bombed out; two were killed and two seriously injured. Casualties were reduced thanks to the anti-blast walls in the air-raid shelter. In Hackney, the main French Hospital building remained intact until the flying bomb V1 attacks in July 1944, and the V2 rocket bombs that followed. At 1:20 a.m. on 2 December the V2 which fell into Wetherell Road smashed the hospital's main doors, windows and window frames, damaged the front of the building and made the steward's quarters uninhabitable. The steward, A.J. Cobden, and his wife, moved to Woking and visited the hospital twice a week until they could move back in a year later.

Owing to the devastation of the East End, the hospital was requisitioned in March 1945 by the War Damage Commission and by the Ministry of Health for its district offices, both bombed out in Ilford. Although by the summer hostilities in Europe had ended, the return of the hospital to normality was far off.

In April 1946, the consensus among inmates was the wish to go back to Hackney and the Littlehampton landladies wanted their rooms back. The Labour MP for Hackney, H.W. Butler,[11] saw that Ministry of Health staff departed in March 1947. Pre-fabricated buildings were put up on vacant land for the day nursery.

1 *PHS*, XV, 1 (1934), pp. 14–15.

2 1 Kings 21.

3 The estate agent was told that he was not their agent, had no authority to act as he had done and 'no claim for commission would be considered under any circumstances whatever'.

4 Frank Hunt later intimated that, Ahab-like, he had been eyeing the hospital for some time.

5 *PHS*, XV, 1 (1934), p. 15.

6 HL H.A1.13.

7 This represented Daniel praying towards Jerusalem and Ahazuerus extending his sceptre towards the kneeling figure of Esther.

8 Robert Nash, in a personal communication, May 2008.

9 She retired in 1946 after twenty years' service.

10 The London Society and the Hackney Borough Council intervened, and both the gates, and for security, the lodge fencing, were saved.

11 He had been a borough councillor when the 50,000 square feet were taken for housing.

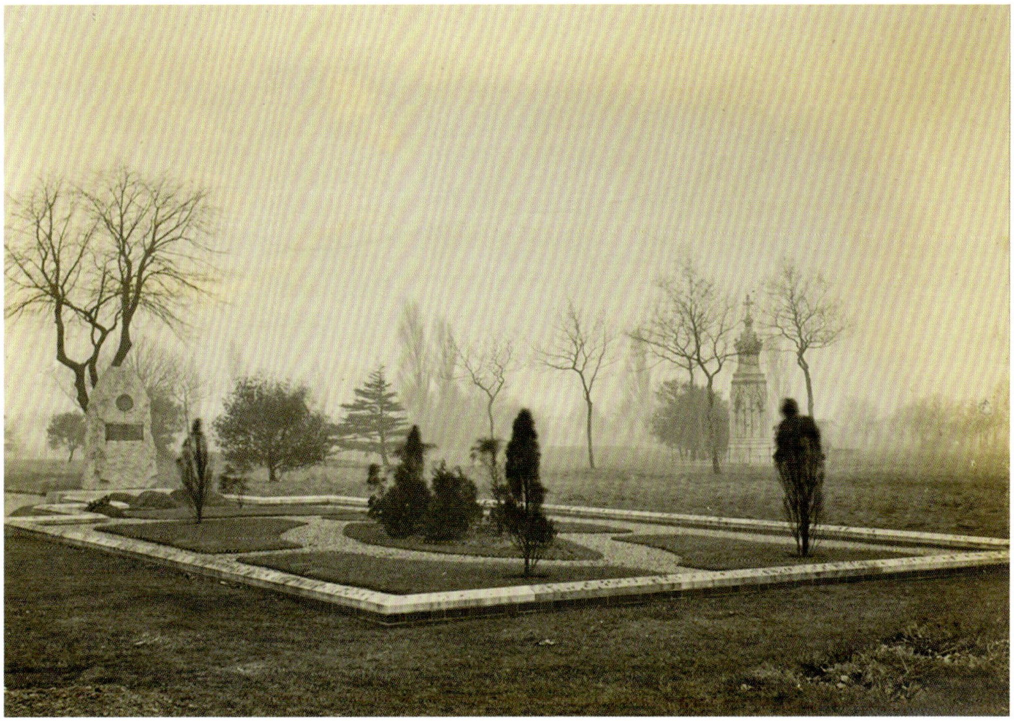

Fig. 87 View of the French Hospital Burial Ground at Little Ilford, c. 1907. *Huguenot Library*

9

Retreat to the country: Compton's Lea, Sussex, 1947–1957

With the consolidation of State health and welfare support by the State under the post-war Labour Government, it was indeed time to reassess the role the French Hospital should play in public health. In September 1946, Major-General C.T. Beckett, a director since 1928 and newly retired from the Army after wartime service abroad, proposed the sale of the hospital, and the purchase of a site 'within easy reach of London'. Most radically he proposed that 'a different class would have to be catered for, owing to the State aid now being so much increased.' Beckett's proposal won the backing of the London Almshouses Committee and the directors thenceforward saw the hospital's future as that of an almshouse in a new location. There was now no objection amongst the directors to the selling of Roumieu's great institutional building and the relocation of its Huguenot collection and library.[1]

The directors swiftly decided in favour of a new hospital, to be 'occupied by inmates to the fullest capacity'. Thanks to a *deus ex machina*, the acquisition of a new building was made possible before the sale of the old one. The Willen Key Company, 'the household name for locks and keys and whose catalogue was the bible for everyone in the trade',[2] bought six of the corporation's Bath and Galway Street houses for £3,575, since their former premises in Bath Street had been destroyed as a result of bombing.

A fine Victorian house a mile from the railway station in Horsham, Sussex, was bought for £7,000. Compton's Lea, with its three reception and sixteen bedrooms, all in very good order, with central heating, and two cottages, standing in ten acres of garden and meadow, was easily and quickly adapted. In mid-August 1947 the residents moved in, and Head Nurse Banks and her ward maid, the cook, kitchen maid, housemaid and 'attendant', joined the head and under-gardener already employed. The Revd H.W. Overs, Vicar of Roffey, was appointed chaplain of the French Hospital, after a gap of five years.[3]

During that time Dr Stephen Duval, deputy-governor, had 'arranged for half the inmates to be near him at Littlehampton, constantly visiting them and seeing to their comfort'. Dr Duval had four churches in his care, as well as the rural diaconate. His sudden death on 12 April 1947 had been 'hastened by overwork', wrote the secretary, Major Aubertin. He was succeeded by his brother Walter John Duval, grandfather of the present deputy-governor, Peter James Duval, elected in 1981.[4]

A good offer of £25,000 for the Victoria Park building and site was made by 'Mr Gelinsky on behalf of a Jewish organization'. It was set aside by the LCC, however, who, again threatening compulsory purchase, acquired the property for £25,000 in 1948. It was rumoured that it was to be used for a Roman Catholic school. The Cardinal Pole Roman Catholic School, named after the Catholic Archbishop of Canterbury in the reign of Mary I, eventually came to occupy the building and grounds, and still does.

All the hospital's treasures taken out of London for safe-keeping during the war years were brought to Compton's Lea: the royal charter and silver from Longford Castle; the hospital's pictures from Dame Margaret in Carmarthenshire and the archives from the solicitor's house in Kent. Marble busts of former Huguenot directors and officers, including that of Richard Hervé Giraud (fig. 52) were also retrieved. The chapel furniture followed in September 1947, when the first Quarterly Committee meeting was held in the new hospital. Lastly, in March 1948, the library was moved to Compton's Lea and 'arranged to the best advantage'.

Life was pleasant enough at Compton's Lea in the late 1940s and the directors after their monthly 'visites de la maison' almost always reported the residents cheerful and contented. But there were too few of them – only ten, nine of them women – to warrant the occupancy of a sixteen-bedroom house standing in broad acres, with cottages and with too large a staff. Three directors warned that 'considerable expense would be called for' if this were to be the permanent home of the hospital.[5] It seemed that Compton's Lea had been a false step.

The directors met for their monthly committee meetings and every three months for the more formal business of their Court. The committee and court meetings distributed the outgifts, pensions, apprenticeship and bursary funds entrusted to them. Only a few 'petitions' for admission to La Providence reached the depths of Sussex.

Compton's Lea ran at a loss from the start, though the deficit – about £400 a year for the first five years – was more than met from revenue, the greater part of it from the sale of Hackney leases and of the field adjoining Compton's Lea House to the Water Board. Much of the directors' time was spent on the administration of the considerable property holdings. By March 1951 the sale of the Finsbury estate was complete, yielding £19,200 1s 9d. The directors decided in 1952 to liquidate what was left of their property holdings in favour of investments in equities and securities permitted by the Charity Commissioners, and the disposal continued.[6] By 1954 the Royal Oak public house and the Galway Street Schools, a Methodist institution, were taken over, under compulsory purchase orders, by the Finsbury Borough Council. As well as lease-holdings, tenancies, and maintenance, the business of War Damage claims went on into the 1950s.

In June 1953, a royal licence was acquired allowing the ownership of Compton's Lea which exceeded the restriction in the Royal Charter of 1718 to land and buildings 'with a yearly value of £500'.[7] A Supplemental Charter was granted in September, 'in the second year of our reign' increasing the allowed value of the Hospital's lands and buildings to £50,000, reducing the quorum to seven (from ten in 1718), and permitting the holding of Courts 'in London or elsewhere'.[8]

The high staffing cost at Compton's Lea was unsparingly attacked in April 1954 by Major-General Beckett. 'Sixteen paid officials or servants, apart from the gardeners, ministered to the needs of twelve inmates'. Thus 'each inmate had a personal attendant, full board and lodging and the equivalent spent on garden amenities which would rent a small but adequate Council cottage'. There was little opposition at the meeting to the general's call for the substitution of annuities for residential care but more from absent directors when canvassed. The Revd E. E. Jourdain felt that 'every attempt should be made to keep the Hospital going' and said, '[I]n addition to the purpose for which the Corporation was founded, in my experience as a parish priest, I do feel that the great need of old people is not so much for money as for care'. Colonel P. A. E. Dumas commented: 'we are losing sight of the "intention" of the French Hospital which is to provide a home in old age'.

The vision of the twin objectives of the French Hospital through the Hackney years – to provide 'not only a peaceful asylum for some of the poor aged descendants of the French Protestants', but also 'to erect a standing memorial of early French Refugees', where 'many rare and valuable books and historical engravings' and 'many portraits of officers and Directors of the Corporation' are displayed, had faded.[9]

The directors at Compton's Lea employed a part-time librarian and were concerned about the value of the hospital's treasures. A visit in 1954 by a well-known Christie's expert, Arthur Grimwade, brought to light the transposing of the covers of the two All Hallows, Thames Street, communion cups when that church's plate had been divided between the French Hospital and St Michael's Paternoster Royal in 1896.[10] The collections continued to increase, with gifts from Miss Susan Minet, and the French Embassy, when, after a visit by the ambassador, M. René Massigli in 1950, a copy of the 1687 Brief by the Catholic James II's calling for assistance to the Huguenot refugees, found in the embassy, was presented by the cultural attaché.[11]

A search for more economical premises in Wimbledon and South Croydon continued. By October 1955 the situation had become critical. Staff problems were acute, better wages and conditions could be found in local factories and canteens, and when the head and under-nurse both left in September 1955 it was agreed that the hospital should close immediately and alternative accommodation be found for the inmates – only eight and all women.[12]

The last male inmate, Louis De la More Mignon, MA, a former solicitor with no pension and of noble French Protestant ancestry, had come to the hospital in Hackney in 1932, suffering from very 'great deafness', died in January 1955 aged 84.[13] The faithful steward, A. J. Cobden[14] and his wife, who stayed on and visited the widespread remaining dependents of the hospital, a cleaner and a gardener were the sole occupants of Compton's Lea.

In near desperation the directors put Compton's Lea on the market.[15] It was agreed that land be found, with or without buildings on it, for a new hospital. The directors held back from the general's urging that 'the library could be handed over to a library in Cambridge, silver and pictures placed in charge of a Club in London and that meetings in future could be held there' to deal with the grants that would replace the residential care. The search went on.[16]

General Beckett's case, supported by several directors,

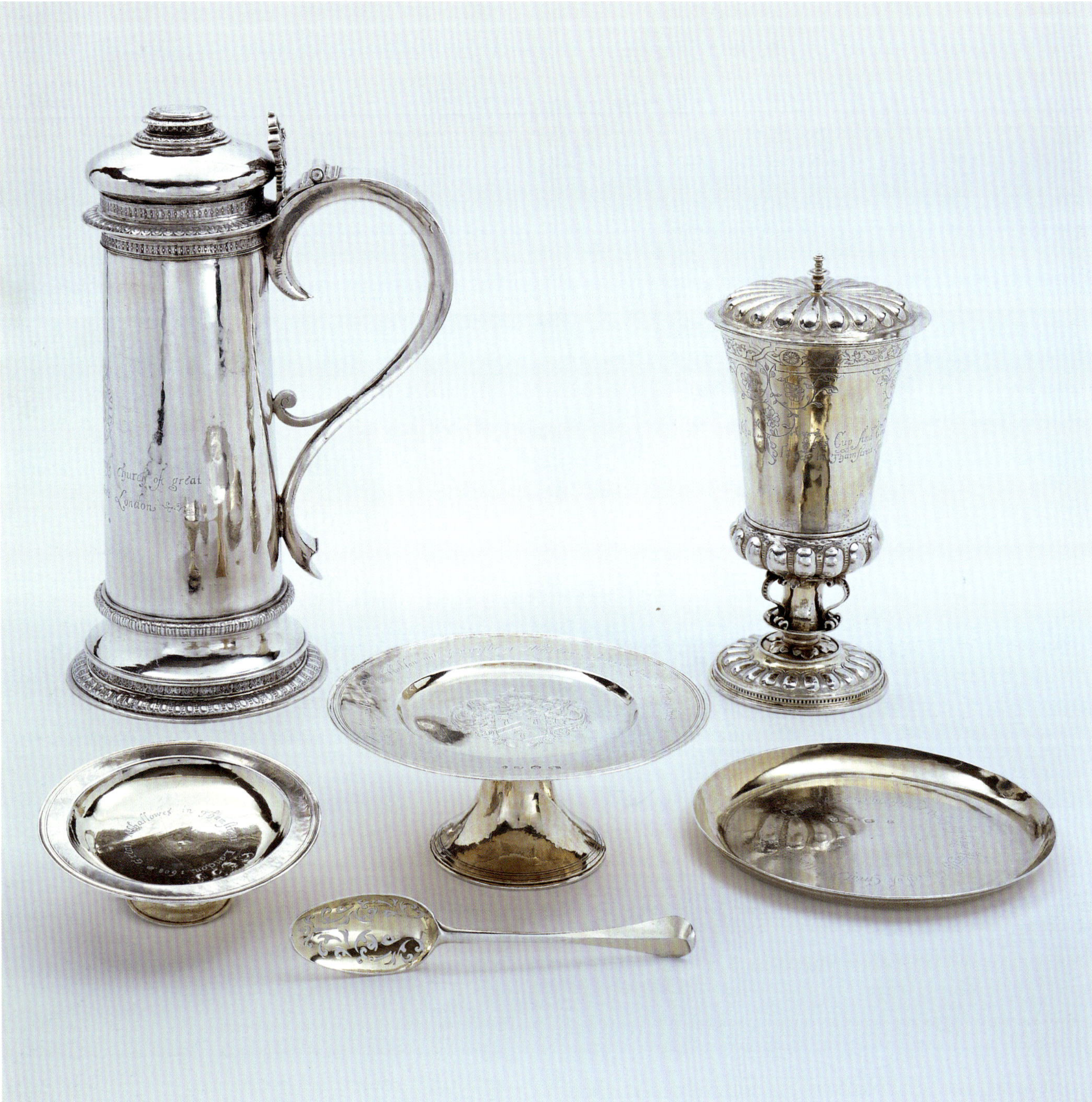

Fig. 88 Communion plate, sterling silver, from All Hallows by the Tower, Thames Street, City of London

Sir Henry Peek, president of the Huguenot Society of London and a deputy-governor of the French Hospital, suggested that one complete service from the communion plate of the recently demolished church of All Hallows should be allocated to the hospital chapel. The Rector and Churchwardens of the United Parishes including the former All Hallows the Great, the Less, St Martin, Vintry, and St Michael Paternoster Royal, agreed, and the decision was sanctioned by the Bishop of London. The plate, 'lodged in a chest in the adjoining City of London Brewery for Security', was accordingly released for use in the French Hospital chapel on 29 April 1896. Placed on the holy table in the French Hospital chapel, the rector, the Revd Thomas Moore, MA, formally presented the sacred vessels to the governor and directors of the corporation commending 'their frequent and reverential use.' A service of dedication in the French Hospital chapel followed. The Order of the Bishop and the Service of Dedication are printed in full in *PHS*, V, part IV, 1896, pp. 431–40.

The plate consists of an Elizabethan paten cover, dated 1575/6, a James I silver-gilt cup and cover, 1608/9, a James I paten and a covered flagon, 1608/9, a Charles I standing paten, 1634/5, and a George I straining spoon, 1719/20. All Hallows, burned to the ground during the Great Fire of London, was rebuilt by Sir Christopher Wren between 1677 and 1683. The Wren tower and north aisle were demolished in 1876 to widen Queen Victoria Street, and in 1893–4, the rest of the Wren church was demolished with the exception of the rebuilt 1870s tower and the vestry on the south side. The furnishings were transferred to St Margaret, Lothbury, and St Paul's, Hammersmith. A contemporary photograph taken by Lambert's of Coventry Street shows the newly acquired group of communion silver. The Elizabethan paten is still regularly used in the communion service at Rochester.

still lay on the table and it was at a crucial Court meeting on 14 January 1956 that he was finally answered and the way forward for La Providence was at last clear. The Charity Commission was represented at the meeting by the Assistant Commissioner, Mr W. E. A. Lewis, who made it very clear that the Commission would oppose 'the substitution of monetary grants for the provision of residential accommodation ... as they regard this as of greater importance'.[17] Independent accommodation for old people of Huguenot descent, near shops and public transport must be made available. 'There would be no objection to the expenditure of charitable funds on the ancillary purpose of the Corporation as the headquarters of Huguenot records and treasures', provided that the amount spent was an 'inconsiderable proportion' of its resources. The new residents should be 'drawn from a wide range of classes', while below the maximum income limit adopted by the National Benevolent Institution and other charities. He suggested reference to the National Association of Almshouses, of which the corporation was a member.

The Court resolved to search for land 'on which to erect a Home for old people', taking the form of 'self-contained accommodation in which the residents would provide their own meals, with the addition of certain communal rooms'.

The assistant commissioner's endorsement of the hospital as the 'headquarters of Huguenot records and treasures' seems not to have been taken up with any enthusiasm, however. The Court resolved that 'the Library and such furniture and other possessions as it was considered essential to retain' would be put into storage. In March 1956 the clerk reported that Mr L. A. Hackett, the general secretary of the National Association of Almshouses had advised that other charities had built almshouses near the south coast.[18]

Some years ago, said Hackett, a scheme had been 'tentatively suggested ... for the conversion into almshouses of a square of small houses off Rochester High Street'. The idea had been 'met with some interest by the Bishop of Rochester' but so far nothing had been done. This was Theobald Square, soon to become the subject of a most favourable report by the clerk, J. O. Attlee, and the surveyor, Cecil Grellier, to the April 1956 Court. Mr Hackett, also present, 'thought that the scheme had everything to recommend it' and the Court agreed that, subject to satisfactory conditions, 'in principle the Hospital should proceed with the project to use Theobald Square as homes for old people'.

1 Ouvry was 80 and handed over as solicitor to his son Romilly in 1948 and A. H. Browning attended less frequently in his seventies.

2 Jim Evans, *A Gazeteer of Lock and Key Makers* (2002), p. 3.

3 He succeeded the Revd Dr S. P. Duval, deputy-governor, who had ministered to the inmates in Littlehampton.

4 *HSP*, XVIII, 1 (1947), p. 29. W. J. Duval was the son, grandson and great-grandson of deputy-governors, all 'members of a great Huguenot family which finds its happiness in serving others'.

5 HL, H.H3; C.H. Jeune, H. E. Greenwood and O. F. Parker, who had inspected the property in February 1947, had considered the hospital 'well advised to secure it – based on the assumption that at present the directors be seeking temporary accommodation ... pending the erection of a fundamentally more suitable type of building'.

6 A licence had been obtained in 1902 for the ownership of sixteen houses in Highbury.

7 The estate at Compton's Lea consisted of 'six acres one rod and twenty perches' and adjoining land. There were also five cottages near Little Hadham in Hertfordshire, given by Miss Susan Minet, with an £850 endowment to the hospital, to be held 'in mortmain' (i.e. by a corporation).

8 *Charter and By-Laws* (2000 and previous editions), pp. 19–22.

9 A. G. Browning, 1892, Blue Book, p. xxvi.

10 A. G. Browning, 'Notes on the Communion Plate lately presented to the French Protestant Hospital, *PHS*, V, 4 (1896), pp. 431–40.

11 The library was a constant worry: five tons of documents had to be moved from the top floor to the basement and a crate of books was found to be damp.

12 Three went into a home in Addlestone, Surrey, three near Epping, Essex, and the others in Bromley, Kent, and Angmering-on-Sea, Sussex.

13 He was buried in the hospital's plot in Roffey cemetery.

14 He was recruited by General Beckett, RA, whose battery sergeant-major he had been at Gallipoli and in France.

15 The Court was told that the Emergency Committee favoured the purchase of a house at South Croydon.

16 In December a house in Caterham which had been considered before Compton's Lea was chosen, again came into view. It could take twenty-five to thirty inmates, though there were now so few to be cared for. Those who had died at Compton's Lea lay with Mr Mignon in the hospital's burial plot in Roffey and had not been replaced. It now seemed doubtful if, in Welfare State Britain, they ever would be.

17 Exemption from tax would continue as funds accumulated after the closure. He confirmed 'without hesitation' that Compton's Lea was 'unsuitable for conversion into flatlets', which was the way forward and the house should be vacated and sold as soon as possible.

18 Mr L. A. Hackett had been asked if there were 'surplus almshouses available elsewhere', Hackett spoke of 'a very lovely block of almshouses near Wokingham' which was probably, like Compton's Lea, 'too far from the town'.

10

Retirement in a cathedral city

In *Great Expectations* Charles Dickens evokes the Rochester of his childhood. When Pip first visits Miss Havisham, the 'large brewery' adjacent to Satis House was disused and had been for a long time'. Pip found the brewery 'empty. The cold wind ... made a shrill noise in howling in and out of the open sides of the brewery ... like the noise of wind in the rigging of a ship at sea'.[1] The forlorn setting of Pip's visit to the embittered, rich old lady of Satis House had changed by the 1840s to a neat open square of nineteen late-Georgian two-storey houses with basements, called, after the former brewer, Theobald Square.

More than a century later the square had 'fallen into a very bad state of repair'. It was still 'a pleasant self-contained close' suitable for housing the elderly and forming a charming backwater in the centre of Rochester under the shadow of the Cathedral'.[2]

Bishop Gundulf's eleventh-century cathedral, the second oldest in England after Canterbury, became the centre of the spiritual life of the French Hospital. The bishop, the Right-Reverend Christopher Chavasse, a man of great energy, dedication and charm, welcomed the directors, and entertained them at Bishopscourt. He established the tradition of holding the Anniversary Evensong in the cathedral in June, followed by a 'strawberry tea' for directors, residents and their families and the Friends of La Providence. Bishop Chavasse was a director of the French Hospital until his death in 1962. The foundation of an organization of Friends in 1960 had marked the end of the fund-raising appeal which achieved £40,000 to help pay for the conversion of the houses, with their old gas lighting and outside lavatories. In 1958, when the Medway District Council agreed to the renaming of Theobald Square as La Providence, the doctor's house at 105 High Street was renumbered 41 La Providence.

The Mayor and Corporation of Rochester supported the French Hospital's move to Theobald Square, assisted with its purchase for £6,000 and that of 105 High Street for £5,000, with the conversion of the houses to 39 one- and two-bedroomed flats and with the re-housing of the remaining tenants. The chairman of the housing committee hailed the 'conversion of an eyesore into a place of which the City can be proud' and anticipated that tourists would 'come to Rochester from far and wide' and would see 'Theobald Square once more as a place of beauty' (figs. 89–91). The bishop planned to provide a chapel in the unusually large crypt similar to the one at Canterbury Cathedral where Walloon and Huguenot refugees worshipped from the 1560s as their descendants and others still do today. The residents of the French Hospital became part of the cathedral congregation.

Rochester was a logical home for the French Hospital because of the long-standing Huguenot links with Kent. Besides the Huguenot congregation who met in the crypt of Canterbury Cathedral there were many Huguenot silk weavers who had settled in Kent and forged links with the growing Huguenot community of weavers in the East End of London.[3] This new location attracted residents whose ancestors had been Walloon or Huguenot settlers in Canterbury, Sandwich, Rye and Whitstable in that county. Proving their descent from French Protestant families of Kent was harder, as the only Huguenot church records in Kent were those for the Canterbury and Sandwich congregations. Over twenty-five Huguenot London churches had kept registers and others survived for Huguenot churches in Bristol, Norwich, Plymouth and Southampton. Of the

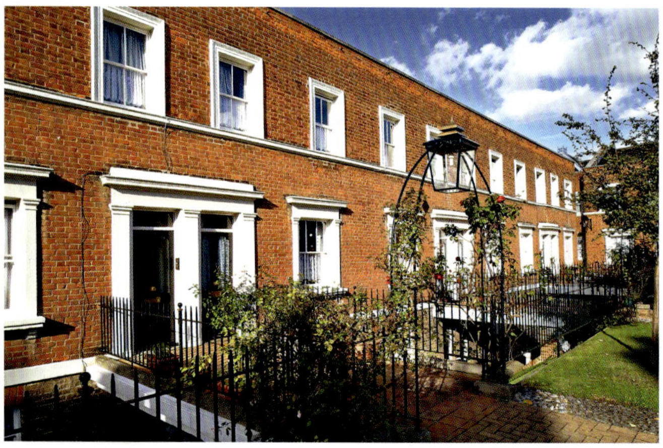

Fig. 89 The French Hospital, La Providence, Rochester, north-western elevation. *Tim Rawle*

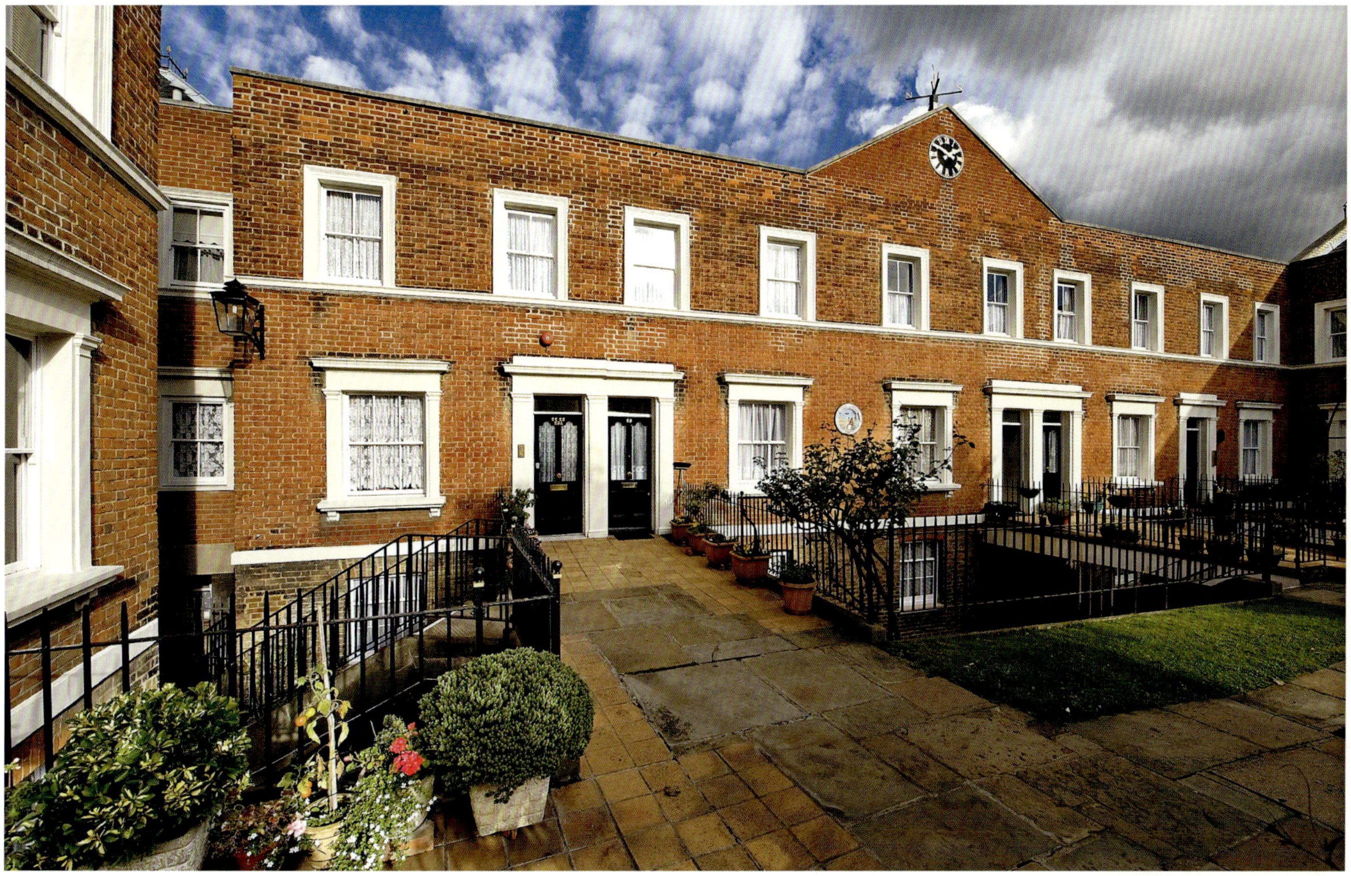

Fig. 90 (*above*) The French Hospital, La Providence, Rochester, main elevation. *Tim Rawle*

steady flow of applicants, some shared Huguenot ancestors with earlier inmates, others were closely related to recent inmates, yet others had recently researched their Huguenot ancestry inspired by the growing popular interest in family history.

In September 1959, the first nineteen flats were filled with new residents including, for the first time, some married couples.[4] The Minister of Housing, the Rt Hon. Henry Brooke, MP, inspected the flats in March 1960 when visiting Rochester, with the MP for Rochester and Chatham, Julian Critchley. In June 1960, the square was officially opened by the Lord Lieutenant, Lord Cornwallis,[5] and directors, residents and guests celebrated with the Bishop of Rochester, who entertained them to tea on the lawn at Bishopscourt.

Princess Marina, Duchess of Kent, Patron of the Friends of the Cathedral, visited La Providence in 1968. She was presented with a piece of lace made by a resident, Mrs Hoppe, a descendant of the Huguenot family of Mummery. The princess died unexpectedly a month later and her memorial service in the cathedral in November was attended by many directors and residents.

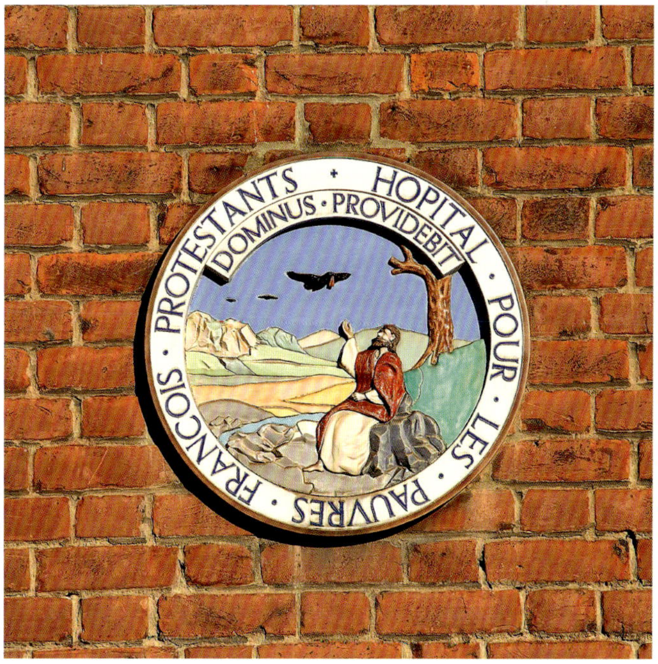

Fig. 91 The French Hospital, La Providence, Rochester, plaque on main elevation showing Elijah being fed by the ravens. *Tim Rawle*

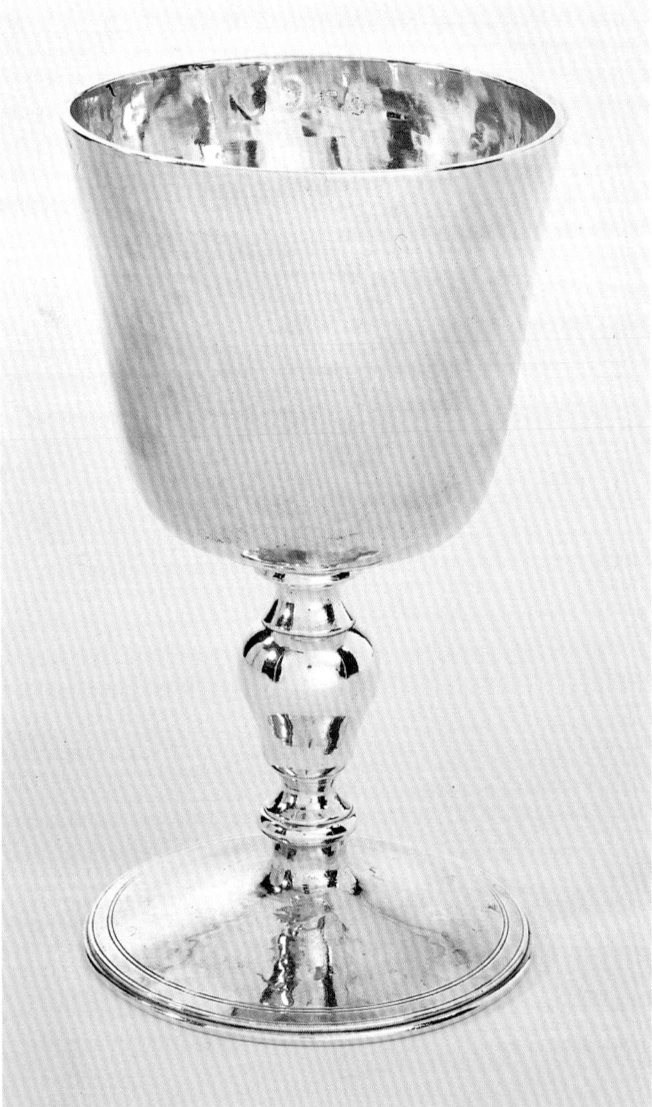

Fig. 92 Communion cup, sterling silver, maker's mark IT, London, 1631/2, inscribed 'I^{B}M A L'eglise vuallonne de Cantorbery 1632'

This is one of twelve similar cups given for the use of the Walloon congregation which met in the crypt of Canterbury Cathedral from the mid-16th century. The initials I^{B}M stand for Jean Bulteel, Pastor of the Walloon Church in Canterbury from 1617 to 1640 and his wife Mary. The commission marked their marriage in 1632. Another member of the congregation, Jaques Santhune, was paid a penny halfpenny each for engraving the twelve inscriptions 'pr marquer le coupes de la ste cene' (Deacon's accounts Cathedral Library, U.47/C.1).

Jean Bulteel, a graduate of Leiden University, opposed Archbishop Laud's attempts to force the Canterbury congregation to adopt the English liturgy and in 1645 he published *A Relation of the Troubles of the Three Foreign Churches in Kent caused by the injunction of William Laud, Archbishop of Canterbury Anno Domini 1634*. The other churches were in Sandwich and Maidstone.

John Duval, deputy-governor, H. E. Greenwood, treasurer and Norman Ouvry, secretary, with John Attlee as clerk, spanned the 1950s and 1960s. W. E. Towne was taken on to collect weekly charges in October 1959 and stayed on as steward until succeeded by Leslie Davies in 1968. Both helped establish La Providence as a community. Cecil Grellier, surveyor, responsible for the transformation of the dilapidated Theobald Square, was succeeded by his son Christopher, who served for twenty-five years before retiring and becoming a director in 1990. By 1988 there were 59 flats for residents.

The spiritual welfare of the residents was well cared for by successive chaplains. The Dean of Rochester, the Very Revd R. W. Stannard, served from 1959 to 1962 and became a director in 1960. Canons Maurice Sharp and Geoffrey Young, both served for ten years each. The present chaplain, the Revd Howard Daubeny, is now in his fifteenth year of ministering to the hospital. The chaplain conducts Divine Service (fig. 92), comforts the sick and reports to the Quarterly Committee. The chaplains' reports start in 1888,[6] when prayers were said daily in the chapel and sermons preached every Sunday. Each Court is opened with the prayer first used in September 1718 and still read in French: 'Since it is of thy favour, O Lord, that we are called to assist and comfort these our Brethren who are in want, grant that we may faithfully discharge our duty.' The records document the last years of three cousins: Caroline Potter, visited when aged 99 ('bedridden, blind, almost deaf ... in good spirits') shortly before her death in 1977; Eliza Jermy (who died in 1962, aged 94), and Mrs Sarah Alice Beazley (who died in 1966, aged 94), all descended from the silk-weaving Toye family of Spitalfields. Clarissa Emily Hoinville is also recorded. She died at 102 and like the others was buried at Roffey. Recipients of outgifts included Caroline Auvache, of Spitalfields silk-weaving stock ('a charming old lady', wrote the clerk), who was cared for in a St Leonard's nursing home when her small capital sum of £800 invalidated her claim for national assistance payments in the 1960s and 1970s.

Though outgifts for specific needs continued, such care was outside the ambit of the directors at La Providence in Rochester. There they provided and continue to provide flats for elderly people of Huguenot descent, or their spouses capable of looking after themselves in 'privacy, [with] their own furniture and belongings around them but with help in sickness and emergency always at hand'.[7]

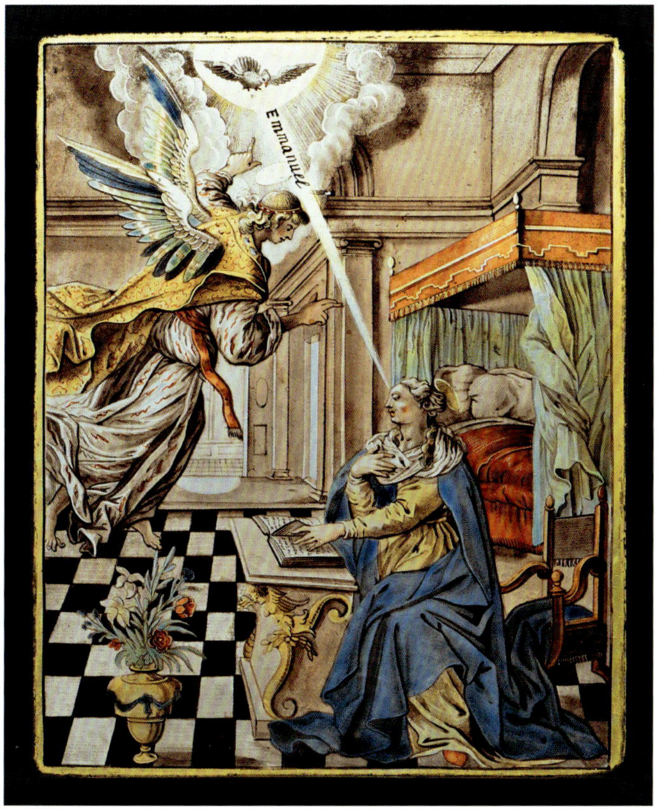

Fig. 93 Annunciation

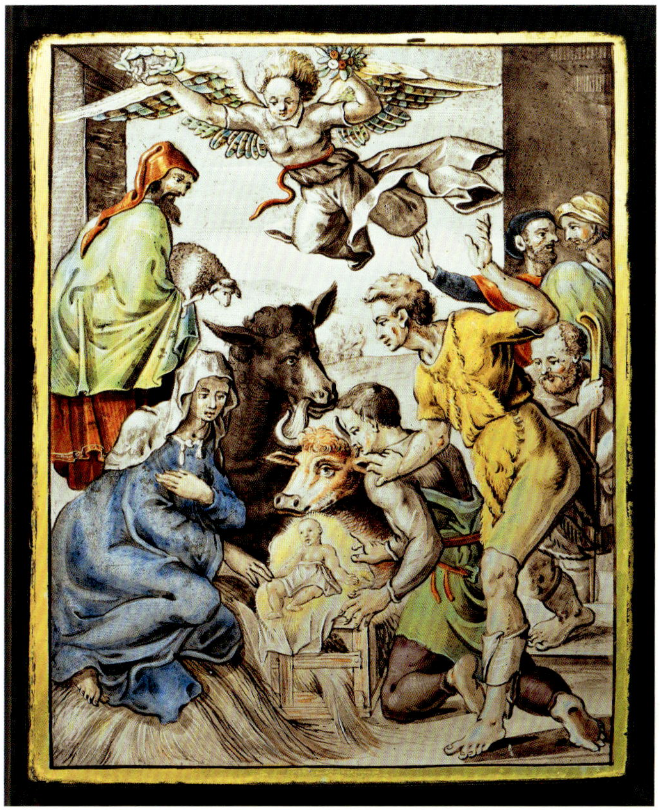

Fig. 94 Nativity

Figs. 93–100 (*this page and overleaf*) Stained-glass panels, Netherlandish, early 17th century, presented by Jacob, 8th Earl of Radnor

The expansion continued. In 1974, nine new flats were created in the former buildings of Rochester's Mathematical School (at which the young David Garrick, of Huguenot descent, attended for a year aged 19 in 1737 tutored by the headmaster) to the rear of 41 La Providence. Four years later, the land lying between the east side of the square and the medieval City Wall was transferred to the hospital for the sum of £10,000 and four new flats built at the High Street end of the site. A common room, with kitchen, and a passage used as the residents' library provide a communal space for Christian worship, where Holy Communion is celebrated weekly by the chaplain. The altar table is placed before a window containing eight seventeenth-century Netherlandish stained glass panels, representing scenes from the New Testament, donated by the late governor, Lord Radnor (figs. 93–100). The room was opened and blessed by the Bishop of Rochester, the Rt Revd Richard David Say, in 1984.

On one side of the common room, the Huguenots' Garden is planted with species associated with Huguenot

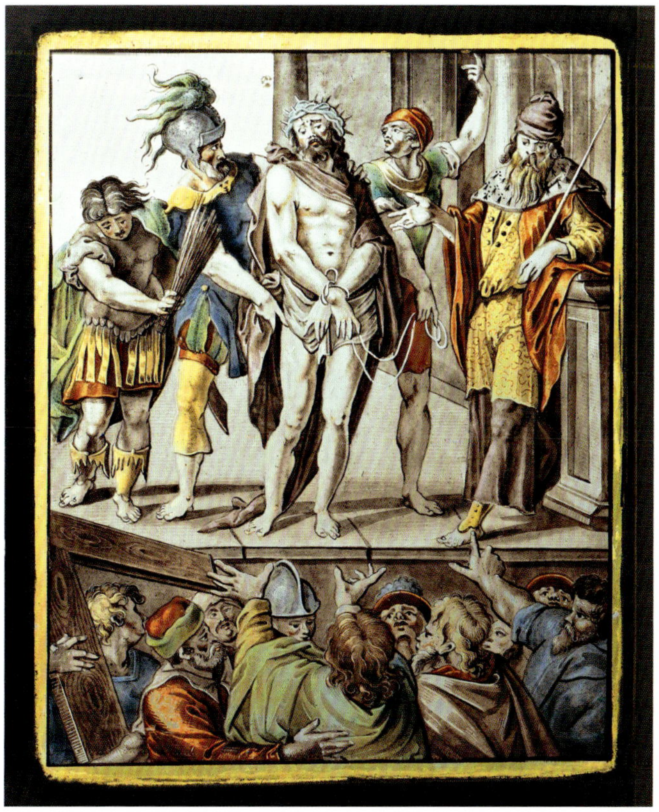

Fig. 95 Scourging of Christ

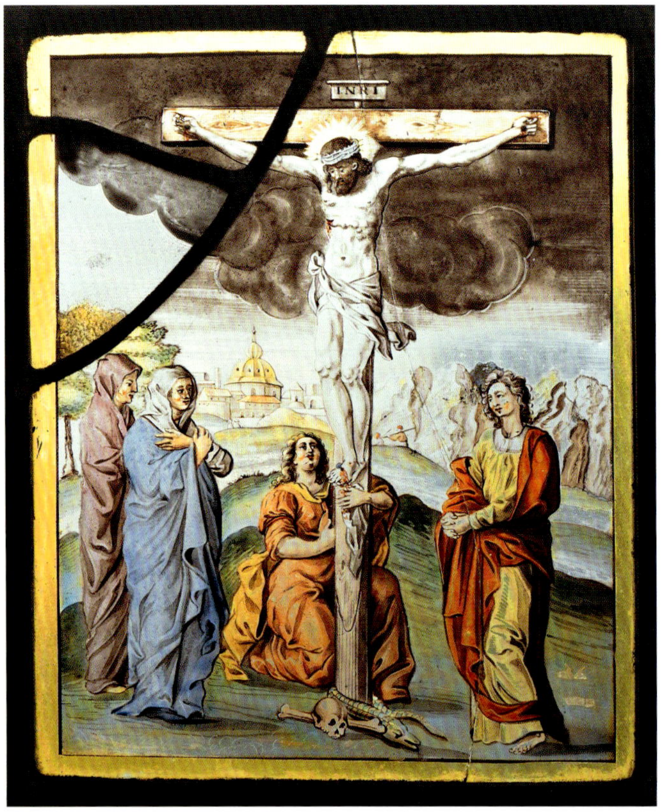

Fig. 96 Crucifixion

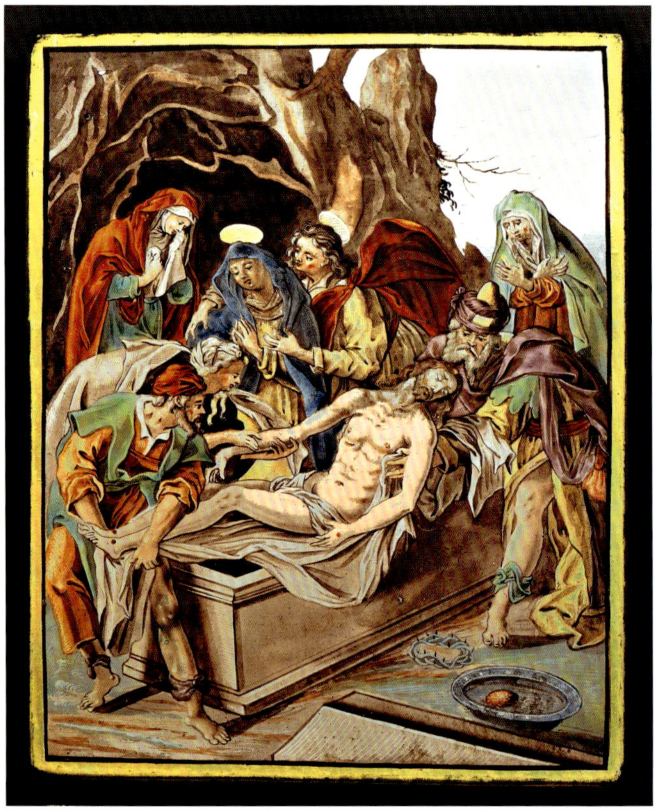

Fig. 97 Entombment

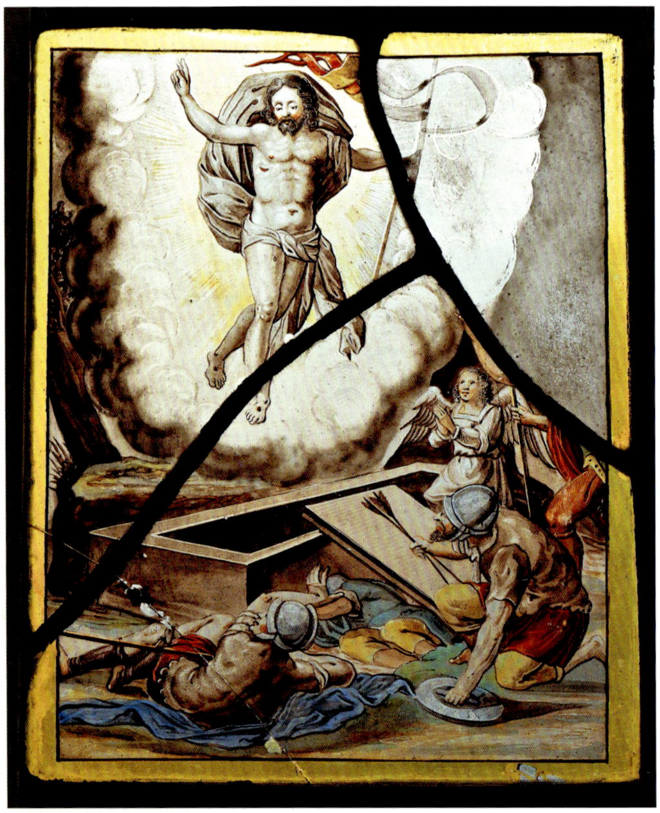

Fig. 98 Resurrection

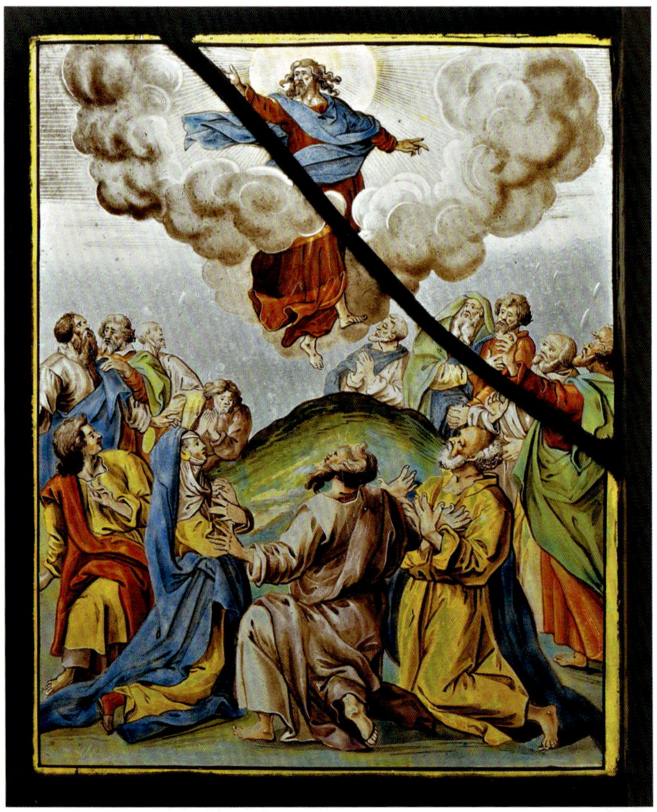

Fig. 99 Ascension

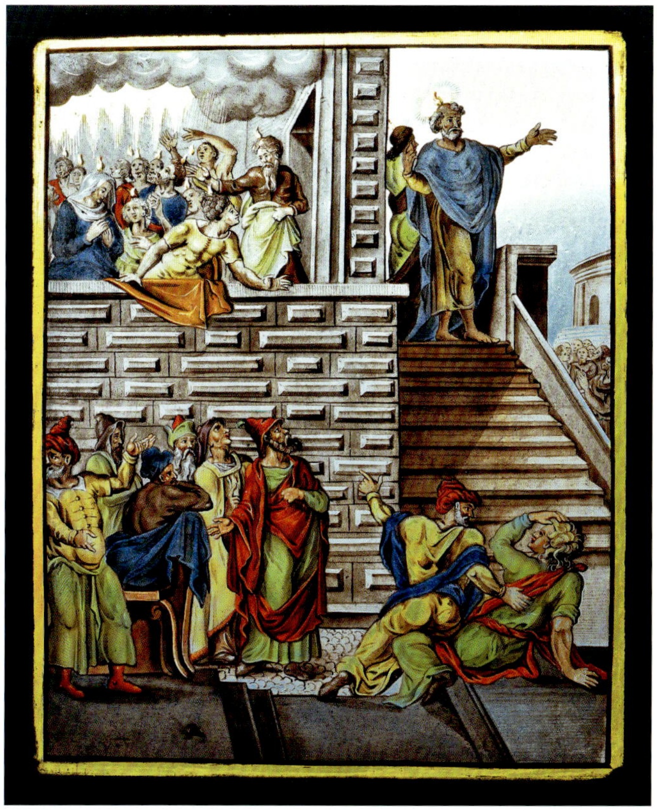

Fig. 100 Pentecost

history and features a bust of Admiral Gaspard de Coligny, the Huguenot leader assassinated in Paris on St Bartholomew's Eve, 1572. The northern side has seating, tables and a sundial supplied by Peter Dollond (fig. 101), optician to George III, and acquired in memory of Jill, Countess of Radnor, wife of the late governor. The hospital also owns a portrait engraving of John Dollond (1706–1761) (fig. 102), a former Spitalfields weaver turned optical instrument maker who set up in business with his son Peter (1731–1820); three later members of the family served as directors.

Fig. 101 (*left, below*) Sundial, brass, inscribed 'DOLLOND', c. 1760

This was probably supplied by Peter Dollond, who was set up in business by his father in Vine Street, Spitalfields, and latterly worked at the sign of the Golden Spectacles and Sea Quadrant near Exeter Exchange in the Strand.

Fig. 102 (*below*) John Dollond, FRS (1706–1761), mezzotint, J. R. Smith after B. Watson

The forbears of John Dollond, the optical instrument maker and inventor of the achromatic telescope, came from Normandy. He worked originally as a weaver, and studied mathematics and astronomy in his spare time. He financed a small optical workshop for his son Peter in Vine Street, Spitalfields in 1750.

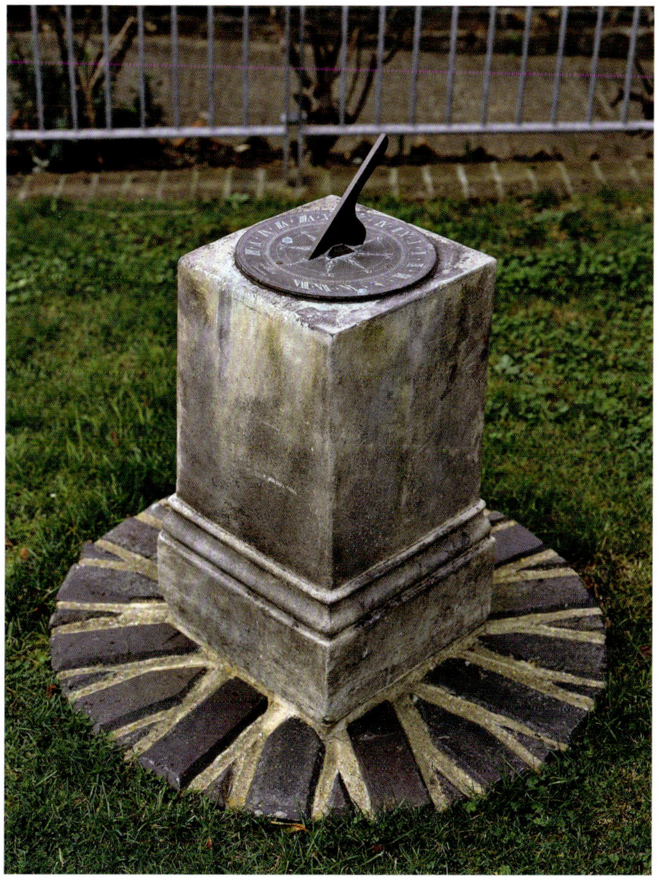

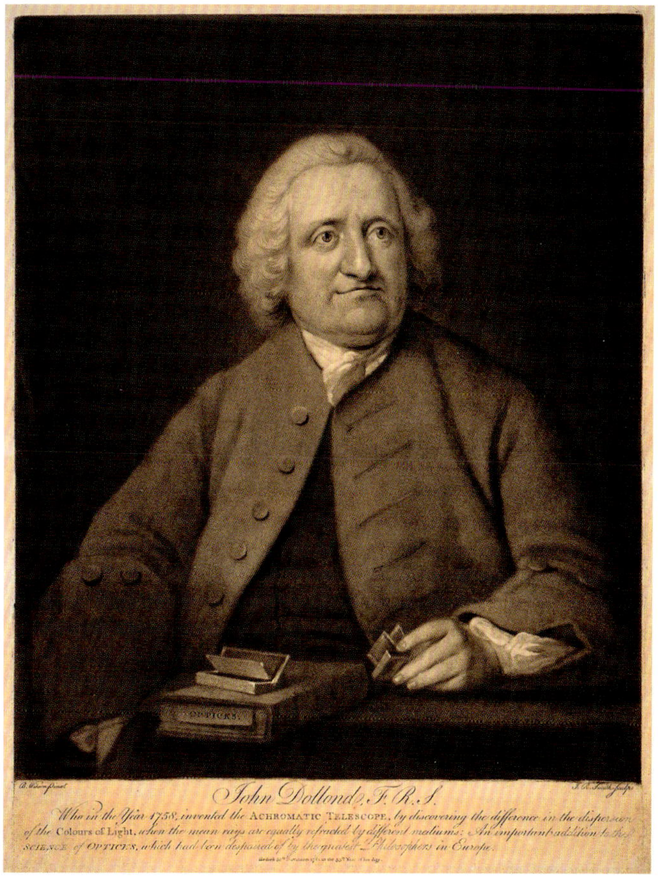
OPTICKS
John Dollond, F.R.S.
Who in the Year 1758, invented the ACHROMATIC TELESCOPE, by discovering the difference in the dispersion of the Colours of Light, when the mean rays are equally refracted by different mediums: An important addition to the SCIENCE of OPTICKS, which had been despaired of by the greatest Philosophers in Europe.

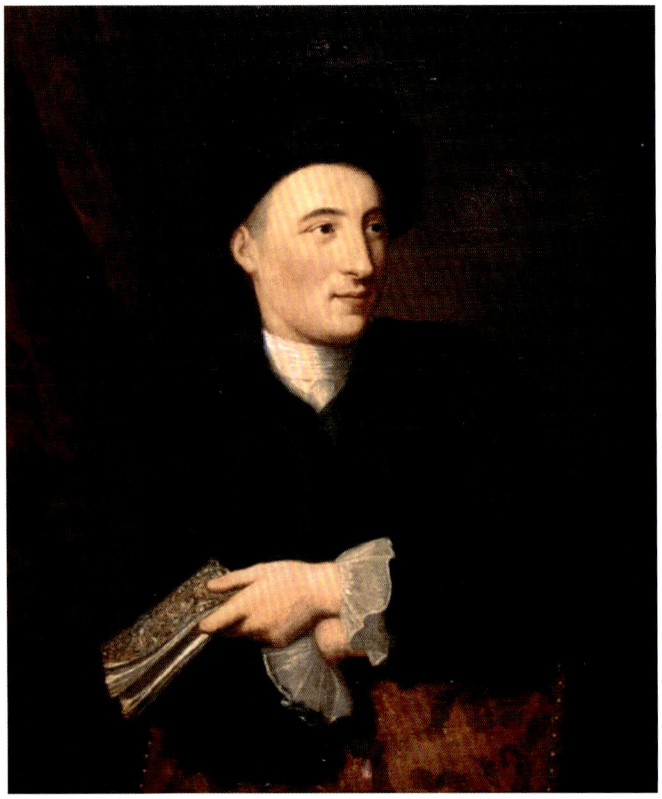

Fig. 103 Dr Matthew Maty (1718–1776), oil on canvas, Bartholomew Dupan, c. 1750. *British Museum*

Matthew Maty was descended from a family of ministers who fled from Dauphiné to Utrecht, Holland. In 1740 Maty moved to England after completing a degree in philosophy and medicine at Leiden. He served as physician to the French Hospital from 1774 to 1776. From 1750 he edited a monthly periodical in French, the *Journal Britannique*. He was elected a Fellow of the Royal Society and appointed principal librarian at the British Museum.

The City Wall site was completed by the building of two more flats, and four flats in the main square were equipped for disabled residents (funded from the sale in 1985 of the remaining property in Hackney – 16 freehold terraced houses in Penshurst Road) and lifts installed adjacent to three main staircases.

The emphasis on expanding and consolidating La Providence as a residence did not encompass the earlier vision of the hospital as the home of Huguenot historic treasures. In the 1970s William Le Fanu and Charles Marmoy revived this once passionately espoused interest. Talk of selling portraits and of sending heraldic shields of armigerous directors (figs. 128–43), originally displayed at dado level around the Directors' Room in Hackney, to the Huguenot Library in London came to nothing. Although the Huguenot Library became the repository for Huguenot records, the valued but limited space in its present home at University College, London, does not offer scope for a museum of Huguenot memorabilia.

The administrative load was lighter. Directors were free of the responsibility for the corporation's properties. The charitable funds benefiting the residents and recipients of outgifts were amalgamated into a single Huguenot General Fund. The Stephen Mounier Apprenticeship Fund, founded in 1777, continues as a separate charity, and directors in turn select young people whose training costs are assisted. The Boislin Trust was created forty-four years after Isaac Bérenger, sieur de Boislin's death in 1709 by the executors of the estate of his sister. Most executors were directors or associated with the French Hospital; one Matthew Maty, 'doctor in physic' to the hospital in 1774, was one of the founding keepers of the new British Museum in 1753 and later its librarian (fig. 103).[8] The Esther Coqueau Charity (known to many poor recipients as producing the 'Cocoa money') had helped 'ten poor maids or widows aged upwards of fifty years' under Esther Coqueau's will, since 1745.[9]

In 1974 Charles Marmoy, the Huguenot Society librarian, asked the directors to transfer to Rochester a large collection of engravings and other unframed pictures. These included photographs of nineteenth-century officers and directors of La Providence and a mezzotint portrait of the first governor, the Earl of Galway (fig. 7). In the process, Paul Minet found 17 portfolios of small water-colours and pen-and-ink drawings by John Colley Nixon (c. 1759–c. 1818), a contemporary and friend of the artist Thomas Rowlandson.[10] Apart from a sketch of a pastor at the Threadneedle Street church (fig. 104), and a water-colour of Dieppe, they were of no Huguenot significance and were sold in a long series of auctions at Christie's, from 1973 to 1986, realizing a total of £150,000,[11] which was of great assistance in funding building costs, especially of the common room.

The directors' belief that the faith of former benefactors should be respected settled a serious debate after an applicant, in 1967, was refused accommodation on the grounds that he was a Roman Catholic. His need was immediate but as there was no flat available the dispute arose over his being placed on the waiting list.[12]

Sir Anthony Wagner, KCVO, Garter King at Arms, was sufficiently persuasive that the restriction of applicants to Protestants 'did not involve the "intolerance"' referred to in the Court minutes. A motion confirming By-law 36 was carried by fourteen votes to seven.

In the early 1980s new directors and officers promoted awareness of the hospital's history and treasures. The tercentenary commemoration of the Revocation of the Edict of Nantes in 1985 promoted this revival. Portraits and artefacts were lent to *The Quiet Conquest* exhibition at the Museum of London, as part of the 'Huguenot Heritage' programme chaired by Lady Monson. Carried out by the Huguenot Society, with Randolph Vigne as its president and the French Hospital's treasurer, the exhibition catalogue compiled by Tessa Murdoch has become a classic of Huguenot scholarship.

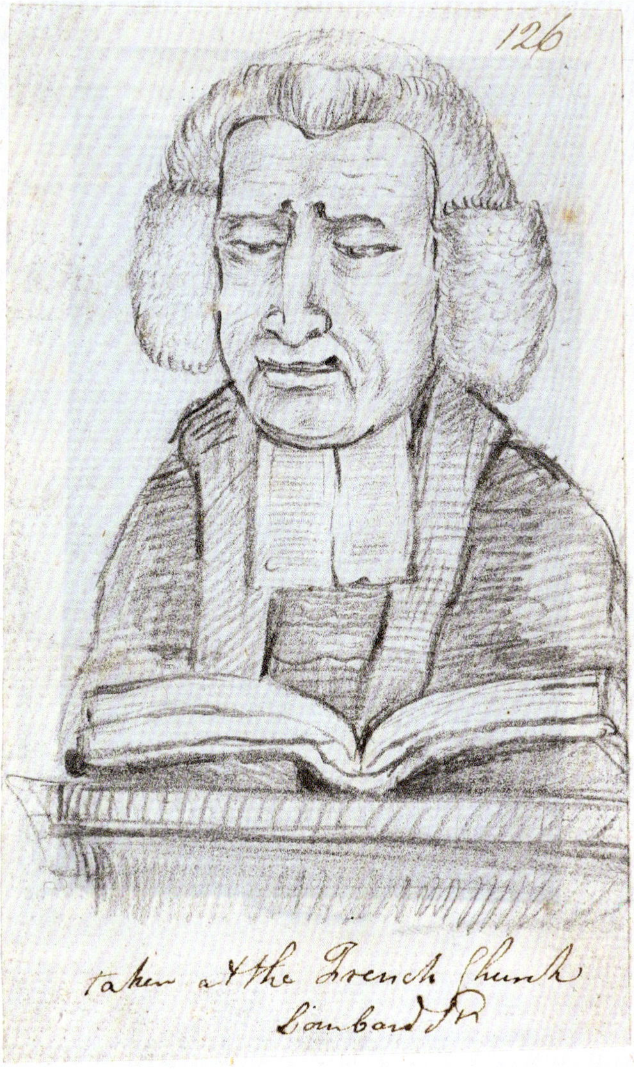

Fig. 104 A pastor of the French Church, Threadneedle Street, pencil drawing, John C. Nixon (c. 1759–c. 1818)

The pastor is reading from the Bible which is open before him on the ledge of the pulpit. The drawing is from a group of water-colours and drawings by John Nixon without Huguenot relevance but for this one which, by the approximate date and the age of the subject, might portray the Revd Louis de La Chaumette, father of three directors of the French Hospital. The rest of the collection was sold.

The governor, Lord Radnor, was, with the Rt Revd Robert Runcie, Archbishop of Canterbury, and the late 9th Duke of Buccleuch and Queensberry, a sponsor of Huguenot Heritage, under the Royal patronage of HM The Queen, who with HRH The Duke of Edinburgh, visited the exhibition in May 1985. On Sunday 29 September of that year, large numbers visited the hospital, after luncheon in the Corn Exchange at which the governor, having toasted 'La Reine' proposed the health of the guests and finally 'The safety and prosperity of Old England'. The day ended with evensong in the cathedral.

At the Museum of London a finely calligraphed genealogy of the Huguenot ancestry of TRH Princes William and Henry was much admired by Her Majesty and the Duke of Edinburgh on their visit to *The Quiet Conquest* (fig. 105). Commissioned by the directors of the French Hospital to mark the tercentenary of the Revocation of the Edict of Nantes, the French Hospital is represented in the pedigree by its first governor, Henri de Massue de Ruvigny, Earl of Galway, from whose cousin Lady Rachel Russell the present Queen is descended through the late Queen Mother, and by Henri Guinand, third deputy-governor, ancestor of the late Diana, Princess of Wales, through her grandfather the 4th Baron Fermoy. It hangs in the reception room at 41 La Providence, where cabinets display historic Huguenot artefacts and documents. These include gifts made following the tercentenary celebrations, which aroused international interest in Britain's Huguenot heritage. Perhaps the most moving is the copy of the Geneva Bible, 1588–90, presented by Madame Jaulmes, which belonged to her ancestors the Fasquest family. During persecution, the Bible was concealed by being baked in a loaf of bread.[13]

The directors' continuing concern for the Huguenot Library was made manifest by the setting up in 1983 of the Huguenot Library Maintenance Fund, with £30,000 available from the sale of the Nixon pictures. Two trustees were appointed by the hospital and two by the Huguenot Society. This unusually large deployment of the hospital's funds was more than justified by the vital importance of the library for research into Huguenot ancestry needed to qualify applicants for residence in La Providence. More recently, in 2005, the hospital agreed to contribute twenty-five per cent of the salary of the project librarian appointed to re-organize and modernize the library and its systems. The contribution continues.

Housed at Hackney and Compton's Lea for nearly a hundred years from its foundation in the 1860s, the nucleus was 'a few books, certainly not more than a dozen, bearing upon Huguenot and Vaudois history' brought from the old hospital in Finsbury.[14] It had grown wonderfully by 1900, when it was amalgamated with the Huguenot Society's own library.

In Hackney it benefited greatly from the expert care of Miss Winifred Turner, Officier de l'Académie. She had begun work in 1926, joined the Huguenot Society in 1931 and the following year was given the additional task of identifying and listing the contents of 'certain large chests of papers' that had lain there 'unrecorded and almost forgotten' since the move from Bath Street in 1866. Judge Dumas and other directors found a mass of documents to do with the French Committee's distribution of the Royal Bounty, from James II's first Brief of 1688 to the Parliamentary grants, up to the death of the last pensioner in 1876.

With the 'letters, receipt forms, loose bills and accounts, with a quantity of account books and records' were several vellum-bound minute books in which 'the eye was at once caught by the honoured names of Philip Ménard and M. de Gastigny ... and many others entirely familiar to all students of our Huguenot church registers and of the history of the French Hospital'. On 10 February 1709, the minutes read: 'Monsieur Philippe Mesnard a remis à la Compagnie la copie d'un article du Testament de feu Mons. Jaques de Gastigny ... Je donne cinq cent livres sterling à la Peste House ...' along with the familiar words that led to the foundation of the hospital ten years later.[15] These Bounty Papers have been much studied, reproduced and computerized, as have their counterpart volumes and documents in the Guildhall archives.

A collection of some thirty consistory minute books (known as *actes*), and other records of Huguenot churches in England were donated by Dr Stacey S. Burn in 1887. His father, John Southerden Burn, had collected, from 1836, non-conformist church registers, for a royal commission, and deposited them in what is now the National Archives. Dr Burn's donation consisted of material J.S. Burn is thought to have acquired from the Revd J.H. Chirol, the last incumbent of the Huguenot church of Le Carré (fig. 38) in its last home in Little Dean Street, Soho. They remained in the Burns' possession as being outside the terms of reference of J.S. Burn's mandate. A priceless item in the 'Burn Donation' is the poor fund account book of 'l'église de la langue francaise en Sanduwits', 1568–72.[16]

The Huguenot pedigrees, almost a thousand of them, many thousands of will extracts and much other research material assembled during his long life by Henry Wagner, a director from 1865, were bequeathed to the hospital in 1924.[17] His correspondence with the father figures of English Huguenot historical studies, the Revd D.C.A. Agnew and R. Lane Poole, members of the Layard family, T.P. Le Fanu and many others, is of great interest.

Other than the Bounty Papers and Burn Donation,[18] the largest of the manuscript collections in the library is that of the French Hospital records.[19] The library's printed books form the most extensive and comprehensive collection in Britain on the Huguenots and their history.

The evacuated parts of the library had been brought back to Hackney only at the end of 1946. The library itself was not transferred immediately to Compton's Lea, when the inmates took up residence there in mid-August 1947, but had remained in the Hackney building until March 1948.

Randolph Vigne, after a long underground and bus journey, the last part through the bombed ruins of the East End of London, found his way through Hackney to the French Hospital in late 1947 and was shown the library in its glass-fronted cases by an elderly, uncomprehending woman attendant. Left free to browse, the Wagner pedigree files opened for him a door to a vast area of research into family history.

It was largely through the efforts of W.R. Le Fanu, a senior and admired figure among librarians and bibliophiles, and later Joseph Scott of University College, London, that the Huguenot Library found its present home. It was providential that the medical librarian at University College was Charles Marmoy, a fellow of the Huguenot Society.

The present directors have taken up the challenge presented by the collections, by commissioning this celebration of La Providence. In recent years, directors have been moved to give or lend family heirlooms which greatly enhance the hospital's additional role as a centre for Huguenot history in England. Gifts include a gold-mounted enamel snuff-box (fig. 106) presented by Frederick the Great of Prussia to a Minet ancestor of the present director, Paul Minet, whose father Peter Minet (fig. 108) was deputy-

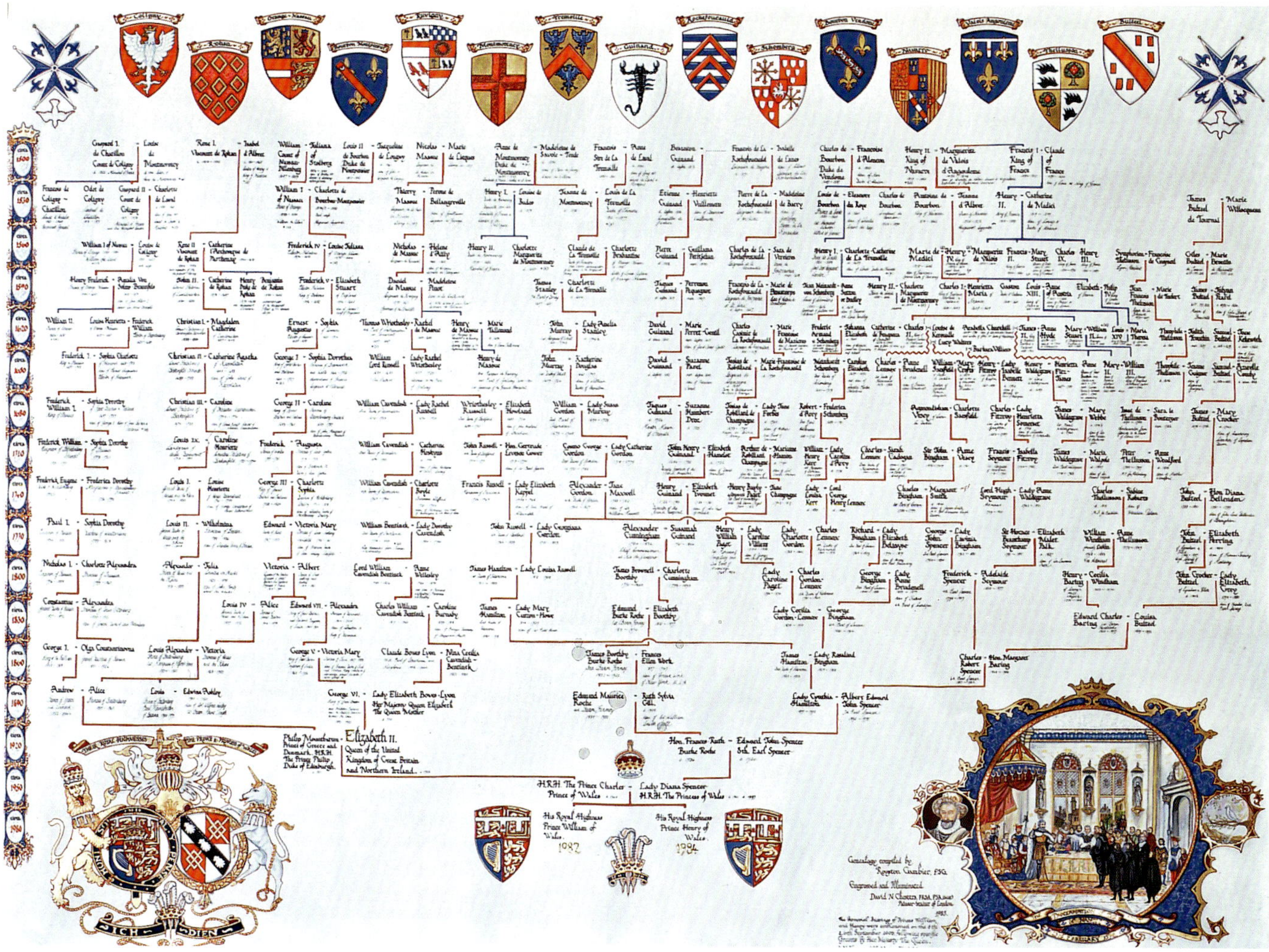

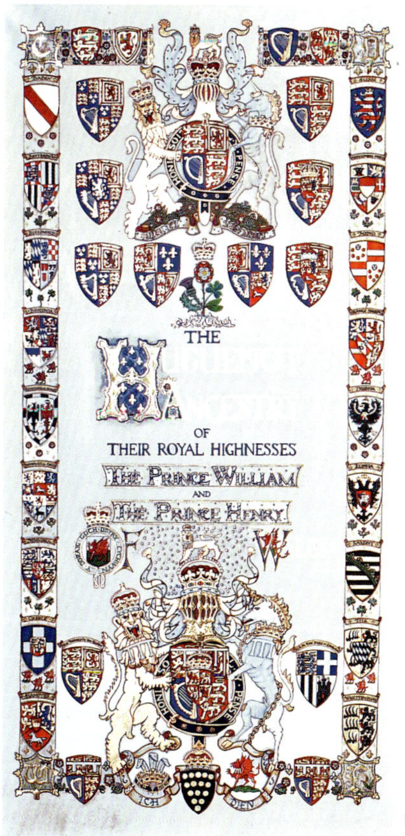

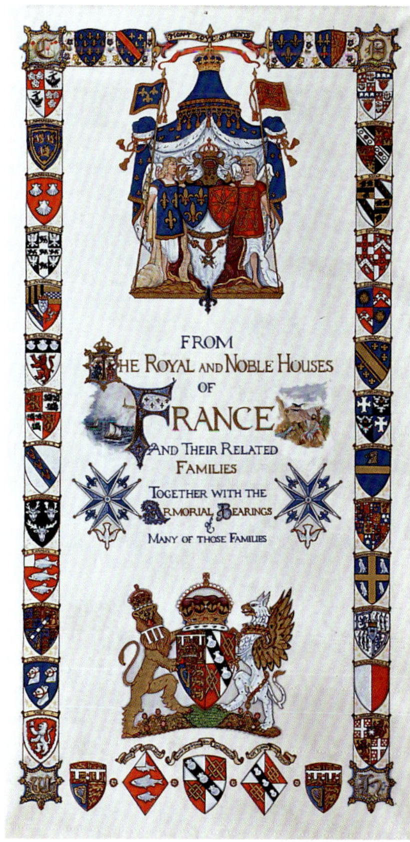

Fig. 105 *The Huguenot Ancestry of Their Royal Highnesses The Prince William and The Prince Henry*, 1985

Compiled by the genealogist Royston Gambier and illustrated by David Chester, painter-stainer, the pedigree was commissioned by the directors in 1985 to mark the tercentenary of the Revocation of the Edict of Nantes. It demonstrates the Huguenot ancestors of the English Royal Family and includes the Guinands (fig. 16), forbears of Their Royal Highnesses William and Harry, through their mother Diana, Princess of Wales.

governor from 1975 to 1978 and the gold watch belonging to Aymé Garnault (fig. 109) donated by the Ouvry family in 2007; the usual numerals on the enamel dial have been replaced with letters spelling the name of the first owner 'AIME GARNAULT'. Garnault (fig. 110) was elected a director in 1762 and was the second of seventeen members of the Garnault/Ouvry/Romilly families to serve in this way. To mark the tercentenary of the founding bequest of La Providence in 2008, the directors acquired a wax medallion portrait of George II by a former director Isaac Gosset (fig. 111).

'Care for those among us who are in distress', as the Court prayer enjoins at each meeting, remains overwhelmingly the prime duty of the directors in the Britain of today, changed for the better from a time when 'distress' could mean the depths of poverty or sickness without treatment. Problems remain and new ones appear. Residents needing constant medical care have to be taken to hospitals or nursing homes. The new requirement of 'care in the community' is presenting challenges to the hospital for those residents who need such care but have no 'community' outside the hospital.

'May they here find that help and comfort of which they stand in need', the Court prayer continues, and 'need' today is interpreted in many different ways. The community provides companionship to ease loneliness. Help is at hand for those who find difficulty in obtaining what the Welfare State provides, financial advantages for those on minimum state benefits, regular visits from a sympathetic steward and deputy-stewards, and from a director during the monthly 'visites de la maison', down to immediate attention in an emergency by means of the 'panic button' with which each flat is provided.

La Providence would give much satisfaction to Jacques de Gastigny and the French Committee of the early eighteenth century in the care it now provides. That proud old Huguenot tradition as exemplified by the thirty-seven refugees who created the French Hospital for those, their brethren, who stood in need, lives on. It is more than a shelter for Huguenot descendants; it is a home for some fascinating treasures from Britain's Huguenot history.

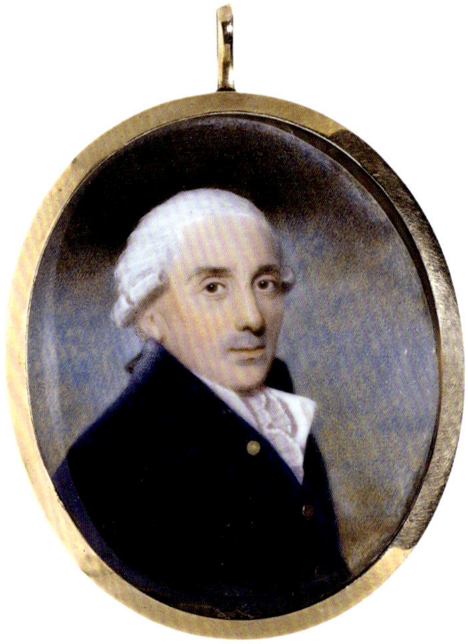

Fig. 107 Hughes Minet (1731–1813), miniature attributed to Samuel Shelley (1750–1808), with hair plaited round the frame and the cipher HM on the reverse, c. 1775

Hughes Minet was the son of the Revd John Minet (1695–1771). His grandfather, Isaac Minet (1660–1745) escaped from Calais to Dover in 1686, where his brother Stephen had already settled. He helped to establish the family's banking business in Dover in 1690. Hughes Minet was brought up in Kent, where his father was vicar of Eythorne and chaplain of Dover Castle and the Cinque Ports. Hughes joined his uncle William Minet (1703–1767) in the family business which had by then a London branch at Austin Friars. Hughes Minet was elected a director of the French Hospital in 1769.

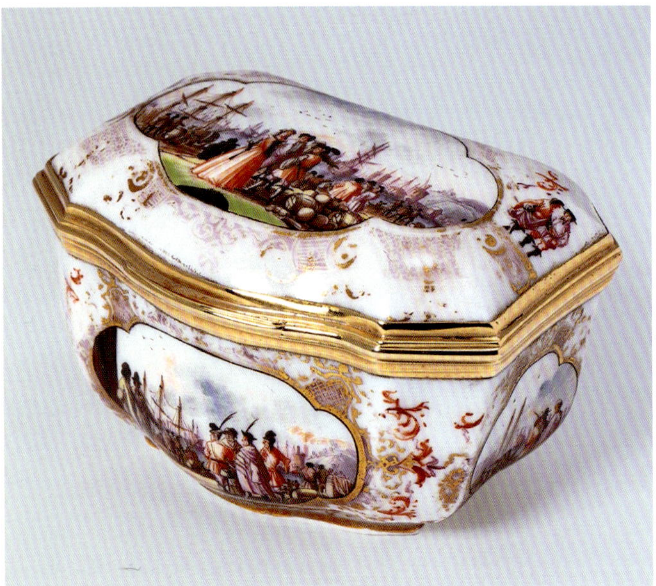

Fig. 106 Snuff-box, gold and enamel, maker unknown, Berlin, c. 1750

Inscribed (on 19th-century parchment label inside the box): 'Snuff box belonging to James Minet, born in Dover in 1698. Died in Berlin in 1774. Said to have been given to J.M by Frederick the Great'.

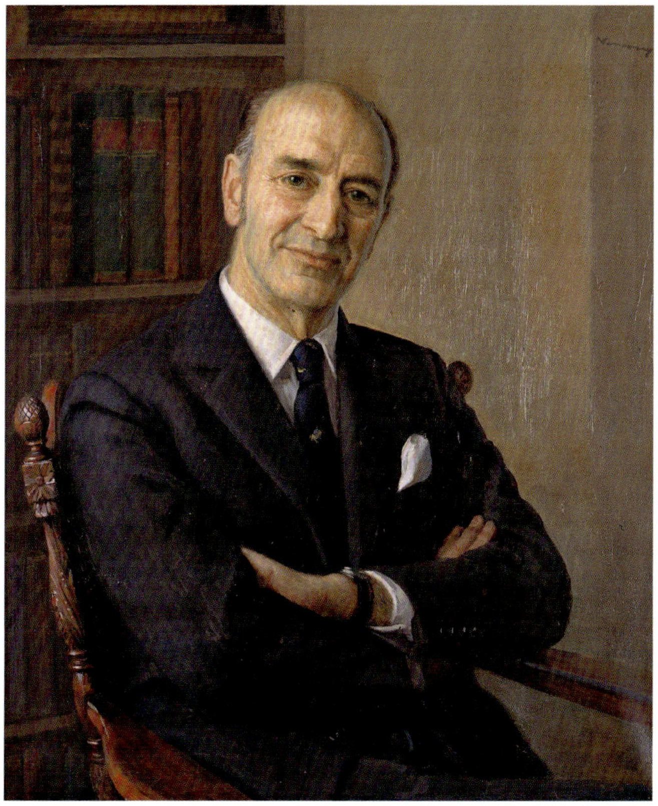

Fig. 108 Peter Brissault Minet (1908–1988), oil on canvas, William E. Narraway, 1977

Descended from Isaac Minet, who fled France for Dover in 1685, Peter Minet was brought up in modest circumstances, the youngest of eight children. In the 1940s Peter Minet became friendly with his cousin Susan Minet of Much Hadham, Hertfordshire, who was descended from Isaac Minet's brother Thomas. Peter became Susan Minet's sole heir. On her death in 1976, Peter Minet inherited a considerable fortune with which he founded the Peter Minet and Idlewild Trusts in 1969 and 1974 respectively. Elected a director of the French Hospital in 1948, he was responsible for building up the membership of the Huguenot Society from 200 in the early 1950s. He strongly supported the society's serious scholarly activities. He served as the hospital's deputy-governor from 1975 to 1978. His obituary (*PHS*, XV, 1989, pp. 97–100) noted that 'Peter Minet's life of early, impecunious toil, leading to affluence, and the respect and influence due to his absolute integrity, was almost a throwback to that of some of his Huguenot forebears.'

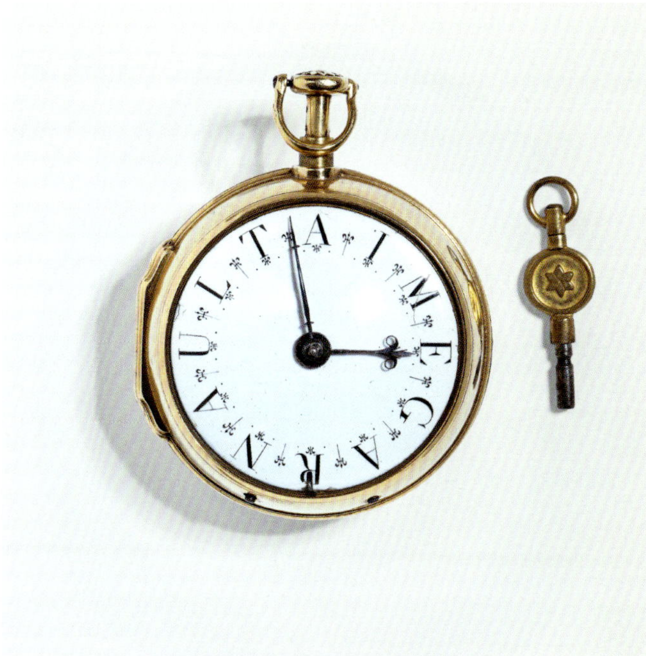

Fig. 109 (*right, top*) Pocket watch, gold case, maker's mark SG inside the outer case (possibly for Samuel Godbehere, London); verge escapement fuse quarter-repeating, striking on a single bell, by Robert Street, c. 1765, with 'AIME GARNAULT' replacing the numbers on the enamel dial

Aymé Garnault (1717–1782), director from 1762, was the son of Pierre, a goldsmith refugee from Chatellerault and the second member of the Garnault/Ouvry/Romilly family to be elected a director of the French Hospital in 1752. Seventeen other members of the family have been or are directors. Aymé Garnault became treasurer of the New River Company which was originally founded by James I to pipe water from Islington to feed the City of London.

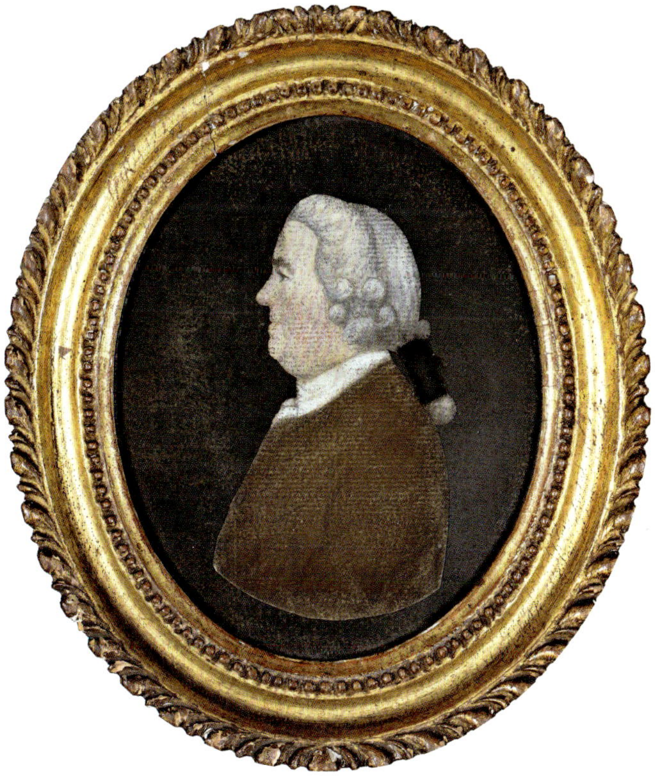

Fig. 110 Aymé Garnault (1704–1782), cut-out miniature in water-colour

Aymé Garnault's family came originally from Chatellerault. His brother Michael was a jeweller of St Peter Le Poor in the City of London and was closely associated with the Berchère and Baril families, who also worked in the jewellery trade. Aymé became treasurer of the New River Company, which supplied the French Hospital with water from 1737/8. He lived in Lincoln's Inn Fields at the time of his death, and still had shares in the New River Company.

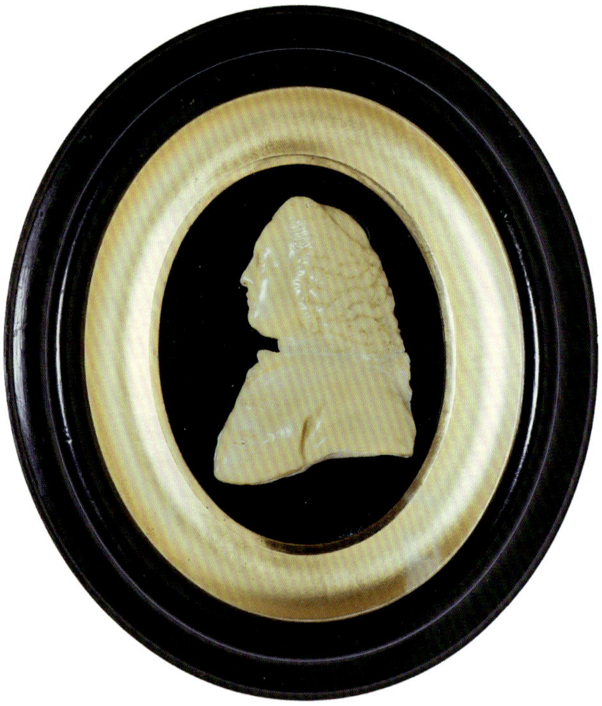

Fig. 111 George II, wax medallion portrait, Isaac Gosset

Isaac Gosset (1713–1799) was elected a director in 1764. The sixth son of Jean Gosset, a Huguenot who settled in St Helier, Jersey, Isaac came to London and was brought up by his uncle Matthew Gosset (1683–1744), a wax-modeller and frame-maker. Isaac became one of the best-known wax-modellers and his likenesses of members of the royal family helped to establish his reputation. His wax portraits were sold as sets for gentlemen's cabinets. The hospital also owns a print after Gosset's medallion portrait of François Duroure, a fellow director (fig. 123).

Isaac Gosset used a special composition of wax in a tint of old ivory, the secret recipe apparently perished with his only son, the Revd Isaac Gosset (1745–1812). Gosset's brother Gedeon (1706–1785) became a director of the French Hospital in 1760. A third brother Jacob (1703–1788) became a director in 1778. In 1773, Isaac became a director of the Society of Artists, and exhibited there regularly from 1760 to 1778. He died in Kensington and was buried in the family vault in Old Marylebone Burial Ground. His portrait by the Genevan artist Liotard is shown in fig. 114.

1 Charles Dickens, *Great Expectations* (1861), chapter 8.

2 Minute Books, 1954–6, 7.4.1956.

3 R. Gwynn, *Huguenot Heritage* (2001), p. 83.

4 *Charter and By-Laws* (1892), By-law 24, p. 31. Times had changed since the framers of the old by-laws had written, with an odd juxtaposition: 'No married persons or such as are afflicted with contagious distempers shall be eligible as inmates'.

5 Lord Cornwallis was a great man of Kent, chairman of innumerable Kent bodies, Colonel of the Buffs and even, in the 1920s, captain of the Kent cricket XI.

6 HL H.C5.1-5, 8.

7 The French Hospital information and application form, 2007 ed., p. 4.

8 Henry Wagner, 'The Trustees of the Original Administration of the Boislin Trust', *PHS*, VIII, 4 (1908), p. 385.

9 *Charter and By-Laws*, (1892), p. 10.

10 Minute Books 1971-8, 3.3.1973; *PHS*, XXI, 3 (1967), p. 168. They had been donated to the hospital in 1890 by Emma Haines, widow of Henry Joseph Rosselloty Haines, elected a director in 1860.

11 The Haines bequest was one of the most munificent in the history of La Providence.

12 It transpired that he did not require this as he had found suitable long-term accommodation.

13 Murdoch, cat. no. 32. The record of births, marriages and deaths in the Fasquest family in the Bible dates back to 1625.

14 Faber, p. vii.

15 Winifred Turner, 'Recent Additions to the Library of the French Hospital', *PHS*, XIV, 4 (1993), pp. 568–9.

16 Being prepared for publication by the Huguenot Society as *HSQS*, LXII.

17 Wagner, *Wills*.

18 *HSQS*, LI.

19 Their listing takes up over half of the 200 pages of the library's manuscript catalogue (*HSQS*, LVI), and 16 of the 64 of its supplement (*HSQS*, LXI).

Directors of the French Hospital
A survey

The inmates or residents of the French Hospital during the first 260 years of its existence in Finsbury and Hackney are well documented, but scant attention has been given to the study of those elected to serve as directors of the corporation.[1] The founding directors were noblemen, merchants and craftsmen, and many of them were subscribers to the foundation fund. They included Pierre Champion de Crespigny, whose direct descendant, Stephen Champion de Crespigny, has served as secretary for over thirty years.

In the first ten years after the granting of the royal charter, a fascinating assortment of professionals, artists and craftsmen from the Huguenot community were elected directors. Among them were: the surgeon Paul Buissiere; the blacksmith and former associate of Jean Tijou, Jean Remy de Montigny; the Paris jewellers Jacques-Louis Berchère and Pierre Marchant, and the minister of the Huguenot Savoy Church, the Revd Israel-Antoine Aufrère (fig. 112). Jean Perigal, the ivory carver from Dieppe, whose vivid account of his escape from France survives and the merchant Charles Lebas were also made directors in that period. Another director elected was Jacques Tabart. Almost certainly the wood carver who had settled first in Dublin where as Jacques Tabary he had worked with his brother Louis on the altar setting for the chapel at the Royal Hospital, Kilmainham, in the 1680s, Tabart may well have been recommended as a director by Ruvigny, the first governor of the French Hospital. There is every likelihood that Ruvigny knew Tabart in Dublin, as Ruvigny's portrait was then and still is in the Hall at Kilmainham. Jacques Tabart's brother Pierre was admitted as an inmate to the French Hospital in 1743 where he died. Lebas, the son of a Huguenot refugee from Caen, Normandy, was a prosperous merchant of Cecil Court, The Strand, with a country residence, Pipewell Abbey, Northamptonshire. He died in 1724, only three years after his election as director. His only daughter and heiress was to marry Viscount Harcourt in 1735.[2] Jaques Gaultier was a major financier, who became a director of the Bank of England in 1728 and Peter Anthony Motteux (fig. 113) traded through the East India Company in porcelain and other exotic goods.

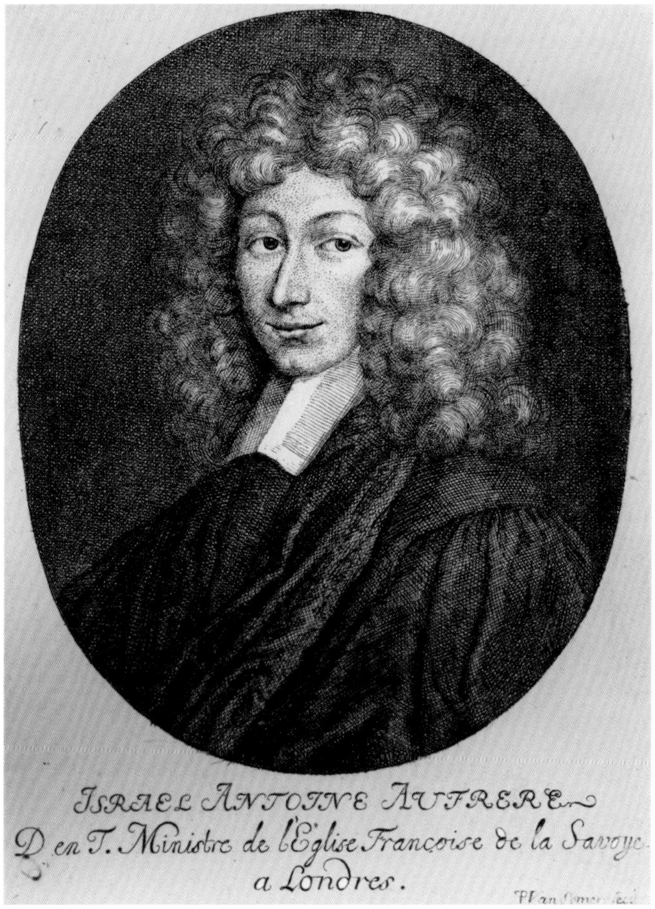
ISRAEL ANTOINE AUFRERE
D en T. Ministre de l'Eglise Françoise de la Savoye
a Londres.

Fig. 112 Israel-Antoine Aufrère (1677–1758), engraving, Paul van Somer, c. 1700. *National Portrait Gallery*

Born in Paris, the son of Antoine Aufrère, marquis de Corville, Israel became a doctor of theology and came to London where he served as chaplain to William III at the Chapel Royal, St James's Palace. He was appointed minister to the French congregation at the Savoy chapel. The silver communion cups and patens, made for the use of his congregation in 1717/18 by the Huguenot goldsmith Louis Cuny are now in the French Hospital collection (fig. 37). Israel built a house in Charles Street, St James's Square, which was inherited by his elder son Anthony. Israel Antoine became a director of the French Hospital in 1725. His correspondence was acquired at Sotheby's in 1908 from the collection of Sir Thomas Phillips under the Browning Trust for the French Hospital Library. His grand-daughter by his younger son George, Sophia, married in 1770 Charles Anderson Pelham, later 1st Earl of Yarborough.

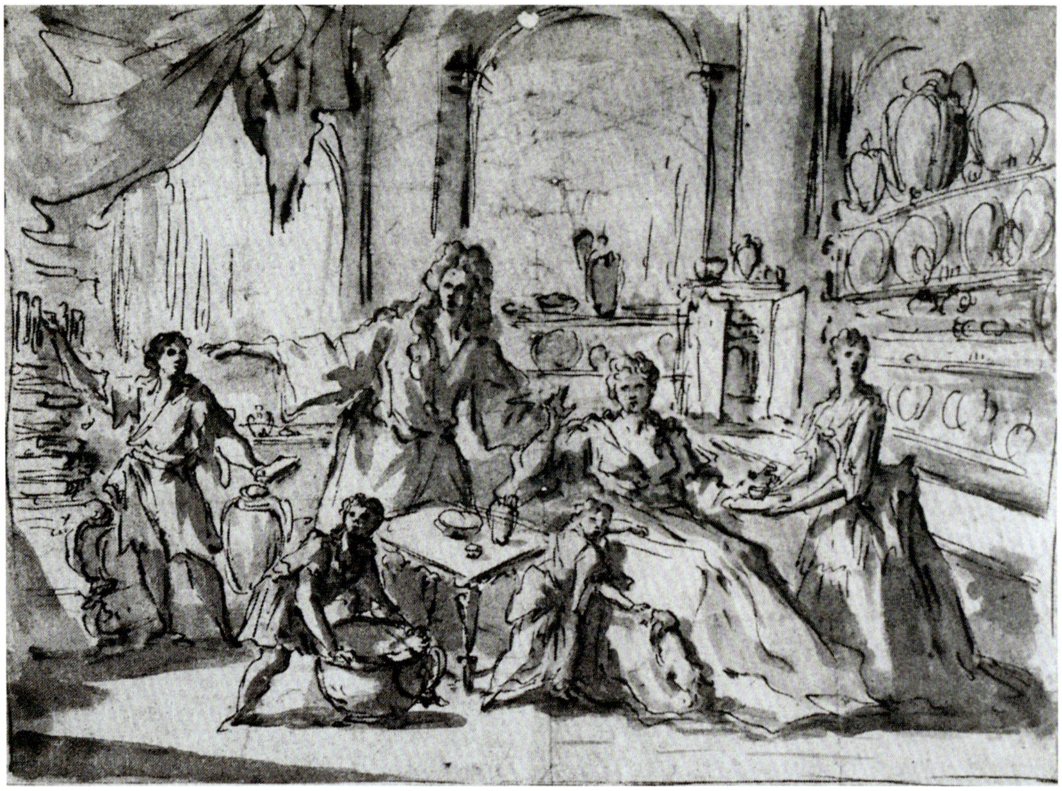

Fig. 114 (*below*) Isaac Gosset (1713–1799), pastel, attributed to Jean-Étienne Liotard, c. 1772. *Private collection*

In 1773, he became a director of the Society of Artists, and exhibited there regularly from 1760 to 1778. See fig. 111 for an example of Isaac Gosset's work and his biography.

Fig. 113 (*above*) Peter Anthony Motteux (1660–1718) and family, drawing, Giovanni Antonio Pellegrini, c. 1713. *British Museum*

Born in Rouen, Motteux came to England in 1685. He had a distinguished literary career as editor of the *Gentleman's Journal* and combined this with his business as an East India Company merchant with premises in Leadenhall Street. His shop was 'At the sign of the Two Fans', near Old India House. Richard Steele described the contents of Motteux's warehouses in the *Tatler* as 'filled and adorned with Tea, China, and Indian Ware. In one place were exposed to view Silks of various Shades and Colour, rich Brocades, and the wealthiest products of foreign Looms'. Both his sons, who are shown as children in the foreground, became directors of the French Hospital. The elder, Peter (1705–1769), a surgeon, was elected in 1758; the younger, Jean (1710–1741), elected in 1729, had a brief but very successful career as a merchant in Hamburg.

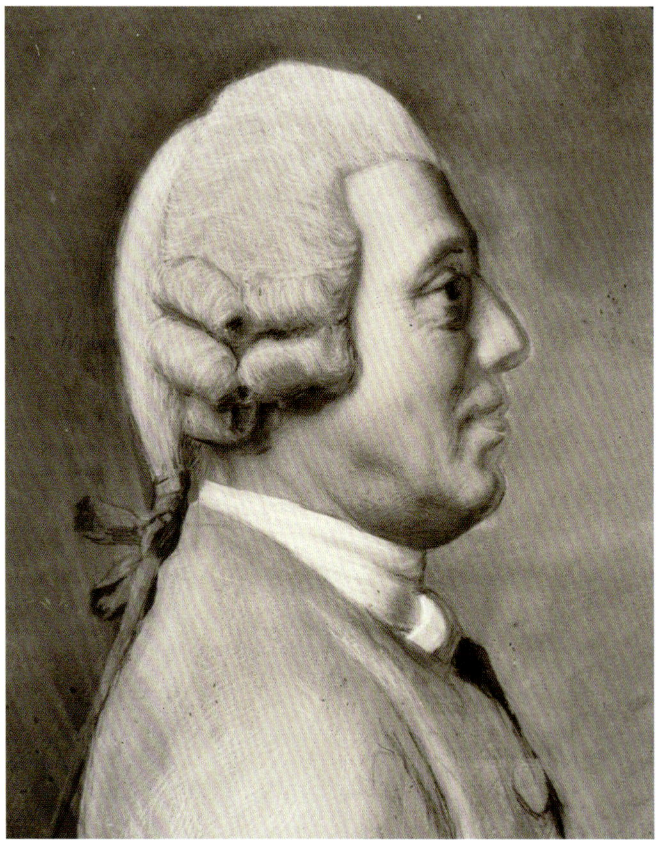

From the earliest years of the hospital a number of Huguenot families known for their philanthropy were among the directors. Jean Bosanquet, belonged to a family from Lunel in the south of France whose munificence is well charted. Jacob Bosanquet presented the Threadneedle Street Church with eight silver communion cups in 1697. The next generation of the family, Claude Bosanquet, also a director, was, with his brother, responsible for the endowment of the Église Neuve in Church Street, Spitalfields, an annexe of the Threadneedle Street church. Besides their directorial links with the French Hospital, members of the de Crespigny, Ducane, Fonnereau, Bosanquet, Lethieullier

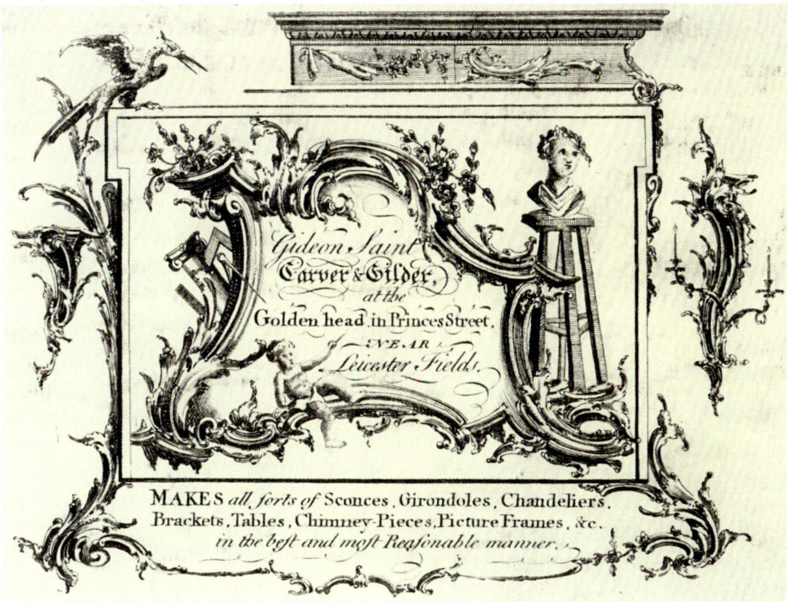
Gideon Saint
Carver & Gilder,
at the
Golden head in Princes Street,
NEAR
Leicester Fields.
MAKES all sorts of Sconces, Girondoles, Chandeliers,
Brackets, Tables, Chimney-Pieces, Picture Frames, &c.
in the best and most Reasonable manner.

Fig. 115 (*right*) Gideon Saint's trade card. *Metropolitan Museum of Art*

Gideon Saint (1729–1799) worked as a carver and gilder at the Golden Head, Princes Street, near Leicester Fields, from 1763. He was apprenticed to Jacob Touzey in 1743. In 1779 he moved to Hoxton, and after his wife's death in 1791, to Groombridge, Kent, where he died in 1799. He was a director of the French Hospital from 1791.

The trade card is pasted into a scrapbook of designs containing 162 drawings and 290 prints pasted in, with a number of drawings done directly into the book. The designs are organized into twelve different sections, and include brackets, shields, clock cases, mouldings, tables and ornaments for chimneys.

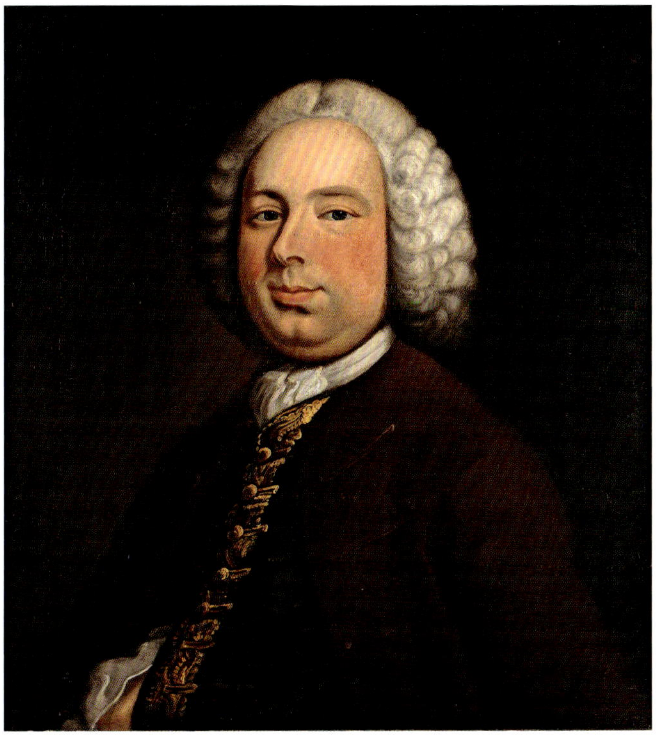

Fig. 116 (*below*) Pierre Ogier (1711–1775), 1761, oil on canvas, artist unknown

The Ogier family came originally from Chassais L'Église in Bas Poitou. Peter Ogier III was one of five brothers, all of whom became master weavers in Spitalfields. His business was based at 4 Spital Square and by 1765 he had £3,000 worth of stock in a warehouse in the City. He became a member of the Livery of the Weavers' Company in 1743 and in 1760 was elected Upper Bailiff.

Pierre became a director of the French Hospital in 1761 and supported the newly founded London Hospital as well. His brother Lewis became a director of the French Hospital in 1771. His younger sister Louisa married the goldsmith Samuel Courtauld and carried on her husband's business after his death, later turning to silk-weaving, her family's trade.

and Delmé families served in the 1730s as governors of the Foundling Hospital, London. Sir Jacob Bouverie, later created 1st Viscount Folkestone, and ancestor of the Earls of Radnor, also served as governor of this infant institution.

In the 1740s and 1750s many of the directors of La Providence were craftsmen. Nicholas Jourdain was a clock-maker, Pierre Dutens was a jeweller, the Gosset brothers Gideon and Isaac were distinguished carvers and gilders and Isaac had a separate career as a wax modeller (figs. 111, 114). Gideon Saint was a carver and gilder (figs. 115). It is surprising to find Sir Estienne-Theodore Janssen, from a papermaking family, elected a director in 1769 since he had served as president of the Anti-Gallican Society.[3] The family came originally from Angoulême although they settled in Holland before emigrating to Britain. Charles Cabrier, who presented La Providence with a long-case clock in 1752 (fig. 29), was not a director, but perhaps he sensed the advantage of conspicuous display of his work in the hope that it would lead to more commissions.

Of the directors of the French Hospital many were connected with the Spitalfields silk trade.[4] Louis Chauvet was one of the most notable weavers of the mid-eighteenth century and employed 450 men in 1750. In addition to serving as a director of the French Hospital he was a governor for life of the London Hospital. Advertisements by the weaving firm of Jamet and Landon of White Lyon Street, Norton Folgate, Spitalfields, appeared in the 1750s; by the 1760s Jacob Jamet was recorded as a weaver of satin. In 1750, the London weaver Jean Sabatier had around 200 men working for him. In 1763 he was listed as a weaver of flowered silk. The Spitalfields weaver Pierre Ogier (fig. 116) was in partnership with Jaques Godin, with an address in Spital Square. Together they offered 60 men to serve the crown in 1745 during the second Jacobite rebellion. Jaques Godin became Upper Warden of the Weavers' Company in 1747. In that year he gave £21 to the building fund for the new London Hospital for which the architect was Boulton Mainwaring, who was also responsible for the extension to the French Hospital. James Godin's son Giles was also a director from 1758. Jaques Godin bequeathed £100 for the poor of the French Hospital. Pierre Ogier's sister Louisa Perina married the goldsmith Samuel Courtauld, thus forging a link with that distinguished Huguenot dynasty, represented in the annals of the French Hospital by Samuel Augustine Courtauld, by then chairman of Courtaulds, the textile company, who was elected a director in 1926. It was Samuel Augustine Courtauld who founded the Courtauld Institute of Art in 1931 and who was largely responsible for bringing the Warburg Institute from Hamburg to London. Samuel Augustine Courtauld found time to be president of the Huguenot Society of London in 1929. He helped the Tate Gallery to buy important works by Seurat and Van Gogh and his own fine collection of French Impressionists including Manet's *Bar at the Folies Bergère* and Cézanne's *Mont Sainte-Victoire* were given to the University of London and form the basis of the Courtauld Gallery collection.

In the eighteenth and nineteenth centuries, a number of directors were distinguished soldiers. One of these was General David Montolieu, baron de Saint-Hippolyte, who served in Piedmont when Ruvigny, Earl of Galway (fig. 7) was Queen Anne's Envoy there. General Louis de Jean (fig. 11) nominated his colleague Earl Ligonier (figs. 9 and 28), who became governor, and General Sir Henry Montrésor. More recently, Major-General Clifford Beckett was descended from Jean Chevalleau, seigneur de Boisragon, who commanded the 33rd Foot under John Churchill, 1st Duke of Marlborough. The Andrés were another distinguished military family to serve the hospital. Major John André became a national hero, having been unjustly hanged as a spy on George Washington's orders in the American War. His uncle and cousin, both named Jean-Louis André, were respectively elected directors in 1786 and 1809, secretaries in 1797 and 1810, treasurers in 1801 and 1820, and deputy-governors in 1808 and 1836. There were more Andrés – seven in all, another secretary and deputy-governor among them, between 1756 and 1868.

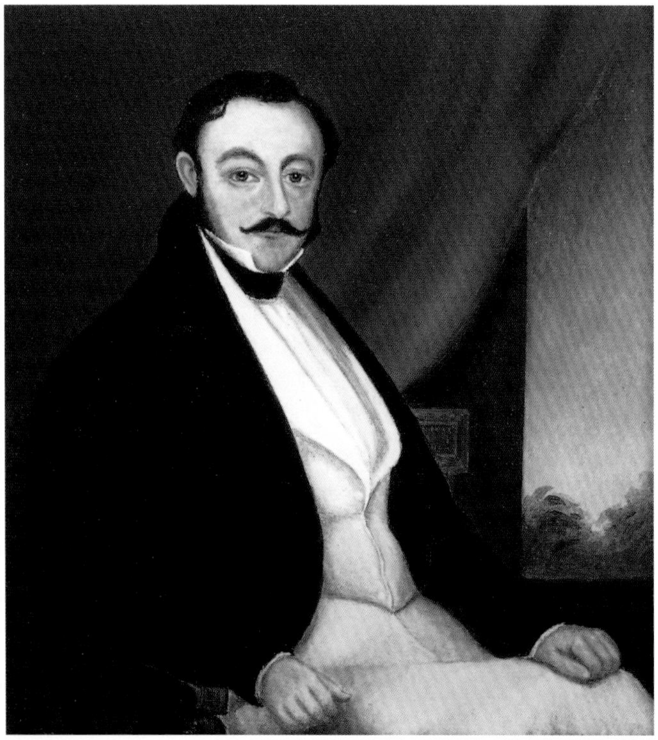

Fig. 117 Hollingworth Magniac (1786–1867), print after portrait, oil on canvas, artist unknown, size not recorded. *National Portrait Gallery*

Hollingworth was the son of Colonel Francis Magniac, a goldsmith supplier of clocks and watches to James Cox for the Chinese market. His elder brother Charles served as Prussian vice-consul at Canton and, aged 25, Hollingworth joined him there. The brothers formed a joint partnership as an agency house and their commodities included Indian opium. After his brother's death Hollingworth formed a partnership with Dr William Jardine in 1825 and by 1828 James Matheson had joined Jardine as the managing partner. The firm became Magniac Jardine in 1841. From 1854 Hollingworth was based at Colworth House, Sharnbrook, Bedfordshire, and his London house in Bolton Row (later Curzon Street), Mayfair.

Hollingworth's collection of medieval art was one of the finest and included portraits, ecclesiastical metalwork, Limoges enamels, ivory and boxwood carvings, faience by Bernard Palissy, glass, and armour. He bought from the sale of Horace Walpole's collection at Strawberry Hill in 1842. According to the diarist Joseph Farington, Hollingworth was adding to a collection which was started by his goldsmith father and his elder brother Charles. Much of his collection was shown in 1862 at the South Kensington Museum. His son Charles commissioned the architect William Burges to design a magnificent monument to his father at Sharnbrook.

Mary Louisa, a daughter of James Peter André, director in 1814, married Richard Grellier (fig. 43), secretary in 1856, whose father Pierre-Paul in 1820 had become a director as his grandfather Leonard Turquand had done in 1770. Mary Louisa's portrait (fig. 44) hangs in the directors' dining-room and a Grellier – Christopher – continues to serve the hospital as a director having previously continued the family's tradition of surveying for 25 years.

A group of directors in the late nineteenth century may have been drawn to the French Hospital by its imposing new building and an awareness of its growing vision as a centre for Huguenot history and memorabilia. Hollingworth Magniac (1786–1867), who became a director in 1843 (fig. 117), was one of these. His father was a goldsmith who had made clocks and watches for the Cantonese market under the supervision of the celebrated London goldsmith and entrepreneur James Cox. In 1805 Hollingworth joined his elder brother Charles in China to oversee the family interests there. They established a business on the river front at Canton, marketing opium amongst other commodities. They sold their opium stock out after prices had increased by a hundred per cent thus making a fortune. Magniac stayed in Canton for twenty years. After his return to London in the 1820s, he married and leased Colworth House at Sharnbrook in north Bedfordshire. His son Charles became a director of La Providence in 1867. Hollingworth Magniac built up a collection of medieval art including historical portraits by Clouet, Cranach the elder, portrait miniatures, ecclesiastical and secular metalwork, Limoges enamels; carvings in ivory and boxwood, and faience ware by Bernard Palissy. He bought many objects from the Strawberry Hill sale in 1842. His collection was sold by Christie's in an eleven-day sale in July 1892 with over 1,500 lots realizing over £100,000.[5]

Henry Wagner (fig. 75), better remembered in Huguenot circles today for his passionate interest in genealogy, helped lay the foundations of early Italian painting in the National Gallery, London.[6]

George Lambert (fig. 68) became a director in 1881. He ran a thriving silversmithing and jewellery business in

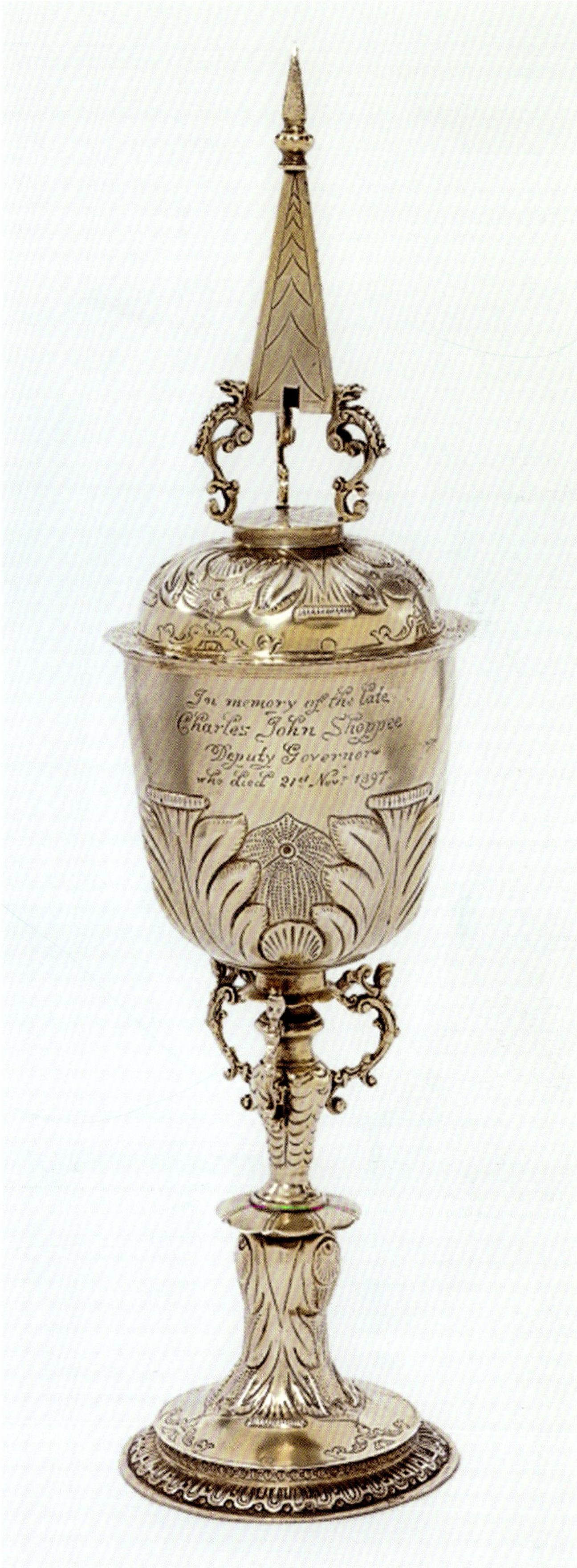
In memory of the late
Charles John Shoppee
Deputy Governor
who died 21st Nov 1897

Fig. 118 Steeple cup and cover, silver-gilt, maker's mark of George Lambert, London, 1898/9

In the James I taste, the cup has a circular foot and bracketed vase-shaped stem, chased with acanthus foliage and fruits; the cover has a triangular steeple finial supported by brackets.

Coventry Street, taking on twenty-two apprentices between 1868 and 1887. In 1887 he became Prime Warden of the Goldsmiths' Company. In that year he presented the Company with a gilt cup modelled on a James I steeple cup on which were recorded the principal events which occurred during the fifty years' reign of Queen Victoria.[7] This makes an interesting comparison with the silver-gilt steeple cup and cover in the James I taste (fig. 118), which Lambert presented to the French Hospital in memory of his fellow director C. J. Shoppee in 1898.

Charles John Shoppee (1823–1897), an architect and surveyor by profession, has been described as 'a cultured, astute, prosperous and sociable professional Victorian gentleman who lived life to the full' (fig. 63).[8] He was very proud of his Huguenot ancestry and assumed the arms of his Lyonnais ancestors. He was a founder member of the London and Middlesex Archaeological Society in 1855. He was elected Master of the Barber Surgeons' Company in 1878. His collection of metalwork, woodwork and antiquities was kept at his home in Mecklenburgh Square and on his death the Victoria and Albert Museum purchased 125 items, including a selection of books from his library.

The eighteenth- and early nineteenth-century directors were seen as the cream of the Huguenot descendants in England. In his *Huguenots: Their Settlements, Churches and Industries in England and Ireland* (1860), Samuel Smiles listed forty-nine names of directors 'well known and highly distinguished in the commerce, politics, science and industries of England'. His list included Blaquière, Boileau, Cazenove, Dalbiac, De La Rue, Labouchère, Majendie, Martineau and Pusey.

Since then members of other leading Huguenot families in England have served as directors, among them: Aubertin, Beaufort, Bourdillon, Cazalet, De Guyon, De La Mare, Faber, Lefroy, Mallalieu, Portal, Roget, Savory, Stallybrass and Tryon.

Interestingly in modern times, the Champion de Crespigny family reappeared when the present secretary was elected a director in 1974 more than two hundred years after Philippe de Crespigny became the second secretary, in 1734 (fig. 26) and Claude became a director in 1760. Mrs Louise Willis, daughter of the present secretary Stephen Champion de Crespigny, was elected a director in 1987, one of the first three women to become directors when they joined the Court in that year, the others being Lady Monson, whose great-uncle, Édouard Majolier, was elected in 1900, and Mrs Lucie Christie, sister of W. R. Le Fanu. Her daughter Mrs Jane Darwin was elected in 1994.

A new departure in recent years has been the election of directors descended from former inmates, the first of these being Charles Marmoy,[9] a descendant of Pierre Marmois admitted in 1761, one of six Marmois or Marmoys who lived at the hospital between 1729 and 1891. More recently Kenneth Bradford, elected a director in 1995 and treasurer in 1999, could recall, as a small boy, visiting his grandmother, a Potier descendant, in the hospital when it was at Victoria Park.

The story of the 728 directors who for nearly three hundred years have maintained this 'monument of the piety of their ancestors' deserves to be told in full. The historian David Agnew hoped that his 'learned friend Henry Wagner' (fig. 75) would produce 'a monograph on the French Protestant Hospital ... containing the Directors' names, with full biographical and genealogical annotations'.[10] It is hoped that the following list will inspire future research on those who have helped to nurture this extraordinary institution.

1 Randolph Vigne and Stephen Champion de Crespigny, *The Directors of the French Hospital, La Providence, 1913–1990*, *PHS*, XXV, 15.2, 1990, pp. 179–83; Henry Wagner, *The Directors of the French Hospital*, *PHS*, X, 10, pp. 137–55.

2 Tessa Murdoch, 'The Inlaid jewel chest on stand made for Rebecca, Viscountess Harcourt, c. 1735', *Furniture History*, XXIII, 1997, pp. 104–8.

3 See Hilary Young, 'Anti-gallican at Chelsea: Protestantism, protectionism and porcelain', *Apollo*, vol. 147, no. 436, June 1998, pp. 35–41.

4 See Natalie Rothstein, *Silk Designs of the 18th Century in the Collection of the Victoria and Albert Museum*, London (1990),

5 See article by Charles Sebag Montefiore on Hollingworth Magniac in the *Oxford Dictionary of National Biography*.

6 Susanna Avery-Quash, 'The Growth of Interest in Early Italian Painting in Britain with particular reference to pictures in the National Gallery' in Dillian Gordon, *The Fifteenth-Century Italian Paintings*, I, National Gallery Catalogues, London (2003).

7 Rosemary Ransome Wallis, *Goldsmiths' Review*, 1973–4, pp. 29–33; *Country Life*, 14 November 1974, pp. 1446–7.

8 Ann Wickham, 'Charles John Shoppee 1823–1897' in the *Barber Surgeons Red Book* (2007), p. 339.

9 Marmoy, *Inmates and Applicants*.

10 Agnew, p. 526.

A list of directors

The year shown is that of the director's first election to the Court. A new director is elected by the Court for life (fig. 119).

G, D-G, T and S denote Governor, Deputy-Governor, Treasurer and Secretary respectively.

E denotes an engraving or etching, M a miniature, P a portrait in oils and Ph a photograph held in the hospital's collection.

An illustration of a director in the book is shown by the figure number.

An asterisk indicates that a director's armorial shield or coat of arms is displayed at the French Hospital.

Until 1834, Christian names of directors were recorded in their French forms.

Adler, Cecil, 1926
Agace, Abdias, 1763
Agace, Daniel, 1788
Agace, Jacob, 1764
Agace, Zacharie, 1758
Alavoine, Pierre, 1761
Albers, James, 1846

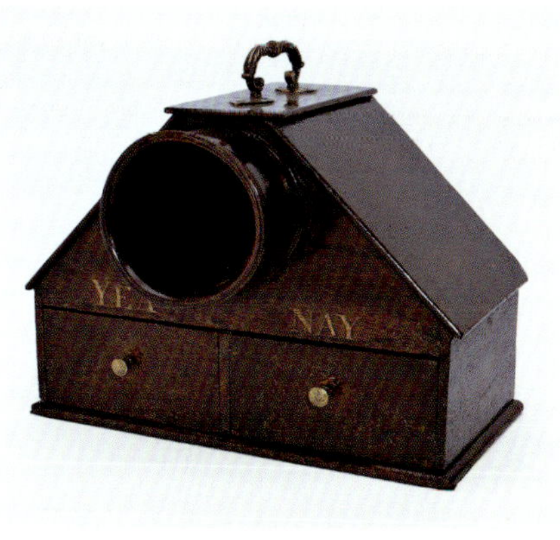

Fig. 119 Ballot box, mid-Georgian
An unusual stained oak pediment-shaped ballot box with two drawers below, inscribed 'YEA' and 'NAY'.

Albert, Jacob,* 1756 (D-G, T)
Amiot, Estienne, 1765
Amyand, Claude, 1723
André, David, 1756
André, David, 1782 (S)
André, Sir Guillaume-Lewis, 1793
André, James Peter, 1846
André, Jaques-Pierre, 1814
André, Jean-Louis,* 1786 (D-G, S)
André, Jean-Louis, 1809 (D-G, S)
Archer, Thomas, 1881
Ardesoif, Etienne, 1789
Ardesoif, Isaac, 1767
Artieres, Joseph, 1765
Auber, Jaques, 1779
Auber, Pierre, 1755
Auber, Pierre, 1767
Auber, Pierre, 1784
Aubert, Antoine, 1773
Aubertin, Pierre, 1771
Aubertin, Thomas, 1911
Aubertin, Thomas Peter, 1933 (D-G, P)
Aufrère, Israel-Antoine, 1725
Auriol, Pierre-Jaques, 1780
Austen-Leigh, Richard Arthur, 1919

Bacalan, Charles, 1729
Barbet, Jaques, 1824
Barbut, Estienne, 1763
Barbut, Jaques, 1772
Baril, Berchère, 1758
Baril, Jaques, 1767
Barnege, Moyse, 1737
Barnouin, Jaques-Henri, 1809
Baronneau, Benjamin, 1718
Barry, Richard de, 1803
Barwell, Revd Arthur Henry Sanxay, 1900
Batten, Stephen Alexander, CBE, 1951
Battier, Jean-Rudolphe, 1771
Baudouin, Jacques,* 1718 (D-G, S)
Beaufort, Daniel de, 1736 (E)
Beaufort, William Morris, 1882
Beckett, Charles John Chichester, 1948
Beckett, Clifford Thomason,* CB, CBE, MC, 1928

Beliard, Louis, 1731
Belloncle, Jaques, 1799 (T)
Benezech, Pierre, 1796
Berchère, Jacques-Louis, 1718
Beuzeville, Estienne, 1774
Beuzeville, Estienne, 1814
Beuzeville, Jaques, 1777
Beuzeville, Pierre, 1776
Binet, Claude, 1740
Binet, Jaques, 1738
Blagny, Jacob de La Motte de, 1718
Blagny, Jean de,* 1732
Blaquière, Jacob, 1763
Blaquière, Jean-Pierre, 1763
Boileau, Charles, 1768
Boileau, Etienne, 1951
Boileau, Sir Francis George Manningham, Bt, 1886
Boileau, Jean-Pierre, 1787
Boileau, Sir John Peter, Bt, 1839
Bonnet, Jean, 1763
Bonnet, Pierre, 1766
Booth, Guillaume-Henri, 1825
Bosanquet, Claude,* 1741
Bosanquet, David Ives, 1965
Bosanquet, Guillaume, 1782
Bosanquet, Guillaume, 1787
Bosanquet, Henri, 1786
Bosanquet, Jacob, 1787
Bosanquet, Jean,* 1735
Bosanquet, Samuel, 1782
Bosanquet, Samuel, 1826
Bosanquet, William,* 1782
Boucher, Jean, 1730
Boucher, Jean, 1760
Bourdillon, Francis William, 1898
Bourdillon, Jaques, 1831
Bourdon, Frederic Armand, 1855
Bouverie, Guillaume, 1st Earl of Radnor, 1770 (G, E)
Boyd, Isaac, 1837
Boyville, Réné de, 1721
Bradford, Kenneth, 1995 (T)
Bredel, Abraham, 1787
Briand, René, 1783 (D-G)
Briggs, Eric Ralph, 1975

Brisac, George, 1774
Broderick, The Hon. Lawrence, 1895
Browning, Arthur Giraud, 1873 (D-G, S, P fig. 59)
Browning, Arthur Hervé, 1901 (T)
Bruse, Isaac de, 1734
Buissiere, Jean, 1741
Buissiere, Paul, FRS,* 1719 (G)
Bureau, Daniel, 1799
Butterworth, Josiah Whitehead, 1875

Cabibel, Pierre, 1718 (G, D-G)
Capper, Frederic William, 1856
Capper, George Herbert, 1910
Carnac, Jean, 1769
Cash, Christopher Keatley, 1965
Cash, James Ouvry, 1960 (T)
Castres, Abraham, 1752
Cazalet, Victor Alexander, 1935
Cazaly, Guillaume, 1800
Chabot, Philip James, 1838 (P)
Chalié, François, 1795
Chalié, Jacques, 1761
Chalié, Jean, 1769
Chalié, Mathieu, 1777
Chamier, Anthony,* 1780 (fig. 120)
Chamier, Jean, 1781
Champion de Crespigny, Alexander Frank Stephen,* 1965 (S)
Champion de Crespigny, Claude, 1760
Champion de Crespigny, Elizabeth Louise (Mrs Willis), 1987
Champion de Crespigny, Philippe, 1734, (S, P fig. 26)
Champion de Crespigny, Pierre, 1718
Charles, Jean Philippe, 1718
Charretié, Jean, 1793
Chassereau, François, 1761
Chavasse, Rt Revd Christopher Maude, MC, 1957
Chauvet, Louis, 1776
Chevalier, Thomas, 1811
Christie, Mrs Lucie Catherine (*née* Le Fanu), 1987
Christie, Thomas Beath, 1887
Clapton, Edward, 1874
Clark, Charles, 1865
Clarmont, Gabriel, 1769 (T)
Clarmont, Mathieu, 1766
Clerembault, Antoine, 1723 (P)
Clerembault, Jean, 1767
Clouseaux, Louis de,* 1718
Collette, Charles Hastings, 1865

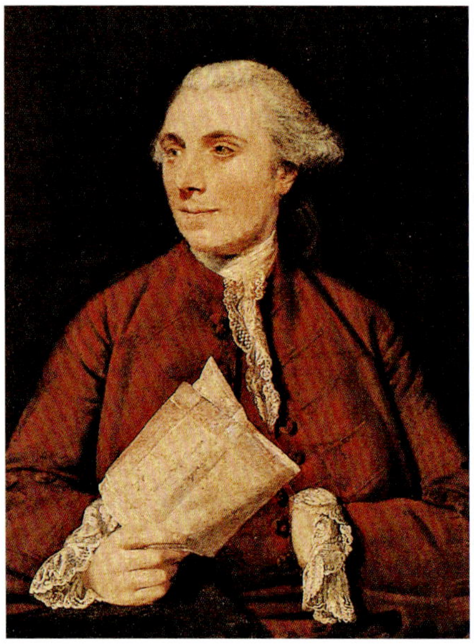

Fig. 120 Anthony Chamier (1725–1780), oil on canvas, Sir Joshua Reynolds, 1777. *Private collection*

The grandson of Daniel Chamier, a minister of the Reformed Church, who sought refuge in England after the Revocation of the Edict of Nantes, he was baptized in the French Church, Threadneedle Street. He became Deputy Secretary of War in January 1772 and Under Secretary of State in 1775. He was elected MP for Tamworth in 1778.

A founder member of the Literary Club and a close friend of Dr Samuel Johnson, Chamier was a friend of Reynolds and sat to him three times for his portrait in 1762, 1767 and 1777.

Collins, Sir William Job, KCVO, 1928
Colombiés, Antoine, 1751
Comarque, René de, 1738
Combrune, Gedeon, 1782
Cosne, Ruvigny de, 1754
Cossart, Jean, 1793
Cottin, Josias, 1770
Courtauld, Samuel Augustine, 1926
Creuzé, Jean, 1767
Cronin, Daniel, 1877
Cronin, Revd Harry Stovell, 1898
Cronin, Walter Daniel, 1896
Curtis, James, 1912

Dalbiac, Simon, 1755
Dalbiac, Simon, 1758
Dargent, Jaques, 1762
Dargent, Jean, 1756
Darwin, Edward Leonard, 1982
Darwin, Mrs Jane Sophia (*née* Christie), 1994
Daubuz, Jean-Théophile, 1794
David, Jean, 1750
Davis, John, 1879
Davy, Robert Manning Matwin, 1935
Debaufre, Joseph, 1783
Debaufre, Richard, 1787
Delafon, Jean, 1731
Delahaize, Philippe, 1769
De La Mare, Francis, 1861
De La Mare, James, 1848
De La Mare, James, 1858
Delamare, Abraham, 1753
Delamare, Andrew James, 1900
Delamare, Isaac, 1762
Delamare, Jacob, 1762
Delamare, Jean, 1757
Delavau, David, 1754
Desbois, Daniel, 1877
Des Carrieres, David, 1794
Deschamps, Jean, 1758
Deschamps, Jean, 1771
Deschamps, Pierre, 1736
Deschamps, Pierre, 1757
Des Clouseaux, Louis,* 1718 (T)
Deseret, Jean, 1795
Deseret, Phinée, 1765
Desert-Dieu, Pierre-Jacques du, 1718
Desmarets, Claude,* 1732 (D-G)

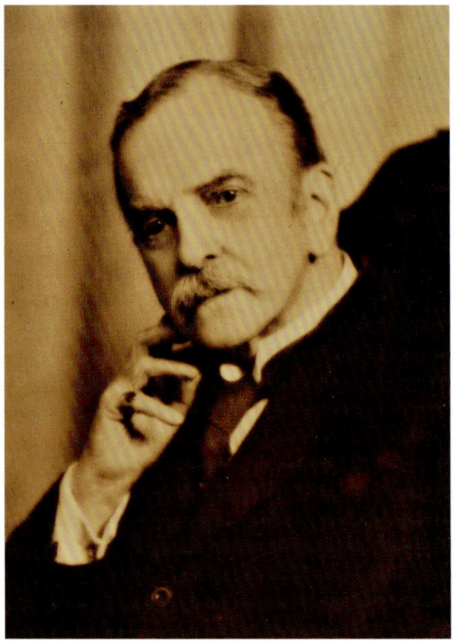

Fig. 121 Sir Robert William Dibdin (1848–1933), photograph

Desmarets, François, 1760
Desormeaux, Jaques Louis, 1798
Devaux, Jaques, 1718
Devaynes, Guillaume, 1770 (E)
Devaynes, Jean, 1760 (E)
Devins, Richard, 1778
Devisme, Gerard,* 1788
Devisme, Guillaume, 1780
Devisme, Pierre, 1765
Dibdin, Charles, 1919
Dibdin, Sir Robert William, 1892 (S, P fig. 121)
Dollond, George, 1819 (E)
Dollond, George, 1853
Dollond, Pierre, 1794
D'Olon, Louis-Benjamin, 1726
Droz, Simeon, 1788
Du Bisson, Jean, 1775
Du Bisson, Thomas,* 1731
Du Boulay, Anthony John Houssemayne, 1985
Du Boulay, Revd Francis Houssemayne,* 1885
Du Four, Paul,* 1718 (T)
Dulamon, Jaques, 1737
Dumaresq, Auguste, 1783
Dumas, Charles Eugene Frederick, CBE, MC, 1950
Dumas, Gerald Piers, 1910
Dumas, Henry John Fairrie, 1892

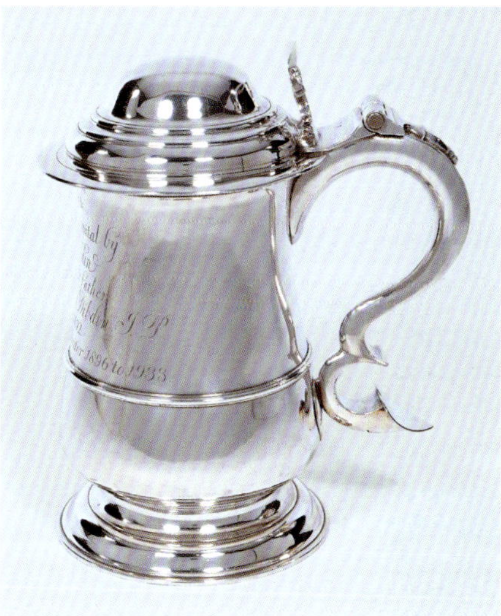

Fig. 122 Tankard, sterling silver, maker's mark of John Langlands, Newcastle, 1760–1768, presented by John Dibdin in memory of his father Sir Robert William Dibdin

Dumas, Henry John Philip, 1884
Dumas, Hugh Charles Sowerby, 1896 (D-G, T, E)
Dumas, Philip Anthony Egerton, 1951
Dumas, Raymond, 1949
Dumas, Rupert Charles Thomas Piers, 1953
Dumaresq, Auguste, 1783
Dumoustier, Jean, 1779
Dupont, Gainsborough, 1794 (P)
Duprat de Charreau, Jean, 1726
Durand, Jean, 1769
Durand, Jean–Charles,* 1824
Duroure, François,* 1742 (D-G, S, fig. 123)
Duroure, Jean, 1781
Dutens, Pierre, 1749
Dutens, Pierre, 1767
Duthoit, Jonathan, 1873 (P)
Duval, Alexander Edward, 2000
Duval, Claude Patrick, 1978
Duval, David,* 1786 (D-G, E, P fig. 33)
Duval, Revd David, 1947
Duval, David Vernon, 1985
Duval, Edward Walter, 1948
Duval, Eleanor Sorel (Mrs Leonard), 1994
Duval, Henry James, 1845
Duval, Herbert Philip, 1908
Duval, Jean, 1786
Duval, John Arthur, 1933 (D-G)
Duval, Louis, 1777
Duval, Louis, 1826
Duval, Michael Edward, 1961
Duval, Peter James, 1973 (D-G, T)
Duval, Philip Smith, 1826 (D-G, P fig. 57)
Duval, Revd Philippe Snaith, 1859
Duval, Robert Michael Lewis, 1981
Duval, Revd Stephen Peachey, 1898 (D-G, S)
Duval, Stephen Smith, 1883 (T, P)
Duval, Walter John, 1908 (T)

Edwards, Revd Richard, 1838
Emly, Henry, 1848
Evans, Edward Prichard, 1877

Faber, Reginald Stanley, 1895
Fâche, Charles James, 1859 (S)
Fâche, Edward Charles, 1904
Fâche, Gordon Lancaster Mountford, MC, 1911

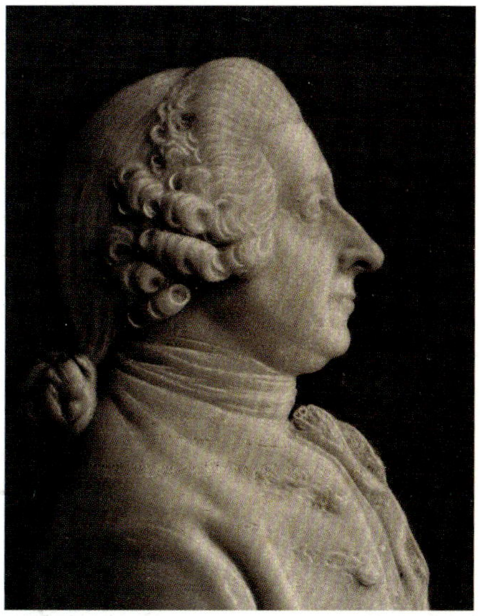

Fig. 123 François Duroure (1715–1808), photogravure by Emery Walker, after a wax medallion by Isaac Gosset

Appointed a director in 1764, Duroure was secretary to the French Hospital from 1765 to 1783 and deputy-governor from 1785 to 1797. The present location of the original wax by Gosset is unknown. For further information on Isaac Gosset see figs. 111 and 114.

Favenc, Abraham, 1782
Favenc, Abraham, 1805 (T)
Fellowe, George Rice, 1826
Fenoulhet, Jaques, 1795
Fenton, Dr William Stewart Rolleston, 1992
Ferard, Jean, 1805
Foissac, Jaques de, 1732
Fonblanque, John Berkeley de, 1951
Ford, Ronald Mylne, 1910
Forrester, Alexandre, 1735
Fosh, Robert Frederick, 1943
Fouace, Gabriel, 1740
Fountaine, Michel, 1769
Fournier, George, 1827
Fremont, Jean, 1776
Frisquet, Pierre-Nicolas, 1771
Fruchard, Jaques, 1749
Fruchard, Philippe, 1718

Gaillardy, Louis de, 1718
Galhié, Robert, 1783
Gambier, Jaques, 1729
Garnault, Aymé, 1762 (M fig. 110)
Garnault, Pierre, 1752

Gastine, Jacques, 1740
Gaugain, Jean Pierre, 1808
Gaultier, Jaques, 1720 (G, T)
Gaussen, Pierre,* 1741 (D-G, T)
Gaussen, Pierre, 1755
Gaussen, Pierre, 1780
Gaussen, Robert George, 1881
Gaussen, Robert William, 1878
Gaussen, Samuel Robert, 1782
Gervis, Henry, 1906
Gignoux, Jean, 1747
Giles, Daniel, 1780
Gilman, Jean, 1811
Girardot-Buissières, André, 1743 (D-G)
Girardot, André,* 1776 (S)
Girardot, Tillieux, 1770
Giraud, Francis Frederick, 1874
Giraud, Richard Hervé, 1829 (D-G, T, S, fig. 52, P fig. 45)
Godin, Estienne-Pierre, 1769
Godin, Giles, 1758
Godin, Jaques, 1742 (T)
Gosset, Gedeon, 1760
Gosset, Isaac, 1764
Gosset, Jacob, 1778
Grace, Oliver Jelf, 1957
Greenwood, Harold Edward, 1929 (G, T)
Grellier, Bernard, MC, 1924
Grellier, Cecil, MC, 1924
Grellier, Christopher Grant Harley, 1990
Grellier, Ernest Francis Waldemar, 1932
Grellier, Norman, MC, 1924
Grellier, Pierre–Paul, 1820
Grellier, Richard, 1837 (S, P fig. 43)
Grellier, William, 1878 (Ph fig. 124)
Griffin, Guillaume, 1795
Griffin, Jean, 1796
Grignion, Claude, 1809
Guillebaud, Pierre, 1787
Guillemard, Daniel, 1810 (T)
Guillemard, Isaac, 1785
Guillemard, Jaques, 1789
Guillemard, Jean, 1769 (S)
Guillemard, Jean, 1793 (D-G)
Guillonneau, George, 1819 (T, S)
Guinand, Jean-Henri, 1721 (D-G, P fig. 16)
Guinand, Henri, 1756
Guinard, Pierre, 1767
Gulhon, Estienne de, 1728

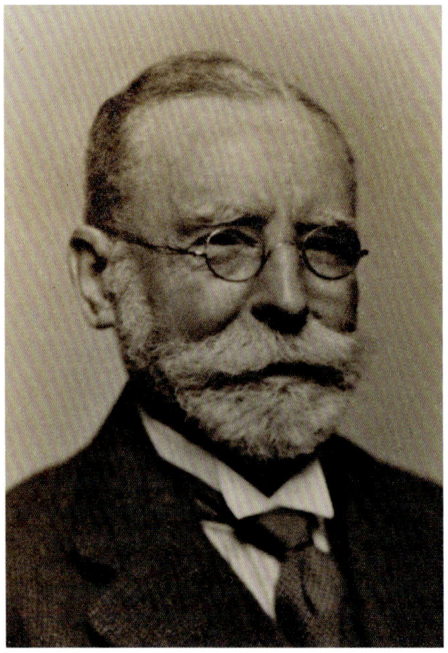

Fig. 124 William Grellier, FRIBA (1847–1934), photograph

Guyon, Estienne, 1756
Guyon, Henri-Guillaume, 1771
Guyon, Jean, 1831
Guyon, Raimond Warwick Debaufré de, 1949

Habberfield, Richard, 1855
Haines, Henry John, 1846
Haines, Henry Joseph Rosselloty, 1860 (E)
Hall, Francis de Haviland, 1912
Hall, Lewis Duval, 1899
Hanbury, Philip, 1843
Hanet, Jean, 1766
Harenc, Benjamin, 1765
Hays, Jaques, 1748
Herisson, Pierre, 1769
Hervart, Guillaume, 1765
Hervart, Philibert, baron d'Huningue,* 1720 (G)
Hesse, Salomon, 1776
Heudebourck-Burford, Alan Reginald, 1995
Hoffmann-Becking, Penelope [*née* Ouvry], 2002
Hovell, Dennis de Berdt, 1866
Hovenden, Robert, 1896

Jackson, Sir Ralph, KBE, CB,* 1986
Jamet, Jacob, 1763
Jamet, Jean, 1787
Janssen, Sir Estienne-Théodore, Bt, 1769
Jaumard, Samuel, 1795
Jean, Louis de, 1740 (P fig. 11)
Jeune, Charles Henry, MBE, 1925
Johnson, Harold Daintree, 1935
Johnson, Harold Jossé, OBE, 1925
Johnson, Sir Louis Stanley, 1920
Jolit, Francis Henry, 1856 (P)
Jolit, François, 1818 (P fig. 50)
Jolit, Thomas Russell, 1836
Jouenne, Louis, 1779
Jourdain, Albert Edward Towle, 1919
Jourdain, Revd Ernest Edward, 1940
Jourdain, Sir Henry John, 1879
Jourdain, Jean,* 1779
Jourdain, Nevill, 1876
Jourdain, Nicholas, 1749
Jourdain, William David, 1834
Jourdan, George, 1794
Jourdan, Jean, 1779
Jullian, Jean, 1748
Julliot, André, 1725

Kent, Arthur Barton, 1902
Kershaw, Samuel Wayland, 1884
Knight, Athro Charles, 1929

Labouchère, John, 1846
Laborde, Josias, 1731
La Chaumette, François-David de, 1791
La Chaumette, Henri-Antoine de, 1798
La Chaumette, Louis-André de,* 1788
La Combe de Cluset, Réné, 1718
Lafone, Alfred, 1890
Lafontaine, Henry Cart de, 1928
Lambert, George, 1881 (Ph fig. 68)
Lande, Albert de, 1718
Landon, Jaques, 1799
Landon, Jean, 1764
Landon, Jean-Luc, 1753
Landon, Philip Aislabie, MC, 1948
Landon, Theodore Luke Giffard,* 1992
Lane, John, 1920
La Neuvemaison, Abraham de, 1767
Langlois, Christophe, 1765
Lapierre, Pierre, 1740
Laporte, Charles, 1738
La Primaudaye, Étienne de, 1787
La Primaudaye, François de, 1761
La Primaudaye, Pierre de, 1740

La Primaudaye, Pierre Henri Alexandre de, 1758
La Rivière, Samuel, 1734
Larminie, Ferdinand Geoffrey, OBE, 1996
Larpent, Sir George Gerard de Hochepied, Bt, 1847
La Rue, Warren de, 1856
La Rue, William Frederick de, 1861
La Sablière, Nicolas de, 1718
Lawrence, Thomas, 1824
Layard, Antoine-Louis, 1780
Layard, Daniel Pierre,* 1775
Layard, Frederick Peter, 1889
Layard, Sir Henry Austen, 1885 (E fig. 60)
Layard, Jean Thomas, 1780
Lebas, Charles, 1721
Le Blanc, Albert, 1719
Le Blond, Robert, 1787
Le Clerc de Virly, Jean, 1718
Le Cras, Noé, 1762
Lee, Henry, 1876
Leeson, Henry Beaumont, 1847
Le Fanu, William Richard,* 1956
Lefebvre, Jean, 1768
Lefevre, Pierre, 1776
Lefroy, Edward Jeffry, 1951
Lefroy, Jeffry Ardern Patrick, MBE, 1961
Lefroy, Jeffry George, 1973
Lefroy, Revd John Percival, 1967
Leglise, Gedeon, 1724
Le Heup, Thomas,* 1718
Le Heup, Michel, 1741
Lemaitre, Pierre, 1742
Le Mann, Michel, 1818 (P)
Le Mare, Geoffrey, 1968
Le Mesurier, Paul, 1794
Le Quesne, Jean, 1736
Le Souef, Jean, 1784
Le Souef, Pierre, 1791
L'Espinasse de Fonvive, Jean, 1721
Letheren, Mrs Teresa Anne, 1999
Levesque, Jean, 1796
Levesque, Pierre, 1813 (D-G, E)
Lichigaray, Samuel, 1777
Ligonier, Jean-Louis, Earl Ligonier,* 1748 (G, P figs. 9, 28)
Lloyd, Richard Harman, 1850
Loubier, Jean-Antoine, 1741
Loubier, Mathieu, 1756
Lucadou, Jacques-Louis, 1788
Lucadou, Jean Daniel, 1769 (T)
Magniac, Charles, 1867
Magniac, Hollingworth, 1843
Magniac, Oswald Cecil, 1912
Maigre, Cyrus, 1775
Majendie, Ashurst, 1845
Majendie, Jean-Jaques,* 1752
Majolier, Édouard,* 1900
Mallalieu, Sir Édouard Lancelot, 1961
Malliet, Jean, 1770
Marchant, Pierre, 1718
Mare, Jaques, 1731
Marplay, Jean, 1790
Marshall, Joseph Irwin, 1940
Martel, Isaac, 1778
Marissal, Jean, 1773
Marmoy, Charles Frank Albert, 1977
Marplay, Jean, 1790
Marriet, Pierre, 1773
Martel, Jaques, 1757
Martineau, Anthony Adeane, 1939
Martineau, Charles Edmund, 2004
Martineau, David, 1799
Martineau, Edward Crispin Akers, 1972
Martineau, Jean,* 1799
Martineau, Richard, 1859
Maseres, François, 1804 (E)
Massé, Jaques, 1741
Massu, Jean, 1785
Masters, Henry William, 1836
Matthews, Edward, 1799
Matthews, Marmaduke, 1847
Matthias, Gabriel, 1787
Matthias, Jacques, 1770
Matthias, Vincent, 1770
Mauger, Josué, 1769
Maze, Jaques, 1782
McCall, Sir Robert Alfred, KCVO, 1928
McCarraher, Mrs Lucy (*née* Wagner), 1997
Ménard, Revd Philippe,* 1718 (S, P fig. 1)
Menet, François, 1780
Mercier, Francis Mitchell Kerr, 1870
Merzeau, Pierre, 1771
Michel, Pierre-Ferry, 1793 (E, P)
Mills, Bernard James, 1927
Minet, Hughes, 1769 (M fig. 107)
Minet, Isaac, 1791 (E)
Minet, Jean Lewis, 1791 (E)
Minet, Paul Piers Brissault, 1969
Minet, Peter Brissault, 1948 (P fig. 108)
Minet, William, 1882
Minier, Charles, 1783
Molinier, Jaques, 1721
Molinier, Charles, 1756
Monckton, Lionel, 1906
Monier-Williams, Monier Faithfull, 1896
Monier-Williams, Randall Herbert, 1933
Monson, Emma (The Lady Monson), 1987
Montagu, Frederic, 1775
Montigny, Jean Remy de, 1723
Montledier, Jean Jaques de Villettes de, 1721
Montolieu, David, baron de Saint-Hippolyte,* 1718
Montolieu, Charles, 1758 (P)
Montresor, Sir Henri Tucker, 1788
Montresor, Jaques-Gabriel,* 1766
Montresor, Jean, 1779
Moore, Daniel, 1815
Moreau, Jaques-Philippe, 1734
Moreau, Philippe, 1721
Motteux, Jean,* 1729
Motteux, Jean, 1763
Motteux, Pierre, 1758
Mouchet, Abraham-Jean, 1812
Mouchet, Jean-Aldebert, 1814
Mounier, Estienne, 1750
Mounier, Pierre, 1784
Moxon, Herbert, 1859
Murdoch, Dr Tessa Violet, 1999
Muysson, Philippe, 1774

Narbonne, Jean, 1726
Nevard, Peter Thomas Charles, 1986
Noguier, Jean Antoine, 1788
Norris, Charles, 1860 (T, E)
Nouaille, Pierre, 1760 (E)
Nouaille, Pierre, 1789

Ogier, Pierre, 1761 (P fig. 116)
Ogier, Louis, 1771
Olivier, Daniel, 1765 (B)
Oulton, Ralph Henry Lefroy, CBE, 1960
Ouvry, Aimé Arthur Carrington, DSC, 1955
Ouvry, Ernest Carrington, 1892
Ouvry, Frederic,* 1869
Ouvry, Jeremy Peter Alderson, 1960

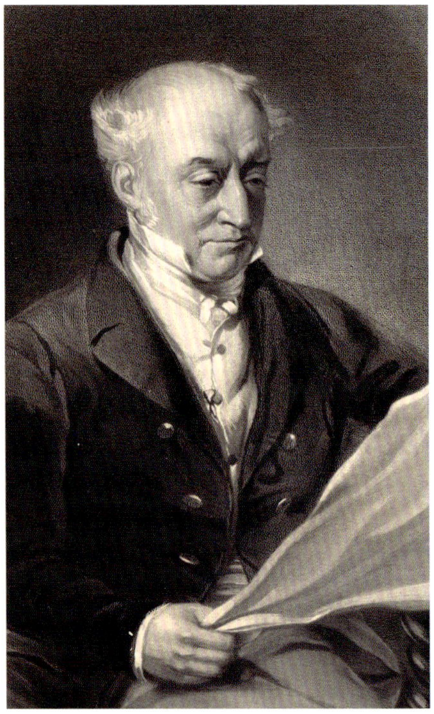

Fig. 125 William Pleydell-Bouverie, 3rd Earl of Radnor (1779–1869), engraving, S.W. Reynolds after a drawing by C.A. Du Val, 1843

Educated largely on the European continent, William was in Paris the day following the storming of the Bastille. He inherited the title in 1828, married twice, and his heir Jacob, was born to his second wife Judith Anne, the daughter of Sir Henry Paulet St John Mildmay. He supported the abolition of slavery. His daughter Jane alluded to her father's 'intense love of the truth and justice' and to his 'ruling sense of duty and veneration for the laws of his country' [H]e had, she wrote, 'a tenderness of heart, hated oppression and wrong doing, and did not shrink from stating his views.' As a Whig, he was a Member of Parliament and active back-bencher. He served as governor of the French Hospital at the time of the hospital's move from Finsbury to Hackney.

Ouvry, Jonathan Garnault, 1960
Ouvry, Revd Lionel Garnault, 1960
Ouvry, Norman Delamain, 1937 (S)
Ouvry, Philippa Cassandra, 2005
Ouvry, Romilly Southwood, 1937 (S)

Panton, Charles, 1859
Parker, Owen Fortrie, 1923
Pechel, Samuel, 1752
Pechell, Sir Paul, Bt,* 1772
Pechell, Sir Thomas, Bt, 1801
Peek, Sir Cuthbert Edgar, Bt, 1886
Peek, Sir Henry William, Bt, 1846 (D-G, Ph fig. 62)
Penny, Solomon, 1718
Perchard, Jean, 1774
Perchard, Pierre, 1794
Perigal, François, 1769
Perigal, Jean, 1718
Perigal, Jean, 1784
Perowne, Edward Stanley Mould, 1901
Petit, Jean Louis, 1773
Petit, Revd Jean Louis, 1858
Petit, Louis Hayes, 1829
Petit, Louis Peter, 1845
Petit, Peter John, 1849
Peyrenc, Jean, 1729
Phené, John Samuel, 1875 (Ph)
Philbrick, Frederick, 1866
Pigou, Jean, 1755
Pilon, Daniel, 1754
Pittar, Parke, 1855
Pittar, Parke Mayhew, 1880
Pittar, William Parke John, 1872
Place, Robert William, 1982
Planck, Pierre, 1766
Planck, Pierre, 1812
Pleydell-Bouverie, Guillaume, 3rd Earl of Radnor, 1803 (G, E fig. 125)
Pleydell-Bouverie, Jacob, 2nd Earl of Radnor,* 1789 (G, E)
Pleydell-Bouverie, Jacob, 4th Earl of Radnor, 1842 (G, E fig. 126)
Pleydell-Bouverie, Jacob, 6th Earl of Radnor, 1900 (G, E)
Pleydell-Bouverie, Jacob, 8th Earl of Radnor, 1960 (G)
Pleydell-Bouverie, William, 5th Earl of Radnor, 1889 (G, E, fig. 127)
Pleydell-Bouverie, William, 7th Earl of Radnor, KG, 1926 (G)
Pleydell-Bouverie, William, 9th Earl of Radnor, 1983 (G)
Pollock, Arthur Becher, 1855
Pontereau, François de, 1718
Portal, Andrew Wallace, 1951
Portal, Bernard Bedwell, 1874
Portal, Burnaby Mark, 1965
Portal, Frederick Welsh, 1881
Portal, Sir William Wyndham, Bt, 1909
Pouchon, Joseph, 1749
Pousset, Pierre, 1799
Pujolas, Moise,* 1718 (G)

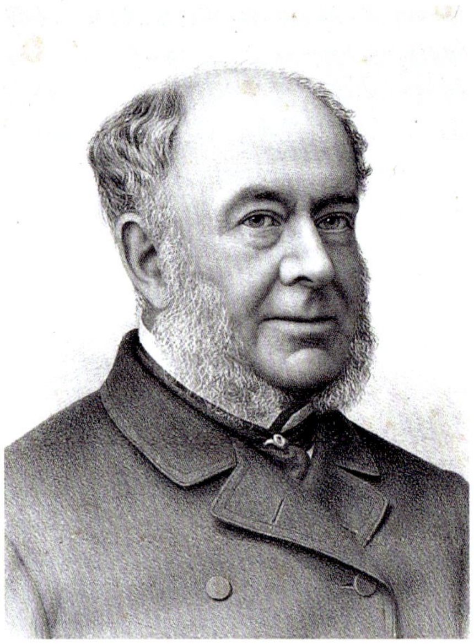

Fig. 126 Jacob Pleydell-Bouverie, 4th Earl of Radnor (1815–1889), engraving after the portrait by George Richmond, dated 1873

The 4th Earl of Radnor was a keen sportsman. He married Lady Mary Augusta Frederica Grimston. At Longford Castle, the family seat, he undertook extensive building work under the direction of the architect Anthony Salvin.

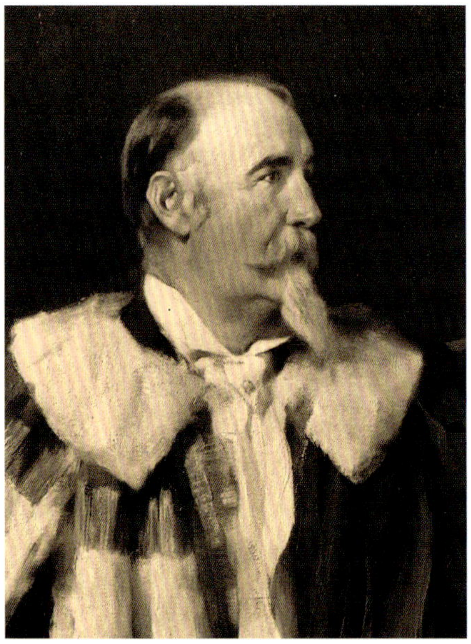

Fig. 127 William Pleydell-Bouverie, 5th Earl of Radnor (1841–1900), photograph after the portrait by Sir James Jebusa Shannon at Longford Castle, 1897

Elected a director of the French Hospital in 1889, the 5th Earl of Radnor served as governor from 1890 to 1900.

Pulley, Guillaume, 1819
Pulley, Guillaume Miles, 1820
Pulley, Henri, 1821
Pulley, John, 1848
Pulley, Joseph, 1820
Pulley, Josias, 1846
Pusey, Hon. Philippe,* 1790

Racine, Jaques,* 1803
Rambouillet, Antonie de, 1725
Ravaud, Estienne-David, 1747
Ravenel, Edouard, 1740
Reignier, André, 1758
Reneu, Pierre, 1718
Renvoizé, Pierre, 1802
Reynous, Isaac, 1725
Richard, Daniel, 1771
Rigail, Moise, 1723
Roberdeau, Isaac, 1751
Roberdeau, Jean-Pierre, 1786
Roberts, Sir George, Bt, 1939
Robethon, Jaques, 1718
Robethon, Jean de, 1721 (G)
Roget, John Romilly, 1953
Roget, Samuel Romilly, 1938
Romilly, George Thomas, 1865
Romilly, Pierre,* 1770
Romilly, Sir Samuel,* 1786 (P fig. 41)
Romilly, Thomas-Pierre, 1779
Romilly, William, 2nd Baron, 1882
Rondeau, Jaques, 1782
Rossieres, Jean de, 1718
Roumieu, John, 1843
Roumieu, Edward Abraham, 1861
Roumieu, Revd John Joseph, 1869
Roumieu, Raymond Lewis, 1878
Roumieu, Reginald St Aubyn, 1876
Roumieu, Robert Lewis, 1856 (T, P fig. 55)
Roussey, Jaques, 1720
Ruffane, Guillaume, 1766
Ruvigny, Henri de Massue de, Earl of Galway,* 1718, (G, E fig. 7)

Sabatier, Jean, 1758
Sailly, Charles de, 1740
Saint, Gedeon, 1791 (fig. 115)
St Colome, Henry de,* 1718
St Leu, Charles de, 1780
St Leu, Charles, 1816
St Leu, Daniel de, 1789
St Maurice, Charles,* 1729
Samson, Pierre-Auguste, 1740
Sapte, Pierre-Antoine, 1790
Saunders, Mrs Miranda Medhurst (*née* Ouvry), 1988
Saurin, Louis,* 1718 (E fig. 6)
Savory, Sir Douglas Lloyd, 1951
Savory, Sir Joseph, Bt, 1884
Scoffier, Claude, 1718
Sebastian, Gerald Noel Boyd, 1907
Sebastian, Lewis Boyd, 1899
Seignoret, Estienne, 1718
Seignoret, Pierre, 1719
Sevestre, Guillaume Denison, 1818
Shoppee, Charles John, 1867 (D-G T, P, Ph fig. 63)
Shoppee, Gerald Augustine, 1887
Silvester, Sir John, Bt, 1811 (E fig. 31)
Simpson, Jean-Vatas, 1818
Smart, James, 1867
Smart, Thomas, 1847
Smith, Edward, 1866
Soulegre, Pierre, 1731
South, Mrs Catherine Evelyn, 1998
South, Charles Philip Bentlif, 1918 (D-G, T)
South, John Charles Bentlif, 1966 (T)
Stallybrass, William Teulon Swan OBE, 1911
Stannard, Rt Revd Robert William, 1960
Stapleton, Very Revd Henry Edward Champneys, 1984
Stone, Thomas, 1860

Tabart, Jacques, 1718
Tanqueray, Charles, 1849
Tanqueray-Willaume, Thomas Butts, 1848
Tascher, Pierre, 1727
Teissier, Charles, 1776
Teissier, Estienne, 1747
Teissier, Estienne, 1781
Teissier, Louis, 1762
Teissier, Henry Brice, Baron de, 1891
Teissier, Revd Philip Antoine, Baron de, 1885
Teulon, Samuel Sanders, 1862
Teulon, Seymour, 1864
Teulon, William Hensman, 1866
Teulon, William Milford, 1863
Thomas, Ivon, 1776
Thomas, Thomas, 1718
Thomas, Thomas, 1766
Thomas, Pierre, 1736
Thouvois, Daniel, 1735
Tiercelin, John Joseph, 1853
Tirel, Pierre, 1735
Tirel-Morin, Jean, 1772
Touray, Michel-Pierre, 1804
Touray, Peter, 1852
Travers, Jean, 1776 (P)
Triquet, Pierre, 1718
Triquet, Pierre, 1756
Tryon, Claude Francis Henry, 1909
Tryon, John, 1899 (T)
Tudert, Louis de, 1718
Turquand, Guillaume, 1825
Turquand, Jean-Louis, 1777
Turquand, Leonard, 1770
Turquand, William, 1849

Vautier, Daniel, 1756
Vere, Pierre, 1794
Vernezobre, Jean-Daniel, 1777
Vialars, Daniel, 1757
Viçouse, Guy de, Baron de la Court,* 1718 (G)
Viçouse, Guy de, 1732
Vidal, Emeric, 1776
Vigne, James Randolph,* 1979 (T)
Vignoles, Charles* 1769
Vigor, Eric, 1965 (D-G)
Villettes, Arthur de, 1753
Villettes, Guillaume-Anne de, 1779
Villettes, Henry Clinton de, 1777
Vincent, Jean-Robert, 1828

Wagner, Sir Anthony Richard, KCVO, 1929
Wagner, Henry, 1865 (P fig. 75)
Wagner, Orlando Henry, 1909
Ward, Allan Ogier, 1912
Ward, Ronald Ogier, DSO, MC, OBE, 1933
Ward, Seth Stephen, 1824
Ware, Thomas, 1866
Waterlow, Sir Edgar Lutwyche, Bt, 1898
White, John Francis, 1857
White, Thomas Armstrong, 1921
Williams, Leonard Llewellyn Bulkeley, 1930
Williams, Robert, 1794
Winsor, Frederic Albert, 1836 (E, P fig. 53)
Wood, Henry James Theodore, 1901
Wyndham, Edouard, 1829

Huguenot heraldry

List of armorial shields of directors of the French Hospital

Many of the shields hung in the Court Room when the hospital was in Hackney. They are all now displayed on the staircase at the French Hospital, Rochester. The dates given indicate first election as director. The arms of the kingdom of France are included. The numbers in parentheses are those on the back of the shields.

Albert, Jacob, 1756 (25), fig. 128: *Azure, a griffin salient or*

André, Jean Louis, 1786 (41): *Argent, in chief two mullets azure and in base a galley her oars in action sable*

Baudouin, Jacques, 1718 (43), fig. 129: *Vert, a lion rampant or armed and langued gules, on a chief or three roses gules voided and barbed vert*

Beckett, Clifford Thomason, 1928 (8): *Quarterly, 1st and 4th, party per pale azure and gules on a fess argent three fleur-de-lis or between four crescents argent all within a semée de spurs, in chief two boars' heads erased or and in base a cross of Malta counter-changed; 2nd, Azure a chevron argent between three crescents or all within a bordure argent charged with three crescents of the first; 3rd, argent, a bordure azure charged with alternate thistles, roses fleur-de-lis and harps or, in chief, three martlets sable, an orle gules*

Blagny, Jacob de, 1718 (15): *Vert, a fess between three escallops or*

Bosanquet, Jean, 1735 (13), fig. 130: *Or, a tree proper, on a chief gules a crescent between two mullets or (intended for) argent*

Buissiere, Paul, 1729 (3): *Vert, three bezants*

Chamier, Anthony, 1780 (22), fig. 131: *Sable (intended for) azure, on a fess or between three roses argent barbed and seeded or, a human heart gules*

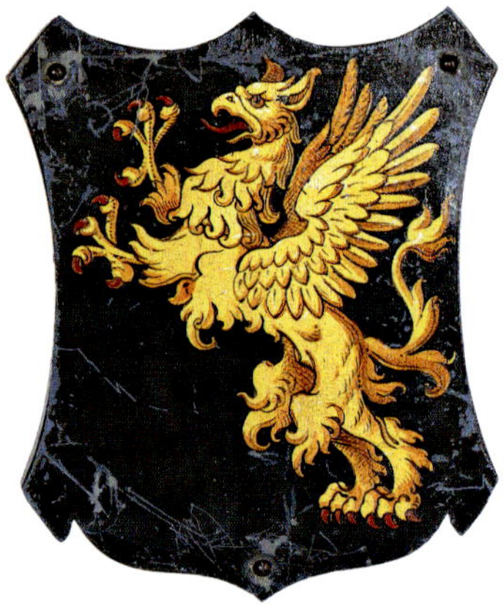

Fig. 128 Arms of Jacob Albert, 1756 (25)

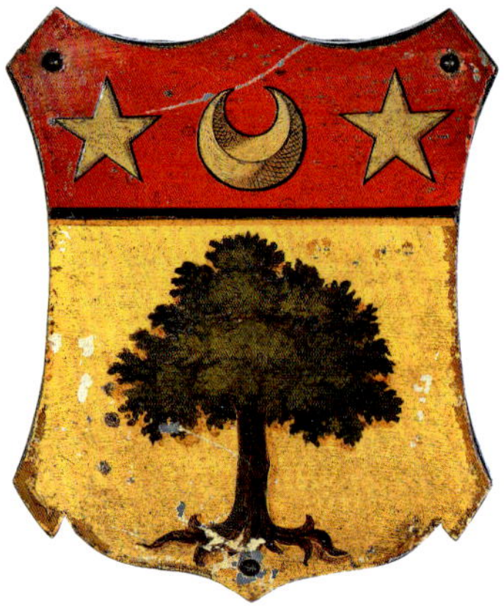

Fig. 130 Arms of Jean Bosanquet, 1735 (13)

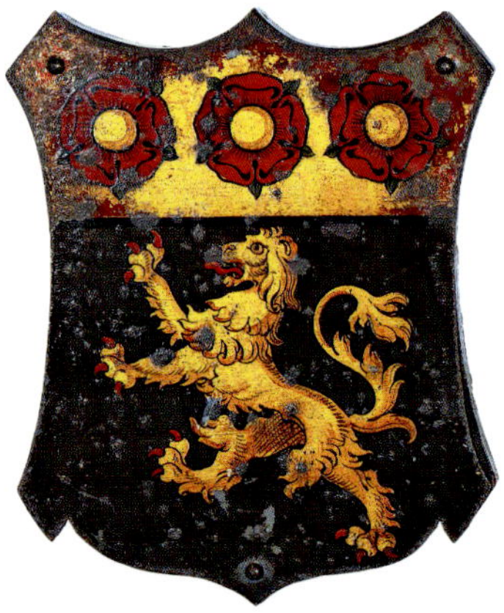

Fig. 129 Arms of Jacques Baudouin, 1718 (43)

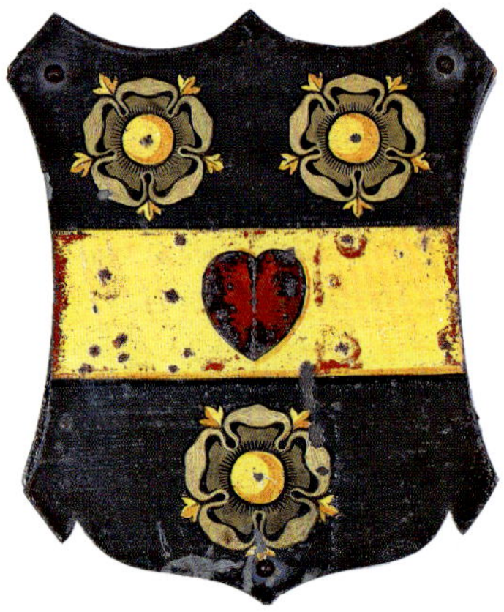

Fig. 131 Arms of Anthony Chamier, 1780 (22)

Champion de Crespigny, Pierre, 1718 (35), fig. 132: *Quarterly, 1st and 4th, argent (intended for) or, a lion salient sable armed and langued gules, in dexter base a fer-de-moulin of the second; 2nd and 3rd, sable, three bars argent*

Clouseaux, Louis de, 1718 (44): *Gules, three pheons or*

Desmarets, Claude, 1732 (4): *Vert, an arm embowed holding a branch of lilies proper*

Du Bisson, Thomas, 1731 (9), fig. 133: *Azure, a lion rampant within a semée of crosses crosslet*

Du Boulay, Revd Francis Houssemayne, 1885 (40): *Argent, a fess wavy gules*

Du Four, Paul, 1718 (5): *Or, on a fess azure a fleur-de-lis argent*

Durand, Jean, 1769 (19): *Gules, a lion rampant or, in the dexter paw a cutlass argent hilted of the second*

Duroure, François, 1742 (11), fig. 134: *Argent, an oak tree proper*

Duval, David, 1786 (37): *Azure, a bend or, three pheons*

France: *Azure, 3 fleurs-de-lis or*

Gaussen, Pierre, 1741 (45), fig. 135: *Azure in base, on a mount vert a lamb passant argent, on a chief of the last three bees volant proper*

Girardot, Andrew, 1776 (18): *Quarterly, 1st and 4th, argent, a lion rampant sable armed and langued gules; 2nd and 3rd, gules, a chevron argent*

Hervart, Philibert, baron d'Huningue, 1721 (33): *argent, an owl gules*

Jackson, Sir Ralph, 1986 (30): *Per chevron gules and argent, on a base wavy azure and argent a tree gules, in chief four piles or issuant from a cloud argent, and two caducei or*

Jourdain, Jean, 1779 (26): *Azure, a lion rampant within a semée of crosses crosslet*

Landon, Theodore Luke Giffard, 1992 (1): *Gyronny of eight or and azure, an inescutcheon argent, on a chief of the first a greyhound courant sable*

Layard, Daniel Peter, 1775 (28): *Quarterly, 1st and 4th, gules, a chevron or between in chief two mullets of six points voided or, and in base a crescent argent, on a chief azure three mullets of six points voided or; 2nd, gules, a cross and in dexter chief a lion rampant holding an anchor or; 3rd, vert, three doves volant*

Le Fanu, William Richard, 1956 (32): *Azure, a swan rousant argent, on a chief or three roses gules*

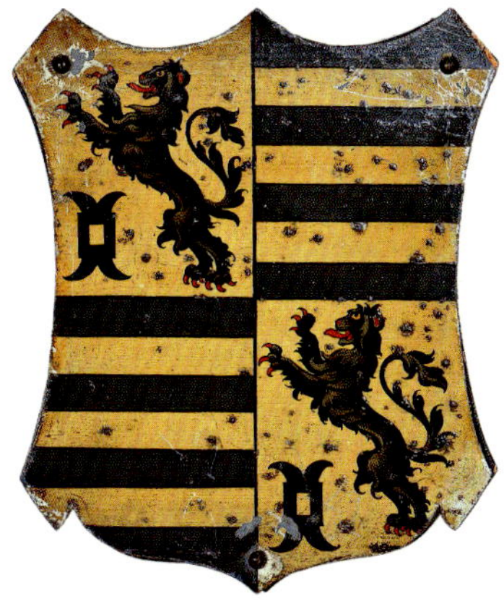

Fig. 132 Arms of Pierre Champion de Crespigny, 1718 (35)

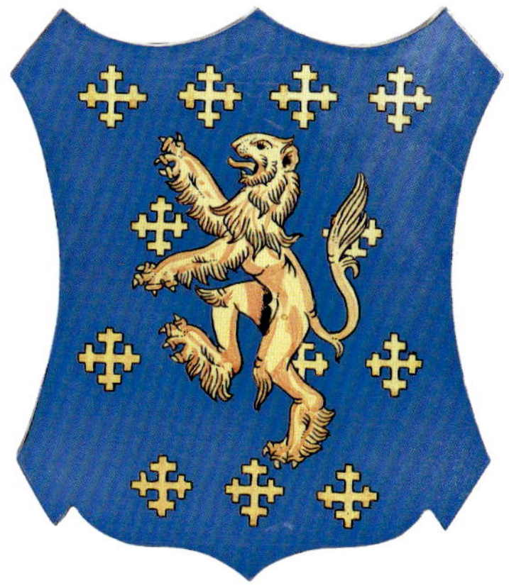

Fig. 133 Arms of Thomas Du Bisson, 1731 (9)

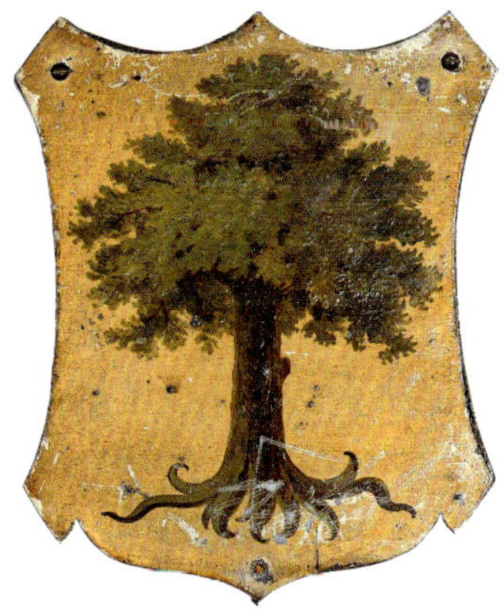

Fig. 134 Arms of François Duroure, 1742 (11)

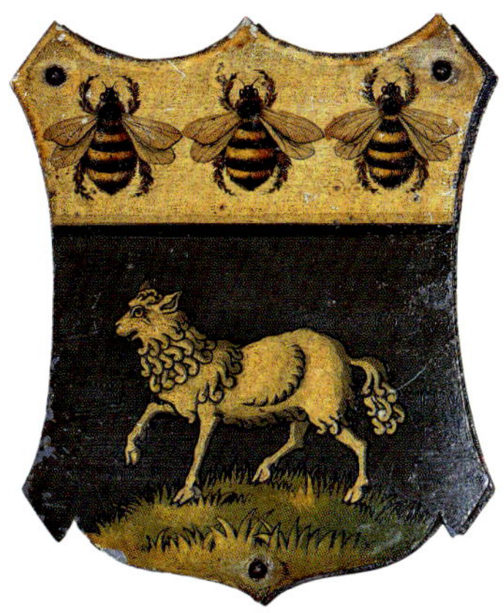

Fig. 135 Arms of Pierre Gaussen, 1741 (45)

Le Heup, Thomas, 1718 (16), fig. 136: *Gules, three beehives between eleven bees volant or*

Ligonier, Earl, 1748 (49), fig. 137: *Gules, a lion rampant or armed and langued sable, on a chief argent a crescent between two mullets*

Majendie, Jean-Jaques, 1752 (50), fig. 138: *Or, in base on a mount vert a tree between to dexter a serpent erect and to sinister a dove close all proper*

Majolier, Édouard, 1900 (34): *Argent, a tree proper and on a chief gules three eastern crowns of seven points or*

Martineau, Jean, 1799 (7): *Paly of six or and gules, on a fess of the last three roses argent*

Ménard, Philippe, 1718 (46), fig. 139: *Or, a lion rampant gules armed and langued sable*

Montolieu, David, baron de Saint-Hippolyte, 1718 (2): *Azure, a fleur-de-lis or between three crescents in chief and as many mullets in base argent*

Montresor, Colonel Jacques-Gabriel, 1766 (29): *Azure, two arms mailed proper holding each a sword erect, on a plate in chief a cross couped gules*

Motteux, Jean, 1729 (17): *Or, three lions passant guardant sinister in pale gules*

Ouvry quartering Garnault (39): *Quarterly, 1st and 4th, argent, a lion rampant sable crowned langued and armed gules,* for Ouvry; *2nd and 3rd, per pale or and azure, barry of six on a chief a pale between two gyrons all countercharged, over all an inescutcheon argent,* for Garnault

Pechell, Sir Paul, Bt, 1772 (23), fig. 140: *Gules, a lion rampant or armed and langued sable, on a chief of the second three laurel branches erect proper*

Pleydell-Bouverie, Jacob Pleydell, 2nd Earl of Radnor, 1770 (36), fig. 141: *Quarterly, 1st and 4th, per fess or and argent, an eagle displayed with two heads sable on the breast an escutcheon gules charged with a bend vair,* for Bouverie; *2nd and 3rd, argent, a bend gules gutté d'eau between two ravens sable, a chief chequy or, and of the last,* for Pleydell

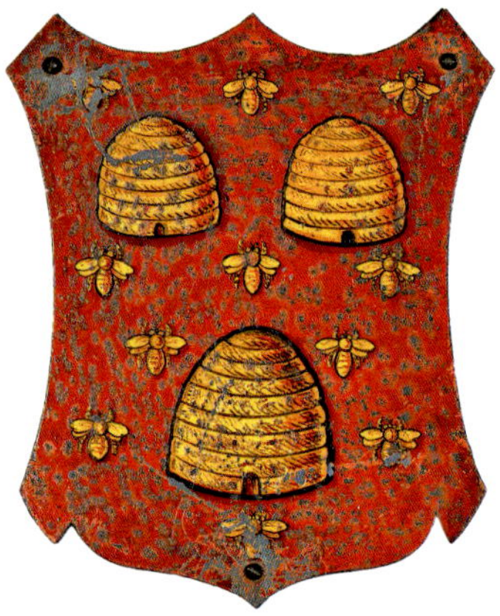

Fig. 136 Arms of Thomas Le Heup, 1718 (16)

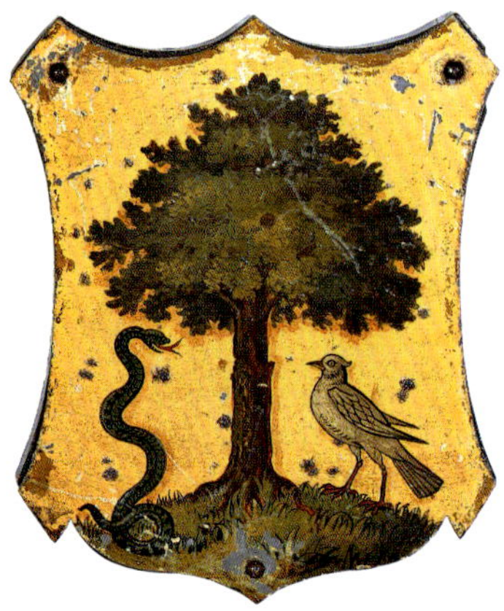

Fig. 138 Arms of Jean-Jaques Majendie, 1752 (50)

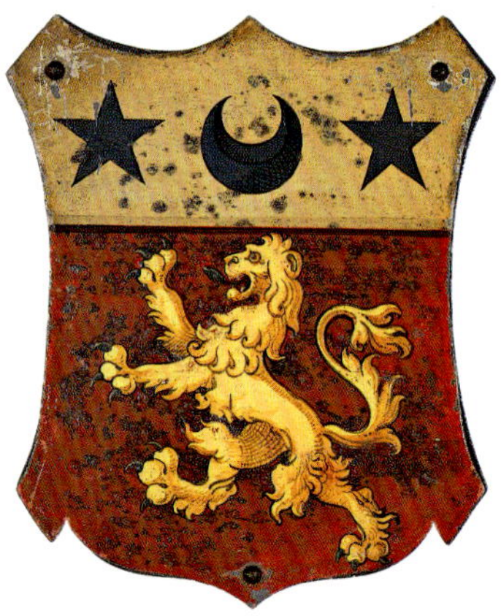

Fig. 137 Arms of Jean-Louis Ligonier, Earl Ligonier, 1748 (49)

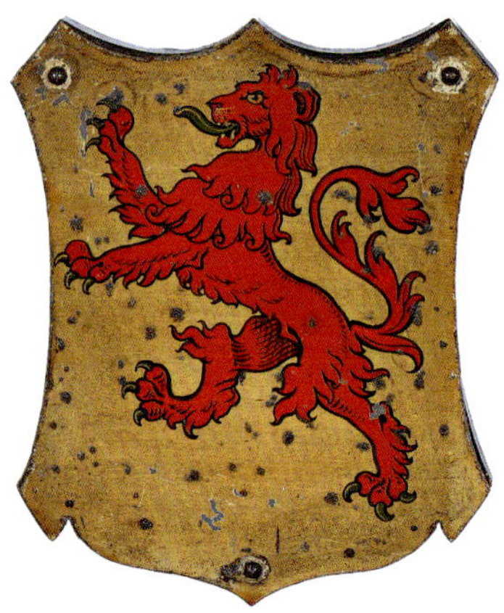

Fig. 139 Arms of Philippe Ménard, 1718 (46)

Pujolas, Moses, 1718 (6), fig. 142: *Per fess wavy azure and argent, in chief three doves proper beaked and membered gules, in base on a mount vert a ram couchant sable horned or*

Pusey, The Hon. Philippe, 1790 (21): *Gules, three bars argent*

Racine, Jaques, 1803 (10): *Vert three dexter hands or*

Romilly, Sir Samuel, 1786 (31): *Argent, in base a lily of three stems issuing from a rock, on a chief azure a crescent between two mullets of the first*

Ruvigny, Henri de Massue de, Marquis de, Earl of Galway, 1718 (38) *Quarterly, 1st and 4th, argent, a fess gules, in chief three martlets sable, on a canton or a battle axe sable; 3rd, argent three mallets gules; 2nd, gules, a chaplet or a chief chequy azure and argent*

St Colome, Henry de, 1718 (14): *Quarterly, 1st and 4th or, a lion rampant gules armed and langued azure; 2nd, vert, four ingots of gold nailed in fret lozengeways: 3rd, gules, three bezants*

St Maurice, Charles, 1729 (47): *Azure, a peacock or displayed, in chief three mullets or*

Sanxay (12), fig. 143: *Argent, a chevron gules [intended for azure] between three coots sable beaked and membered of the second*

Saurin, Louis, 1718 (48): *Gules, on a fess or a lion passant guardant sable*

Viçouse, Guy de, baron de la Court, 1718 (20): *Party per pale gules and vert, an eagle displayed or ducally crowned and langued vert and armed counterchanged*

Vigne, James Randolph, 1979 (42): *Gules, three savages' heads affrontée erased argent*

Vignoles, Charles, 1769 (27): *Or, a fess azure, between three saltires couped gules*

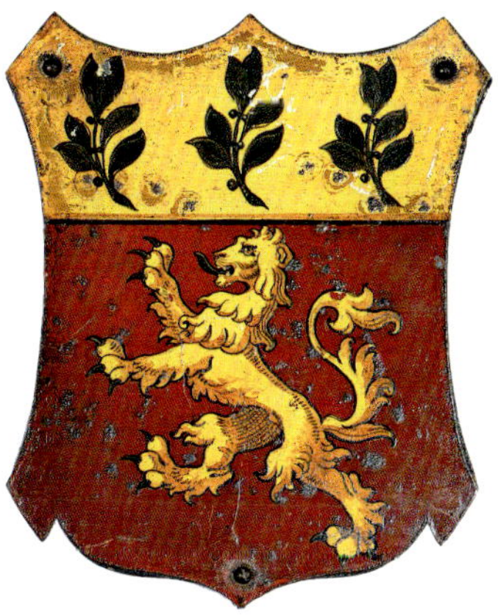

Fig. 140 Arms of Sir Paul Pechell, Bt, 1772 (23)

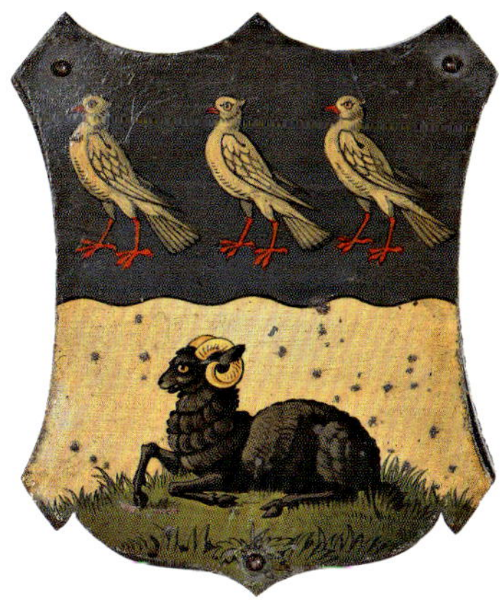

Fig. 142 Arms of Moses Pujolas, 1718 (6)

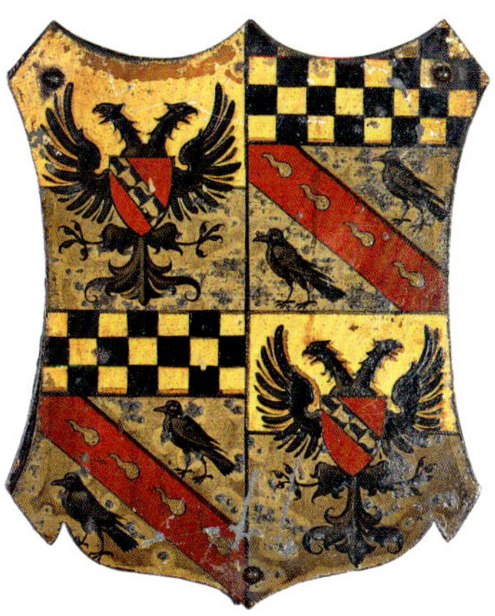

Fig. 141 Arms of Jacob Pleydell-Bouverie, 2nd Earl of Radnor, 1770 (36)

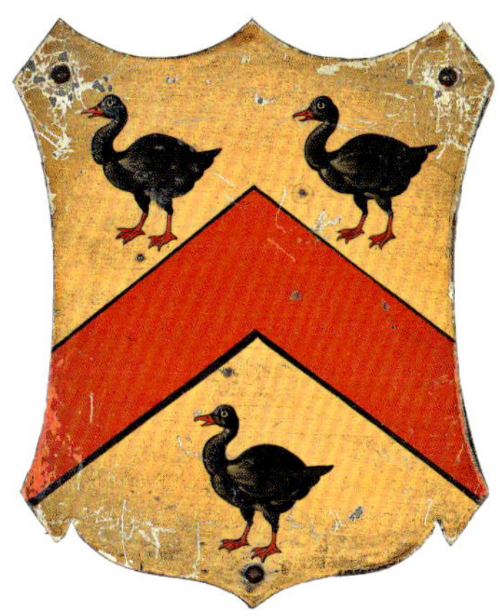

Fig. 143 Arms of William Sanxay (12)

Book-plates in the French Hospital and their heraldry

In the eighteenth and nineteenth centuries book-plates, often printed from engraved copper plates, were prerequisites of ownership for any serious book collector. Set styles were followed and there were myriad designs mostly based on heraldry. While the styles give an idea of date, the designs show how the owner thought of himself and how he wished to be regarded. Many of the eighteenth-century engravers of book-plates are now well known, although only a few of the book-plates here indicate who engraved them.

The book-plates in the collection belonged to Huguenots associated with the hospital, many as directors. Adoption of the English style of the period betokens the loyalty of these Huguenot refugees to their adopted country and reflects their integration. Although some of the heraldry and mottos may point to a French ancestry; the recorded engravers are English.

References:

Names of the book-plate owners are given as they appear on their book-plates.

Chippendale refers to a style, dating from about 1740 until the 1790s, which features exuberant and imaginative embellishments on a rococo theme. Engravers had their favourite stock patterns which were altered slightly to incorporate heraldry and sometimes family emblems.

F with a number refers to an entry in the Franks Bequest catalogue (Howe).

Jacobean refers misleadingly to a style dating in fact from the early 18th century. It is characterized by the use of fish-scale ornament on the solid-looking, dignified design. The scales can look more like bricks or hung tiles and the whole effect is reminiscent of some of the carved furniture and house decorations of the time. The style has nothing to do with the Jacobean period.

W with a number refers to an entry in the manuscript list compiled by Henry Wagner, FSA, now in the Huguenot Library.

Julius Caesar Bernard [not a director]

Arms: *A bear rampant and muzzled*

Crest: *A demi-bear rampant muzzled*

Motto: 'Malo mori quam foedari' [I would rather die than be disgraced] (a traditional Roman proverb)

Armorial, W1

W. Bosanquet [William Bosanquet, director from 1782]

Arms: Bosanquet impaling Ives: *Or, on a mount vert a tree, on a chief gules a crescent between two mullets argent*, for Bosanquet, impaling: *Argent, a chevron sable between three Moors' heads couped*, for Ives

Crest: *A demi lion rampant gules*

Spade-shield armorial, F3118, W3

Peter Castelfranc [not a director]

Arms: *Waves of the sea in base, thereon a ship three-masted in full sail, on a chief gules three cross crosslets argent*

Crest: *Out of a ducal coronet a cross flory*

Armorial, W12

John de Chair [not a director]

Arms: *On a chevron or between three trefoils slipped two mullets* engraved by J. Kirk, St Paul's Church Yard

Chippendale armorial, F8340, W11

Anthony Chamier [Antoine Chamier, director from 1780]

Arms: *Azure on a fess or between three roses two and one argent barbed and seeded, a human heart gules*
A mullet as a mark of cadency for the third son

Crest: None

Motto: 'Patriæ quid debeat, et quid amicis' [The country to which I am indebted and which I love] (Horace, *Ars Poetica*, l. 312)

Armorial, F5531, W19

The eagle wings extended are part of the design; the Chamier crest is quite different.

Philip Champion Crespigny [director, 1734]

Arms: Champion de Crespigny impaling Fonnereau: *Quarterly, 1st and 4th, a lion salient in the dexter base a fer-de-moulin pierced; 2nd and 3rd, azure, three bars argent*, for Champion de Crespigny, impaling: *gules, three chevrons argent on a chief azure a sun in splendour or*, for Fonnereau

Crest: *On a chapeau turned up ermine, a cubit arm mailed erect holding a broad sword*

Motto: 'Mens sibi conscia recti' [A mind aware of its own integrity] (Virgil, *Aeneid*, I. 604)

Jacobean armorial; F7329

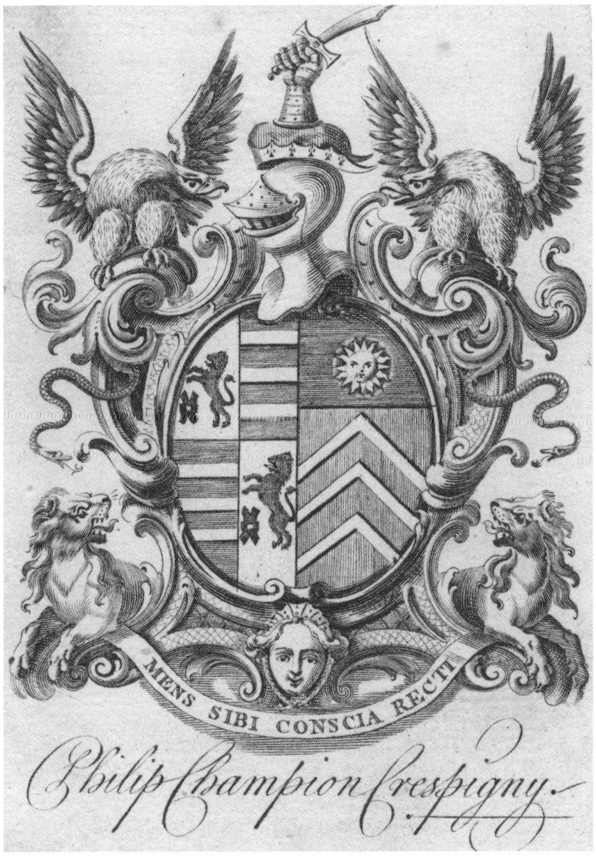

Fig. 144 Philip Champion de Crespigny's book-plate.
Geoffrey Vevers

Henry Daniel Cottin [not a director]

ARMS: *Azure, two chevronels between three boars' heads erased or*

CREST: *A boar's head erased*

SUPPORTERS: *Two boys the dexter holding a caduceus and standing on a musical instrument and the sinister an armillary sphere and standing on a globe*

Chippendale pictorial armorial, F6976, W14

John Theophilus Daubuz [Jean-Théophile Daubuz, director from 1794]

ARMS: *Ermine, a chevron gules between three acorns slipped and pendant*

CREST: *A demi-griffin*

Wreath-and-ribbon armorial, F8306, W2

S. Dayrolles Esq [not a director]

ARMS: *Azure, a chevron or between in chief three mullets or, and in base a porcupine passant*

CREST: *A five-pointed mullet inverted over a sovereign's helmet*

Early Jacobean armorial, F8264, W5b

Anonymous for Solomon Jeissonniere Dayrolles, FRS (1709–1786) [not a director]

ARMS: *Two rolls of paper in chevron between three baker's rolls*

CREST: *A demi-doctor of divinity or lawyer holding a roll of paper in both hands. On the right-hand side a blighted tree with shoots and on the other flowers and a smoking cannon*

Pictorial armorial, W5a

Geo Delavaud [not a director]

ARMS: *Argent, on a mount in base a tree, in front thereof a lion passant gules, in chief azure three mullets or*
A crescent as a mark of cadency for the second son

CREST: *Out of a count's coronet, a lion rampant*

Armorial, F8420, W18

G. De Visme [Gerard Devisme, director from 1788]

ARMS: *Argent, a chevron gules between two mullets in chief and a crescent in base or*

MOTTO: 'Virtute duce comite fortuna' [With Virtue in command, Fortune follows] (Cicero, *Epistulae ad familiares*, x, iii)

Festoon armorial, F8562, W13

According to Henry Wagner the mullets should be estoiles and the crescent should be gules.

D'Olier [not a director]

ARMS: *Quarterly 1st and 4th, or, on a chevron gules between three bunches of grapes a crescent surmounted by a bezant, all within a bordure azure semée de lis; 2nd, azure, three Corinthian columns in fess each surmounted by a dove close; 3rd, gules, on a bend or three martlets sable within a bordure ermine*

CREST: *A dove close holding in its beak an ear of wheat*

MOTTO: 'La bonté de dieu' [The bounty of God]

Armorial, F8820, W36

Thomas du Buisson [Thomas Du Bisson, director from 1731]

ARMS: *A lion rampant holding between its paws a mullet of six points pierced*

Armorial, F9166, W10

Andrew Coltée Ducarel LL.D., Doctor's Commons [not a director]

ARMS: *Argent, three lozenges gules*

Jacobean armorial, F9174/5 (Franks does not make a distinction between two plates), W33

John Dupré Putney Surry [*sic*] [John Dupré, not a director]
ARMS: *Three pales each charged with a fleur-de-lis*
CREST: *A lion sejant, guardant*
Jacobean armorial, F9371, W34
These arms differ from other du Pré arms

John Coles Fourdrinier [not a director]
ARMS: *Party per bend gules and argent, two anchors dexter erect, sinister reversed*
CREST: *On a cap of maintenance an unicorn's head*
MOTTO: 'Toujours fidèle' [Always faithful]
Armorial, F11104, W20

Geo. Garnier [not a director]
ARMS: *Azure, a sword bendwise point downwards, between in the sinister chief a fleur-de-lis, and in the dexter base an oak branch fructed*
CREST: *A lion's head erased gorged with an oak wreath*
Jacobean armorial, F11695, W4

Lewis Andrew de la Chaumette [Louis-André de La Chaumette, director from 1788]
ARMS: *Argent, three doves volant and in base three bars wavy*
CREST: *A squire's helmet plumed*
Armorial, F8382, W28

Alexander La Milliere [not a director]
ARMS: *Gules, three roses*
MOTTO: 'Inter aspera carpiae' [Choose between the rough]
Jacobean armorial, F17496, W32

R. La Touche Junr [not a director]
ARMS: *Party per fess argent and gules in chief two mullets of six points pierced and in base a pomegranate*
MOTTO: 'Quid verum atque decens curo et rogo' [I care for and ask what is true and befitting] (Horace, *Epistulae*, I, 1, line 11)
Crest: A mullet of six points pierced
Wreath-and-ribbon armorial, F17675, W30

Samuel Lichigaray [director from 1777]
ARMS: *Azure, three coots or sans beaks sans legs*
CREST: *Lion rampant holding a poignard in the dexter paw*
Festoon armorial, F18288, W31

Henry Lewis Majendie [not a director]
ARMS: *Or, on a mount in base a tree between dexter a serpent erect and sinister a dove*
A crescent as a mark of cadency for the second son
CREST: *An arm in armour embowed, holding a scimitar*
MOTTO: 'Qualis ab incepto' [The same as from the beginning] (Horace)
Armorial, F19532, W22

Lewis Montolieu [not a director, son of baron de Saint-Hippolyte]
ARMS: *Azure, a fleur-de-lis, between three crescents in chief and as many mullets in base*
CREST: *A fleur-de-lis between two wings erect*
MOTTO: 'Deo et principi' [For God and the prince]
SUPPORTERS: *Two eagles regardant, wings expanded* (as for a baron of the Holy Roman Empire)
Armorial spade shield with supporters, F20943, W7

Daniel Olivier London [Daniel Olivier, director from 1765]
ARMS: Olivier impaling Daubuz: *Argent, an olive tree*, for Olivier, impaling: *Azure, a chevron argent between three acorns slipped and pendent*, for Daubuz
CREST: *A squire's helmet*
SIGNED: 'Stent sculp Gutter Lane.'
Chippendale armorial, F22314, W23
Howe suggests that the arms are Olivier impaling Massé for Susannah daughter of J. Massé whom Olivier married in

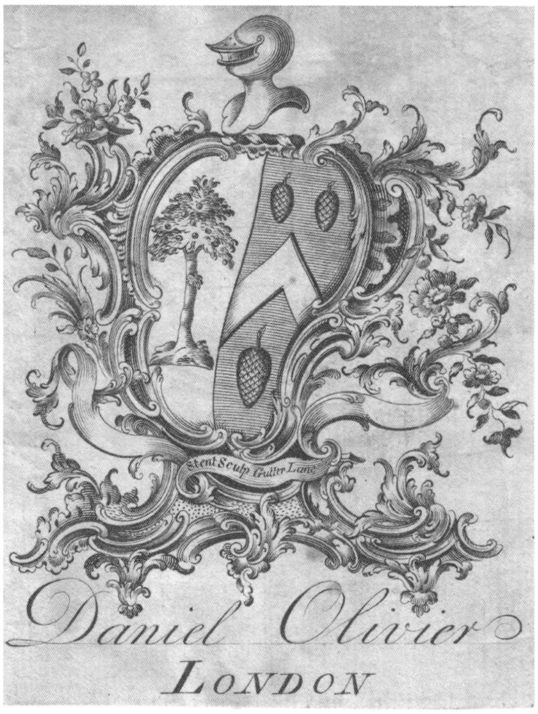

Fig. 145 (*right*) Daniel Olivier's book-plate. *Geoffrey Vevers*

1750; Henry Wagner thought the impalement was of Daubuz but with the wrong tincture. He wrote that the Daubuz arms should be: *Ermine, a chevron gules between three acorns slipped pendant proper*.

Lt. Colonel Pechell [not a director]

ARMS: Pechell with Brooke quartering Wilmot in pretence: *A lion rampant on a chief three laurel branches erect*, for Pechell: *A crescent as a mark of cadency for the second son In pretence quarterly 1st and 4th, a cross engrailed per pale sable and gules*, for Brooke: *2nd and 3rd, on a fess between three eagles' heads erased an unicorn lodged between three escallops*, for Wilmot

CREST: *A lark*

Chippendale armorial, F23071, W25

Lieutenant-Colonel Pechell (1724–1800) was created a baronet in 1797. He was a second son and married Mary Brooke in 1752. She was an only child and heiress to the Brooke and, through her mother, the Wilmot fortunes.

Alexander Pelissier, MD [not a director]

ARMS: *Argent, on a cross a roundel between four fleurs-de-lis, and on a chief gules a lion passant guardant*

CREST: *A fleur-de-lis or issuing from a bezant between a pair of falcon's wings per fess argent and azure*

MOTTO: 'Victrix fortunae sapientia' [Wisdom the conqueror of fortune] (Juvenal, *Satires*, xiii, 20)

Wreath and-ribbon armorial, W15

Jn Lewis Petit MD Coll. Regal. Med. Lon. Soc. S.R.S. & S.S.A. [not a director]

ARMS: quarterly 1st and 4th, *gules, a dexter hand issuing from a cloud in sinister, holding a Roman fasces in pale, between two mullets; 2nd and 3rd, gules, a saltire argent between four cinquefoils, and in pretence, azure, on a chevron argent between three crosses flory two leaves*

CREST: *A demi griffin's head erased*

Wreath-and-ribbon armorial, F23400, W8

Frederick Pigou [not a director]

ARMS: Pigou impaling Wilson: *Or, three spearheads gules two and one*, for Pigou impaling: *Argent, a wolf rampant on a bar in chief three mullets pierced*, for Wilson

Chippendale armorial, F23626, W16

Johann de Ponthieu Esq., Portland Place [not a director]

ARMS: *Quarterly, or and gules*

Crest: *A tree*

MOTTO: 'Plutôt rompre que plier' [Rather break than bend]

armorial, W27

For de Ponthieu the crest should be an olive tree.

Isaac Reynous [director from 1725]

ARMS: *Or, on a bend azure between two eagles displayed, three mullets of the first*

CREST: *A demi-griffin segreant regardant holding a banner or charged with a mullet azure*

MOTTO: 'Spernit pericula virtus' [Virtue despises danger]

Chippendale armorial, F23474, W24

Peter Romilly [director from 1770]

ARMS: *Argent, in base a lily of three stems issuing from a rock, on a chief azure a crescent between two mullets of the first*

MOTTO: 'Persevere'

Wreath-and-ribbon armorial, F25463, W35

Romilly

CREST: *Upon a rock a crescent*

Coronet for a baron

Crest and coronet, F25461, W26

For Sir John Romilly (1802–1874), who was created Baron Romilly in 1866.

William Sanxay [not a director]

ARMS: Sanxay impaling Clerk: *On a chevron azure between three coots close*, for Sanxay impaling: *Argent on a bend gules between three roundels as many swans close, or a canton sinister azure a demi-ram rampant over all a baton*, for Clerk

CREST: *A duck close*

MOTTO: Nec spe nec metu [Without hope, without fear]

Armorial, W9

Sir John Silvester [director from 1811]

ARMS: *A sea lion couchant ducally crowned*

CREST: *A lion couchant*

MOTTO: 'Nec Degener.' [Nor loss of worthiness]

Chippendale armorial, F26929, W21

Charles Dymoke Willaume [not a director]

ARMS: Willaume impaling Lukin: *Argent, on a fess embattled vert between three damask roses four ermine spots*, for Willaume impaling: *A lion rampant debruised by a bend company*, for Lukin

CREST: *On a mound a pineapple*

Armorial, F31827, W17

Notes to the Huguenot book-plates illustrated on the end-papers[1]

William Bosanquet (1757–1800), director from 1782

This spade-shield armorial book-plate shows the arms of Bosanquet impaling those of Ives for William Bosanquet, who married Charlotte Elizabeth Ives in 1787. The Bosanquets became major financiers. Armorial spade-shield designs like the wreath-and-ribbon and festoon styles are found from 1770 until well into the nineteenth century. The device of a tree in earth is found in several Huguenot book-plates and may symbolize the family thriving in its new country.

Anthony Chamier (1725–1780), director in 1780

A major financier, Chamier's advice was sought by Newcastle's government during the Seven Years' War. He served as under-secretary of state for the southern department under Lord Weymouth (fig. 120). A founding member of the Literary Club, Chamier was a frequent host to Dr Johnson at his country house. One of his ancestors had helped to draft the Edict of Nantes for Henri IV. Chamier died shortly after becoming a director of the French Hospital. His Chippendale-style plate with its dramatic eagle comes in two sizes; the larger is shown here.

Gerard Devisme, director from 1788

The Devisme or de Visme family claim descent from the eighth-century sovereign counts of Ponthieu. Even after the main family escaped to England the title comte de Visme was recognized by successive French governments. In France the family used the *cri-de-guerre* 'Montjoye St Denis' as their motto, whilst in England they also used 'J'aspire'. This book-plate is in the wreath-and-ribbon design with a strong three-dimensional shield.

Lewis Andrew de La Chaumette, director from 1788

De La Chaumette, a London merchant, was the son of the pastor of the Église de l'Artillerie in London. This eared-shield armorial dates from the early nineteenth century when his first names were anglicized.

Samuel Lichigaray (d. 1812), director from 1777

Samuel Lichigaray's father, Samuel Peter Lichigaray had come from Orthes in the Pyrenees and settled in Exeter, marrying a lady from Tiverton. Like the wreath-and-ribbon style, the festoon armorial on this book-plate was popular between 1775 and 1800.

Daniel Josias Olivier (1722–1782), director from 1765

Olivier's book-plate, engraved by Stent of Gutter Lane in about 1760, is an exuberant example of the Chippendale style. Olivier was a descendant of the Revd Jourdain Olivier of Pau and was said to have been 'the most influential of all the eighteenth-century financiers with a Huguenot name'.

Peter Romilly (1712–1784), director from 1770

This handsome book-plate is in the wreath-and-ribbon style. Romilly wed Margaret Garnault, also of Huguenot descent, and worked as a jeweller in Frith Street, Soho, where, according to his son Samuel, he 'delighted in his library'. He also had an anonymous book-plate, a Chippendale armorial with the arms of Romilly impaling those of Garnault. Chippendale book-plates mostly date from 1735 to 1780. His son, Sir Samuel Romilly (1757–1818, fig. 41), became Solicitor General and was a director from 1786.

Sir John Silvester, FRS, FSA (Bt. 1812) (1745–1822), director from 1811

Silvester was Recorder of the City of London 1803–1822 (fig. 31). His two book-plates in Chippendale style and engraved by G. Terry of Paternoster Row, St Paul's (*fl.* 1760–1780), are based on the book-plate used by his father, Sir John-Baptist Silvester (1714–1789), who was physician at both the London Hospital and the French Hospital and wed the Huguenot Aletta Catherine Everardina D'Aulnis de La Lande in The Hague in 1740. Sir John Silvester continued to use book-plates of old-fashioned design.

1 Information drawn from Howe under the entries for Bosanquet F3119; Chamier F5531; de La Chaumette F8382; de Visme F8562; Lichigaray F18288; Olivier F22314; Romilly F25463; Silvester F23399.

Inventory of the contents of the French Hospital, 1742

Londres le 26e. Octobre 1742.-

Inventaire fait selon l'ordre de la Corporation, par Messieurs Guinand, Marchant & Desmaretz des Meubles & Effets qui Sont aujourd'hui en nature dans l'Hopital François, lesquels ont été remis a la charge de Mr. & Made. Roumieu, a leur entrée comme Economes dans ledit Hopital.-
Lesquels Meubles ou Effets Sont sous la garde des Personnes ci apres nommées, Sçavoir

Anne Cheré, Servante de l'Econome dans la Chambre No. 3 –

1 Lit garni
2 pres. Draps de Lit d'un Lé[1] & demi

Louise Collet & une Servante dans 11 Chambres comme Suit No. 4 & 5, No. 8, No. 31 a 35, No. 38 & 39 outre la Loge des –Portiers No. 58. contenant en tout

41 Lits garnis, y compris les 2 qui Seront remis dans la chambre No. 8 –
1 Ditto pour elle & son Mari
53 pres Draps de Lit d'un Lé & demi
4 — Do. de 2 Lés
12 Ecuelles } d'Etaim
12 assietes } d'Etaim
39 Pintes } d'Etaim
39 Cuilleres } d'Etaim
40 Pots de Chambre } d'Etaim
5 Baricots[2] p Chaises percées } d'Etaim
6 Lampes de cuivre
6 Cheminées garnies

Ester Gentet & une aut femme dans leur Chambre No. 9 –

2 Lits garnis
3 pres Draps de Lit d'un Lé & demi
nul { ~~2 Ecuelles~~ } d'Etaim
nul { ~~2 assietes~~ } d'Etaim
2 Pintes } d'Etaim
2 Cuilleres } d'Etaim
2 Pots de Chambre } d'Etaim
1 Chandelier de Cuivre[3]
1 Cheminée garnie

la Veuve Carcin dans Sa Chambre No. 10

2 Bois de lit garni de rideaux & une Courte pointe
2 pres Draps de Lit, dun Lé & demi
1 vieux Chest of Drawers
3 Chaises de Paille
1 Pot de Chambre d'Etaim
1 petite grille de Cheminée

Marie Latour, dans l'autre chambre No. 10 –

2 Bois de lit garnis de Rideaux
2 Matelas
1 Traversin
1 Oreiller
1 Couverte blanche
1 Do. . de couleur
4 pres. Draps de Lit d'un Lé & demi
7 assiètes } d'Etaim
1 Pinte } d'Etaim
1 Salliere } d'Etaim
1 Cuillere } d'Etaim
1 Cheminée avec la garniture, excepté les Pincettes - un Chandelier de Cuivre
une Table

Jeanne Williame, 4 Chambres No. 11. 12. 14. 15 –

22 Lits garnis
25 pres. Draps d'un Lé & demi
2 — Do. . de 2 Lés
18 Ecuelles } d'Etaim
18 Assietes } d'Etaim
20 Pots de Chambre } d'Etaim
4 Baricots } d'Etaim
1 Bassin à Lit } d'Etaim
19 Pintes } d'Etaim
20 Cuilleres } d'Etaim
4 Lampes de cuivre
4 Cheminées garnies

Susanne Henry, 4 Chambres N°. 13, 22, 23, 24 –

28 Lits garnis
35 p^{res} Draps de Lit d'un Lé et demi
18 Ecuelles
18 Assietes
6 Baricots
1 Bassin a lit } d'Etaim
25 Pots de Chambre
27 Pintes
27 Cuilleres
5 Lampes de Cuivre
5 Cheminées garnies

Messrs. Duplessis & Delouches, dans leur Chambres N°. 15

2 p^{res}. Draps de Lit de 2 Lés
2 — D^{o}. - d'un Lé et demi
6 Serviettes
3 Nappes
6 Assietes
2 Cuillères } d'Etaim
2 Ecuelles
la Cheminée garnie

Marie Fauché, 7 Chambres N°. 17 a 21 - N°. 25 & 26

30 Lits garnis
45 p^{res} Draps de lit d'un Lé & demi
18 Ecuelles
8 assiètes
29 Pintes } d'Etaim
29 Cuilleres
27 Pots de chambre
4 Baricots
6 Lampes de Cuivre

Jean David Brun & sa femme dans la Boulangerie

1 Lit garni sans rideaux
2 p^{res}. Draps de Lit de deux Lés
1 Pot ou Tankard
2 Cuilleres } d'Etaim
nul ~~2 Ecuelles~~
1 Pot de Chambre
Outre les Utenciles. mentionnez ci après dans l'article de la Boulangerie

Daniel Aubertin au dessus de la Blancherie N°. 35. –

2 p^{res}. Draps de lit d'un Lé & demi
1 Cheminée garnie
24 Couteaux a manches d'yvoire
8 Lampes de Cuivre & 4 de fer blanc

Sur la Loge des Portiers, les 3 Blanchisseuses, N°. 36.

2 Lits garnis Sans rideaux
2 p^{res}. Draps de lit d'un Lé & demi
2 — D^{o}. . . . de 2 Lés
3 Pots de Chambre
3 Pintes } d'Etaim
3 Cuilleres
1 Cheminée garnie

Anne Fonteneau femme du Jardinier & 2 Servantes sous elle, au nouveau Batiment N°. 45 a 56 inclus –

10 Chambres & 2 Cabinets, contenant en tout - –
69 Lits garnis
89 p^{res} Draps de Lit d'un Lé & demi
4 — D^{o}. - - - - de 2 Lés –
18 Serviettes
24 Ecuelles
24 Assiètes
72 Pintes
72 Cuilleres } d'Etaim
72 Pots de Chambre
7 Baricots
2 Bassins de lit
1 D^{o}. p^{r}. laver les mains
12 Lampes de cuivre
9 Cheminées garnies Sans conter celle de Sa Chambre

Dans les Petites Maisons: Antoine Colin & Sa femme

31 Matelas
4 D^{o}. . . petits
44 p^{es}. Draps de Lit d'un Lé & demi
2 — D^{o}. - - - de 2 Lés
31 Ecuelles
33 Pintes } d'Etaim
31 Pots de Chambre
3 Baricots
2 Cheminées garnies avec leurs Cages de fer

Entre les mains de la Veuve Carcin

8 Napes de plusieurs grandeurs
7 D^{o}. . . petites
12 Serviettes neuves
7 D^{o}. moyennes, 15 D^{o}. mauvaises
8 D^{o}. - grosses
30 Napes p les refectoires
12 Essuye mains
1 Nape & 2 Serviettes } p^{r}. l'usage de la
1 Pot, 2 Coupes et 2 assietes d'Etaim } Communion

Poids –

Poids		
59^{oz} 4–	2 Douz^{nes}. Cuilleres a Soupe -	d'Argent
47–5–	2 ——— Fourchettes	d'Argent
14–10–	2 grandes Cuilleres a Soupe	d'Argent
1–8–	8 petites D^{o}. p le Sel & la moutarde	d'Argent
16–10	2 Sucriers	d'Argent
	2 Douz^{nes}.	Plats d'Etaim
	9 Douz^{nes} assiètes	Plats d'Etaim

11 fevrier 1743/4
5 Cuilleres a Soupe
4 D^{o}. petittes a Tea
} remises a la Charge de M^{r}. A. Roumieu les 5 Cuilleres pes 9 oz-17 les 4 petites 4

Dans la Chambre de Mad^{e}. Marin

1 Lit de plume
1 Couverte blanche
1 Courtepointe
1 p^{res} Draps de lit de 2 Lés

Dans le Magazin

N°. 1. 25 V^{es}. Drap oliveatre[4]
" 2. 10 D^{o}. rougeatre
" 3. 11½ D^{o}. Brun
" 4. 58 environ, Toile rayée p Matelas
" 5. 3 p^{res}. Crokus ou Toile p Paillasses & un reste
" 6. 8 aunes[5] Toile crüe p doubleure
" 7. 56¼ au Toile de Suisse large
" 8. 56¾ D^{o}. –
" 9. 56¼ D^{o}. –
" 10. 43 au D^{o}. etroite, en 2 Morceaux
" 11. 41¾ V^{es}. Toile de differentes Sortes, en 4 Coupons
" 12. 6¼ V^{es}. Couty
" 13. 10½ V^{es}. Serge flanelle
" 14. 20 V^{es}. Toile a careaux bleu & blanc, en 2 coupons
58 Draps de lit étroits
8 D^{o}. . . . . larges
2 D^{o} – appartenant à M^{r}. Duplessis, dans un Paquet
40 Chemises d'Homme
47 D^{o}. . . p femme
13 Napes
2 Essuyemains
8 Oreillers
13 mechantes Serviettes
23 Couvertes neuves, de laine blanche
3 D^{o}. . . . D^{o}. . . de couleur rayées
7 Matelas neufs
Plusieurs Lits de plumes vieux, vieilles Hardes[6] p homme & femmes &c^{a}.

Dans une Armoire audit Magazin

1 Douz^{ne}. Chapeaus ~~neufs~~.
2 D^{o}. . . Bas de femme
1 D^{o}. . . . D^{o}. p homme
1 D^{o}. . . . Chemises p homme
1 D^{o}. . . . D^{o}. p femme
1 D^{o}. . . . Draps de lit Etroits
} tous neufs – Sous la garde de la Veuve Carcin

Suite de l'Inventaire du Magazin
Dans l'Armoire qui appartient a Mad^{elle}. Bussiere
les 23 Articles Suivants

un Corps de Moire blanc
une Robe & Jupe de Damas rouge
une D^{o}. . & D^{o}. - de Satin bleu
une Jupe de Soye verte piquée
une Robe de Satin rayé rouge et blanc
une Robe & Jupe de Soye blanche
une Jupe de Calamanque rouge piquée
une Jupe de Taffetas rouge, le haut blanc, doublée
plusieurs Coifures a Dentelles
une paire Bas de Soye verts
+ les Articles apartenant a Mad^{lle}. Buissiere ont eté donné a sa Mort, qui est arrivee le 22eme. Mars 1746. a Marie Latour la Servante, par l'ordre de Monsieur Buissiere. [in a later hand]
16 Chemises . .
14 Tabliers . .
6 Coifes de nuit
1 Tablier de Taffetas rouge
10 Mouchoirs de poche
7 Essuye mains
1 Camisole
1 p^{re} Caleçons
2 morceaux de Soye
3 Jattes des Indes japonnées & une Boite a poudre
une Tablette garnie d'argent
une Tabatiere a pompe garnie d'arg^{t}. & une autre petite d'Ecaille
un petit Livre de Pseaumes avec des Crochets d'argent

23 Articles, dans l'armoire de Mad^{elle}. Bussiere

Dans la Chambre a coté du Magazin & au Parloir de l'Econome

25 Ecuelle neuves
18 Mogs de pintes moitié neuves
3 Douz. Assietes neuves
2 Bassins de Lit
4 Barricots
15 Pots de chambre
20 Assiètes vieilles
8 plats de differentes grandeurs
1 D^{o}. chez la Fonteneau
2 Bassins a laver les mains -
3 D^{o}. - a Barbe
1 Passoir ou Bassin troüé
} d'Etaim
1 grand Chauderon de Cuivre & son trepié
2 Lanternes de Corne

Suite de l'Inventaire des 2 Chambres ci contre

une Bassinoire
une Marmitte
sept Poilons differentes grandeur
deux Cuilleres a Pot
une Ecumoire
cinq Chandeliers
trois Pots p de la Biere
} de Cuivre
un Mortier & Son Pilon - -
un porte Mouchette & Mouchettes
} de Leton
une Casserole & une Poile de fer
3 p^{res}. de Balances, 2 grandes & une petite
2 Porte huiliers, Tunbridge Ware
1 grande Pendule
2 petits Horloges, un dans la Cuisine
3 grands Miroirs a Cadre { *Xme. 1743. Rendu a Marie Latour un de ces Mirroirs apartenant a Ma.^{le}. Buissiere – par Ordre des Messieurs* [in a later hand]

Dans la Cuisine

11 Douz^{ne}. Assiétes
10 D^{o}. . . Ecuelles
3 grands Pots a Biere
2 Passoirs
2 Bassins a Beure
} d'Etaim
3 Marmites
4 Casseroles
6 Poilons, diff^{tes}. grandeurs
6 Cuilleres a Pot
1 Ecumoire
1 Lechefrite
} de Cuivre
1 D^{o}
2 grandes fourchettes
5 Broches a rotir
1 Tourne Broche
4 grilles a grille
} de Fer

2 pots de Cuivre p^{r}. chaufer la Bière
2 grands Coppers garnis de plomb avec leur Couvert de Cuivre
la Grille de la Cuisine & ses appartenances
une grande Table & divers Dressoirs

Dans le Refectoire des Hommes

4 Tables mediocres & une longue
11 Bancs & un long D^{o}.
2 Lanternes
la Grille de la Cheminée garnie
une Lanterne au Bas de L'Escalier

Dans le Refectoire des Femmes

3 Tables
6 Bancs

Dans la Sale des Directeurs & les Cabinets

4 Tables carrées & une Ovale
38 Chaises garnies de Cuir rouge
4 Portraits en Cadre
1 Tableau p les aprentiss
la Grille de la Cheminée avec ses appartenances, le garde Cendre de ~~Leton~~
un Chaufe assiétes de ~~Leton~~
un Miroir avec une Inscription
quatre grandes Serrures de Leton completes
une Armoire a tenir les Livres
un grand Pot de Chambre d'Etain
le Cofre des Archives
un Panier a Charbon ~~de cuivre~~

Dans la Cave des Provisions

25 Fromages de Chester
7 Barils de Beure dont deux Sont entamez
4 D^{o}. de Savon, - de méme
1 petit Baril de Vinaigre
Environ d 20. de Chandeles
13 Sceaux a Cercles de fer
plusieurs Douz^{nes}. de Bouteilles vuides

Dans la Cave a la Viande

des grandes Balances avec environs d 200. depoids

Dans la Voute a Vin

2 Bariques de Vin rouge
1 D°. - - de Vin blanc
10 Douz^{es}. Bouteilles de Vin rouge
5 D° & 1 Bouteille D°. blanc

Dans la Cave a Biere

37 Tonneaux p^{r}. la Biere, de differentes grandeurs avec leurs appartenances
Environs 60 Chaldrons de Charbon
une grande Cuve & une moyenne a coté du reservoir a Biere
6 grands Brocs de Cuir p la Biere

Dans la Blancherie

une grande Chaudiere de Cuivre montée

Dans la Brasserie

une grande Chaudiere de Cuivre montée, une Pompe de plomb,
les Cuves & autres appartenances, necessaires a la Brasserie

Dans la Laverie

une Chaudiere montée,
une Pompe & tuyau de plomb

Dans la Boulangerie

un grand four,
une Chaudiere montée & son Couvert de cuivre
un Puisoir de Cuivre
des Balances avec environ d 250 . de poids
un grand Coffre a Sel
une grande Huche a pêtrir
une Table & autres utensils necessaires
~~20 Sacs de farine & une Poulie p les descendre de la Chambre~~

Au dessus de la Boulangerie dans une Chambre

20 sacs de farine & une Poulie p les descendre

Dans une autre Chambre

72 Boisseaux qui font 9 Quartiers de Dreche ou <u>Malt</u>
1 Moulin
2 quintaux Houblon en 3 Sacs
une Grüe avec Ses appartenances
1 Poids a la Romaine

Dans le Sechoir au dessus de la Cuisine

un Fourneau de fer & sa Cage
une Seringue a feu avec 30 Sceaux de Cuir

Notes des Effets qui appartiennent a diverses personnes comme Suit .

a la Veuve Carcin, Domestique dans la Maison

1 Lit } de Plumes
2 Oreillers } de Plumes
1 Traversin } de Plumes
1 Matelas
4 Couvertes, 2 blanches & 2 Vertes
1 Chest of Drawers
1 Table –
9 Chaises
1 metier p faire des Matelas
1 Poilon } de cuivre
1 Casserole } de cuivre
2 Chandeliers de fer
1 Miroir
7 Draps de lit
14 Serviettes
7 Napes
2 Essuyemains
1 Grille & ce qui en depend
Environ 6 d Poids de plomb
2 Tours de lit, un jeaune & un vert
1 grande Armoire de Chêne

a Marie Fauché, Servante dans la Maison

1 Lit } de plumes
1 Chevet } de plumes
1 Oreiller } de plumes
11 Draps de lit
3 Napes
12 Serviettes
5 Essuyemains
1 Bible
1 Pot a Thé } d'Etaim
1 Bassin } d'Etaim
1 grand miroir
1 petit D°
1 Chest of Drawers
1 Cofre
2 Boites
1 Table
1 Fer a Boite } p^{r}. repasser
1 D°. a feu } p^{r}. repasser
1 Garniture de Lit, gofré bleu
1 Courte Pointe

a Fonteneau Jardinier & a Sa femme
Dans leur chambre

1 Bois de lit garni de rideaux verts
1 Lit } de Plumes
3 Oreillers } de Plumes
3 Traversin } de Plumes
1 Matelas
1 Blanket
2 Couvertes vertes
1 Armoire
2 Tables
2 Cofres
6 Chaises de paille & une a Bras
Pincettes, fourgon & Souflet
1 grille p griller
2 petits Miroirs
3 Chandeliers de Cuivre
1 Chauderon a Thé

Note de 17 Articles que Mad^{e}. Marin a remis a M^{r}. Roumieu apparten^{t}. a Jeanne Harpin, dans les petites Maisons

En argent, trois chelins & Sept Sols
1 Mogue de Pinte
1 Coupe
1 Tabatiere ovale
1 petite D^{o}. ronde
5 Cuilleres a Soupe
1 D^{o}. p Enfant
5 D^{o}. a Thé
1 fourchette a 2 Dents
1 p^{re}. Pincettes a thé, defaites
1 petite Boucle
1 piece de 30 Sols de france
1 Ditto de 4 Sols
1 Mogue de demi Pinte

} <u>21 pieces d'argenterie</u>

Jeanne Harpin est decedee le 22e. Aout 1743. Une partie de cette Argenterie a été mis parmy celle a l'usage des Messieurs & le reste jay vendu & aye mis le produit sur le Debit de mon Conte le 15e. Fevrier 1743/4 a fol. 19. [in a later hand]

1 Crochet doré
1 Bague d'or unie
1 P^{re}. Boutons de Cristal
1 Bague d'or sans pierre

NB il y a plusieurs autres Articles de ladite Jeanne Harpin mentionnez dans l'Inventaire que M^{r}. Vitrac en a donné a Mad^{e}. Marin, dont on n'a pas pris Connoissance

Memoire de l'argent que Mad^{e}. Marin a remis a M^{r}. Roumieu & qui appartient aux personnes suivantes pour le leur delivrer lors qu'elles le lui demanderont

\+ a Marie Margas, Six Livres Sterling & deux Chelins
± a Isaac Bauchet, Imbecille, dix Chelins
NB o a Elizabeth Maniché dans les petites maisons, huit Chelins
* a Susanne Delaunay en Enfance, treize Chelins six Sols
∓ a Henry Giraudeau, une Bague d'Emeraude

1742
9bre. 23° Mis sur mon Conte les 8. Chelins q'Elizabeth Maniché~~e~~ a laissée.

1745^{+}
8bre. 16 Mis sur mon Conte £3 „ – „ 6. Quy est tout ce quy me restoit en Main, a son decez. *N.B. apartenant a Marie Margas.* [in a later hand]

1747/8
Mars 22∓ Mis ce jour le produit de la bague de Henry Giraudeau defunt a fol^{o} 28. sur mon Conte.

1748/9.
Mars 11* Mis sur mon ^{Conte} 13^{s} · 6^{d} apartenant a Susanne De Launay, defunte. a fol^{o} 40.

1753
7bre. 15± Mit sur le Debit de mon Conte £.10. apartement a Isaac Bauché a fol^{o} 79.

1 Breadth of cloth between the selvedges.
2 Kegs.
3 It is more likely that the chandelier was made of brass rather than copper.
4 Ves: probably the plural abbreviation of *verge*, a cloth measure.
5 An *aune* is an old French measure of length.
6 The expression 'vieilles hardes' may be translated here as 'old clothing'.

Picture notes

Items belong to the French Hospital unless otherwise stated.

Frontispiece (a) Jacques de Gastigny (d. 1708), oil on canvas, circle of Pierre Mignard, c. 1680, 29⅞ × 23⅝ in. (76 × 60 cm), in late 17th-century giltwood frame

Frontispiece (b) Gastigny's signature from a letter. Add MS 83701. *British Library*

Title page *Elijah being fed by the ravens*, detail from a silver-gilt alms-dish, maker's mark of George Lambert, London, 1897/8
PROVENANCE: Gift of the deputy-governor, Sir Henry William Peek, 1898

Fig. 1 Philippe Ménard (d. 1737), oil on canvas (much over-painted), French School, c. 1700, 29½ × 22⅞ in. (75 × 58 cm), contemporary English frame

Fig. 2 The Temple of Charenton, engraving, reprinted in London by members of the Société des Parisiens, 1708, 8¼ × 8⅛ in. (21 × 20.5 cm)
INSCRIPTION: 'Le Temple de Charenton proche de PARIS Ma Maison sera appellée Maison d'Oraison. Ce Temple a été rebati par la permiss^{n}. de Louis XIII l'An 1624. Et démoli par l'Ordre de Louis XIV 22 Oct. 1685.'

Fig. 3 The Royal Bounty, printed accounts, published by Paul Vaillant (1671–1739), 1710. *Huguenot Library*

Fig. 4 *Trinity Almshouses at Mile End*, engraving, Simon Gribelin, 1696, 16 × 24 in. (41 × 65 cm). *British Museum*
INSCRIPTION: 'This View of an Almes-house Built by the Corporation of Trinity-House in the year 1696 at Mile=end near London, wherein Twenty-eight decay'd Masters of Ships and Pylots, or the Widows of Such are by the said Corporation maintain'd – As are Fifty nine Persons more of the Like quality, at Deptford in Kent.'

Fig. 5 Receipt for 58 peppercorns representing the rent due to the Worshipful Company of Ironmongers for the lease of the land on which the French Hospital was built, 1774. *Huguenot Library*

Fig. 6 Revd Jacques Saurin, engraving, Thomas Trotter, 1787, 6 × 5 in. (15.2 × 12.7 cm)
INSCRIPTION: 'Saurin from an original picture'

Fig. 7 Henri de Massue de Ruvigny, Earl of Galway (1648–1720), mezzotint, John Simon, c. 1705, after painting by Philip De Graves, 9⅞ × 14⅜ in. (25 × 36.5 cm)
INSCRIPTION: 'His Excellency Henry Earl of Galway &c General Commander in Chief of all Her Majesty's Forces, that are to act in conjunction with the Portuguese in Spain / Philip De Graves pinx. I. Simon fec. Cum Privilegio; Sold by E. Cooper at ye 3 Pidgeons in Bedford Street.'

Fig. 8 Paten, silver (Britannia standard), maker's mark of Robert Hill, London, 1716/17, diameter 9½ in. (24.2 cm)
INSCRIPTION: 'The Gift of Lewis De Tudert Esqr: to y^{e}: French Congregation at Hoxton y^{e}: 25th: March 1717.'

Fig. 9 Sir John, later Field-Marshal Earl Ligonier (1680–1770), oil on canvas, Philip Mercier, c. 1738, 29½ × 24⅜ in. (75 × 62 cm), in contemporary giltwood frame
PROVENANCE: Samwell of Upton House, Northamptonshire; William Butlin Sale, Christie's, London, 28 March 1898, lot 86; presented to the French Hospital by Sir Henry Peek in 1898
LITERATURE: John Ingamells and Robert Raines, *A Catalogue of the Paintings, Drawings and Etchings of Philip Mercier*, The Walpole Society, LXVI, 1976–8, 1978, p. 27

Fig. 10 Louis Montolieu, baron Saint-Hippolyte (c. 1761–1822), oil on canvas, signed 'Joseph Clover pinxit, 1806', 29½ × 24½ in. (75 × 62 cm)

Fig. 11 Lieutenant-General Louis de Jean (1706–1764), oil on canvas, formerly attributed to Philip Mercier, 1730s, 29⅛ × 24 in. (74 × 61 cm), in contemporary carved and gilt frame
INSCRIPTION: 'Major of his Maj^{ties}. [*sic*] first Troop of Horse Guards / Sold by I. Faber at the Golden Head, Bloomsbury Square'
PROVENANCE: Upton House, Northamptonshire, by 1822 as by Mercier; William Butlin Sale, Christie's, London, 28 March 1898, lot 95, presented by Sir Henry W. Peek Bt, deputy-governor, 1898
LITERATURE: John Ingamells and Robert Raines, *A Catalogue of the Paintings, Drawings and Etchings of Philip Mercier*, The Walpole Society, LXVI, 1976–8, 1978, under no. 26, p. 19
The French Hospital also owns an impression of the mezzotint by John Faber II based on this portrait.

Fig. 12 *The French Protestant Hospital, Old Street* from Maitland's *History of London*, engraving, 1756, 6¼ × 10 in. (16 × 25 cm)

Fig. 13 Affidavit signed by Paul de Lamerie for James [Jacques] Ray, 1737. *Huguenot Library*

Fig. 14 *The French Hospital, Old Street, Finsbury*, oil on canvas, artist unknown, c. 1860, 23¼ × 35½ in. (59 × 90 cm)

Fig. 15 David Le Marchand (1674–1726), oil on canvas, Joseph Highmore, c. 1723, 48¾ × 39¼ in. (124 × 99.7 cm). *National Portrait Gallery*

Fig. 16 Jean-Henri Guinand (1686–1755), oil on canvas, circle of John Theodore Heins, c. 1735, 28¾ × 23⅝ in. (73 × 60 cm), in a later frame c. 1765
Jean-Henri's daughter Susanna married Joseph Fry, MD, in the early 1750s.
PROVENANCE: Presented by Henry Ambrose Fry and his son

Edward Alexander M. Fry, both of Birmingham, descendants of Jean-Henri Guinand, April 1896

Fig. 17 Francis Calvert's bill for oil, 1743. *Huguenot Library*

Fig. 18 Joseph Kilpin's bill for sugar, 1743. *Huguenot Library*

Fig. 19 Benjamin Knott's bill for linen, 1741. *Huguenot Library*

Fig. 20 J. Perchard's bill for pewter, 1739. *Huguenot Library*

Fig. 21 Joseph Holt's bill for ironware, 1748. *Huguenot Library*

Fig. 22 Trade card of Elizabeth and Martha Baker, 1757. *Huguenot Library*

Fig. 23 Set of three-pronged forks, sterling silver, maker's mark of William Scarlett, London, 1722/3, 7⅞ in. (20 cm)
INSCRIPTION: (on each) 'French Hospital'

Fig. 24 Sugar castors, silver (Britannia standard), maker's mark of Thomas Bevault, London, 1714/15, 7¼ in. (18.4 cm)
A pair of plain octagonal pear-shaped castors, on moulded feet with a rib round the bodies; the pierced covers with octagonal baluster finials (one of the covers has been repaired)
INSCRIPTION: (on both) 'FRENCH HOSPITAL'
LITERATURE: For Bevault see Joan Evans, 'Huguenot Goldsmiths in England and Ireland', *PHS*, XIV, 1933, p. 528.
The weight of the castors was recorded as 16 ounces 8 penny-weights in both the 1742 and 1766 inventories.

Fig. 25 Looking-glass, walnut with inlaid inscription, c. 1733, the frame with scrolled fretted cresting; the glass plate a later replacement, 42 × 27 in. (106.7 × 68.6 cm)
INSCRIPTION IN MARQUETRY: 'TO THE WORTHY MANAGERS.OF THIS CHARITABLE CORPORATION FROM A WELL WISHER TO THE SAME AUGUST 1733'

Fig. 26 Philippe Champion de Crespigny (1704/5–1765 [?]), oil on canvas, British School, c. 1745, 29½ × 24⅜ in. (74.9 × 61.7 cm). *Kelmarsh Trust*

Fig. 27 Pierre Daudé (1653–1733), oil on canvas, signed and dated by 'Jos Highmore, pint.', 1733, 49 × 39⅞ in. (124.5 × 101 cm)
PROVENANCE: Presented to the French Hospital as part of Pierre Daudé's substantial bequests to the hospital
LITERATURE: Judge Dumas, 'Huguenot History written in the Portraits and Pictures at the French Hospital'. *Proceedings of the Huguenot Society*, vol. 14, pp. 326–33

Fig. 28 Field-Marshal Sir Jean-Louis Ligonier, KCB (1680–1770), oil on canvas, Bartholomew Dandridge, c. 1745, 4⅞ × 39 in. (124 × 99 cm), in original contemporary frame
PROVENANCE: Presented by the sitter, 1 July 1752
When C.H. Collins Baker visited the French Hospital, Victoria Park, Hackney, in 1947 he noted that the portrait was given by the sitter in 1752 as by Dandridge (note in National Portrait Gallery archives from C.H. Collins Baker, 2 January 1953).

Fig. 29 Eight-day long-case clock, walnut case, Charles Cabrier, London, c. 1752, 98 × 21½ × 11 in. (249 × 64.5 × 28 cm)
A George II burr-walnut veneered long case, cross-banded and inlaid with chequered stringing, the arcaded hood surmounted by a fretted pediment, with three sphere finials; the arched dial with 11½-inch circular chapter-ring, the spandrels cast and chased with urns and dolphins, with strike silent movement and date aperture
The gift of this clock is recorded in the minute book of the Corporation in April 1752. It is listed in the contents of the Directors' Meeting Room in 1766.

Fig. 30 *The Rake's Progress, Scene 8, The Rake in Bedlam*, engraving, William Hogarth, 1735, 14 × 15¾ in. (35.5 × 40.5 cm). *Victoria and Albert Museum*

Fig. 31 Sir John Silvester (1745–1822), engraving, T.L. Busby, 1824, 17½ × 14 in. (44.5 × 35.5 cm)

Fig. 32 William Bouverie, 1st Earl of Radnor (1724–1776), oil on canvas, Thomas Gainsborough, dated 1770, 50 × 39 in. (127 × 99 cm). *Private collection*

Fig. 33 David Duval (1751–1836), oil on canvas, artist unknown, c. 1830, 31½ × 27¼ in. (80 × 69 cm)

Fig. 34 Library chair, mahogany, c. 1765, 42 × 25 × 25¼ in. (107 × 64 × 63.5 cm)

Fig. 35 *La Malheureuse Famille Calas*, engraving, C. de Carmontelle, 1765, 16⅝ × 13⅝ in. (42.3 × 34.5 cm)
INSCRIPTION: 'La Mere, les deux Filles, avec Jeanne Viguiere, leur bonne Servante, le Fils et son ami, le jeune Lavaysse
Qualibus in tenebris vitae quantisque peric[u]lis
Degitur hoc aevi quodcumque est. Lucret'

Fig. 36 *Les Adieux de Calas à sa famille*, engraving, signed: 'inv. peint & Gravé par D. Chodowiecki à Berlin', c. 1765, 12⅛ × 16⅜ in. (30.6 × 41.5 cm)
LITERATURE: Randolph Vigne, 'The Killing of Jean Calas: Voltaire's First Huguenot Cause', *PHS*, XXIII, 5, 1981, pp. 280–94

Fig. 37 Silver communion cups for the French Church, Hoxton, maker's mark of Robert Hill, London, 1716/17, 8 in. (20.4 cm)
INSCRIPTIONS: (one cup) 'The Gift of Mrs Rachel Ribeaut to the French Congregation at Hoxton, The 25 March, 1717'; (the other) 'The Gift of Mr Stephen Romilly to the French Congregation at Hoxton, The 25 March, 1717'
PROVENANCE: Given by Rachel Ribeaut and Stephen Romilly to the French congregation at Hoxton 25 March 1717; given to the French Hospital by Pierre Fargues, 1791
Born at Montpellier in 1684, Stephen Romilly went to Geneva in 1701, where he met the minister Jacques Saurin (fig. 6), and then came to England and founded a bleaching business at Hoxton. He married Judith de Monsallier and had four sons. His third son Peter became a prosperous jeweller of Frith Street, Soho, and father of the eminent lawyer Sir Samuel Romilly, who served as a director of the French Hospital from 1786. Stephen Romilly died in 1733 in poverty. Rachel Ribeaut may be identified with the lady of that name who received monthly external assistance from the French Hospital from April 1743 to July 1749 after making an application in February, 1742/3, aged 75, 'estropiée ne pouvant pas marcher' (Marmoy, 1977, II). She was then living in Holland Street at the sign of Noah's Ark. She originally came from La Rochelle. The earliest reference to a French church at Hoxton occurs in 1714, though its exact site is unrecorded. Worship was

non-conformist and was led by Isaac Babault, minister. The church closed in 1785. The plate from Hoxton was given to the French Hospital in 1790 by Pierre Fargues, who ran an academy in Hoxton. His nephew attended the French Protestant School at Westminster (see *PHS*, XV, p. 28).

Fig. 38 Alms-dish, silver (unmarked), London, attributed to Jonah Clifton, c. 1720, diameter 11¼ in. (28.5 cm)
ENGRAVING: Lamb in the centre
INSCRIPTION: 'Bien-heureux Sont Ceux Qui Sont Appellez [*sic*] au Banquet Des Noces De L'Agneau'.
EXHIBITED:: *The Quiet Conquest*, Museum of London, 15 May–31 October 1985, no. 81
LITERATURE: W. Minet, 'The Communion Plate of the Church of Le Carré', *PHS*, XIV, pp. 101–3; Murdoch, no. 81, p. 74

Fig. 39 Alms-box, mahogany, mid-Georgian, width 12 in. (30.5 cm), on later stand

Fig. 40 Communion plate for the Savoy Chapel, 1717/18
A pair of communion cups, silver (Britannia standard), London, maker's mark of Lewis Cuny, 1717/18, both 9 in. (22.8 cm)
With bell-shaped bowls on circular moulded feet and baluster stems, the bowls with slightly everted lips one with the original scratch weight 26=18
A pair of patens, silver (Britannia standard), London, maker's mark of Lewis Cuny, 1717/18, both 10 in. (25.4 cm) in diameter
Each on circular moulded foot, with a rosette of cut-card work at the junction with the top, and moulded rims; one of the patens is inscribed on the base with the original weight: 24 =12

Fig. 41 Sir Samuel Romilly, KC, MP (1757–1818), oil on canvas, Sir Thomas Lawrence, 23½ × 19½ in. (59.7 × 49.5 cm). *National Portrait Gallery*

Fig. 42 Jacob Pleydell-Bouverie, 2nd Earl of Radnor (1749–1828), oil on canvas, Nathanial Dance, 49 × 39 in. (124.5 × 99 cm). *Private collection*

Fig. 43 Richard Grellier (1801–1863), oil on card, unknown artist, c. 1855, 6⅛ × 4¾ in. (15.5 × 12 cm)

Fig. 44 Mrs Louisa Grellier, *née* André (c. 1811–1879), oil on canvas, circle of George Henry Harlow, 1830s, 29½ × 24⅜ in. (75 × 62 cm), in contemporary frame
PROVENANCE: Presented by her grandson G.H. Capper

Fig. 45 Richard Hervé Giraud (1800–1886), oil on canvas, signed W. Fyfe, 1874, 32⅝ × 39¾ in. (83 × 101 cm)
PROVENANCE: Presented by Arthur Giraud Browning, 1874

Fig. 46 The Revd Thomas Hervé, drawing, A. B. Connor, Wandsworth, 1904, after a miniature in the possession of Francis Frederick Giraud Esq. of Faversham, 9½ × 7¾ in. (24 × 19 cm), in a labelled frame by W. M. Power, Westminster

Fig. 47 The Revd Joseph Claude Meffre (1766–1845), oil on canvas, artist unknown, 1830s; 29 × 24 in. (73.5 × 61 cm)
LITERATURE: Dom Aidan Bellenger, 'Another French Community in England: Refugees of the French Revolution', *PHS*, XXVII, 4, 2006, pp. 473–80

Fig. 48 A Petition: a printed application form submitted in 1845. *Huguenot Library*

Fig. 49 Waiter, sterling silver, maker's mark of Edward Jay, London, 1791/2, 10¾ in. (27.3 cm)
With reeded rim on four feet, engraved on the front with a crest, and on the back 'Francis Jolit'
PROVENANCE: Francis Jolit

Fig. 50 Francis Jolit (c. 1754–1836), oil on canvas, John Opie, c. 1805, 35 × 27⅛ in. (89 × 69 cm)

Fig. 51 Salver, sterling silver, maker's mark of William Peaston, London, 1754/5, diameter 11¼ in. (28.6 cm)
With shaped shell and scroll border on three hoof feet, engraved on the front with a later monogram and on the back 'Francis Jolit'
PROVENANCE: Francis Jolit

Fig. 52 Richard Hervé Giraud (1800–1886), photograph by H. Dixon of marble bust by J. Lawlor, 1882, 6 × 4⅜ in. (15.2 × 11.2 cm)
INSCRIPTION: 'PHOTOGRAPH OF A MARBLE BUST OF RICHARD HERVÉ GIRAUD, ESQ^RE^. DEPUTY GOVERNOR OF THE FRENCH PROTESTANT HOSPITAL. PRESENTED TO THE CORPORATION BY HIS FELLOW DIRECTORS AT THE GENERAL COURT, 1ST. APRIL, 1882, IN RECOGNITION OF HIS VARIED SERVICES TO THE INSTITUTION DURING A PERIOD NOW EXTENDING TO 53 YEARS.'

Fig. 53 Frederic Albert Winsor, oil on canvas, follower of Louis-Leopold Boilly, c. 1800, 20¼ × 19½ in. (51.5 × 49.5 cm), in an 1830s frame

Fig. 54 Frederic A. Winsor (1763–1836), lithograph, J.A. Vinter after Dupont, 13⅞ × 11⅝ in. (35.3 × 29.6 cm)
INSCRIPTION: 'Originator of Public Gas-Lighting Founder of the Gas Light and Coke Company Incorporated by CHARTER AD 1812', 'with printed signature and annotation: F. A. Winsor', 'Died 11th May 1836 aged 68'

Fig. 55 Robert Lewis Roumieu (1814–1877), oil on canvas, signed 'J. Desanois Eques p 186[?]', 35⅞ × 27½ in. (91 × 70 cm)

Fig. 56 The French Hospital, Victoria Park, Hackney, from the south-west, water-colour, attributed to R. L. Roumieu, c. 1876, 36¼ × 41½ in. (76.5 × 105.5 cm)

Fig. 57 Philip Smith Duval (1837–1878), oil on canvas, artist unknown, English school, 1860–70, 35⅜ × 27½ in. (90 × 70 cm)

Fig. 58 Communion flagon, sterling silver, maker's mark of Edward and John Barnard, London 1866/7, 10¾ in. (27.3 cm)
PROVENANCE: Presented in 1867 by Philip Smith Duval, deputy-governor, for the use of the new French Hospital chapel at Victoria Park, Hackney

Fig. 59 Arthur Giraud Browning, FSA (1835–1907), oil on canvas, signed by A. B. Connor, c. 1900, 42½ × 35½ in. (108 × 90 cm), in original composition frame

Fig. 60 Sir Henry Austen Layard (1817–1894), lithograph, S.W. Reynolds, published by P. & D. Colnaghi, 1850, 19⅛ × 13⅞ in. (48.5 × 35.3 cm)

Fig. 61 Certificate of the Huguenot Society of London, 1885, 21 × 15 in. (53.5 × 38 cm)

Fig. 62 Sir Henry William Peek, Bt, MP (d. 1898), photogravure, 13½ × 10¼ in. (34.5 × 26.2 cm)

Fig. 63 Charles John Shoppee (1823–1897), photograph, Fradelle & Young, The Photo-Mezzo-Tint Gallery, 246 Regent Street, London, 6⅝ × 4 in. (17 × 11 cm)

Fig. 64 Armchair, oak, 17th-century style, 50 × 27½ × 28½ in. (127 × 70 × 72.5 cm)
PROVENANCE: Presented by C. J. Shoppee, for the use of the governor

Fig. 65 Tankard, sterling silver, maker's mark SL in monogram, London, 1685/6, 6½ in. (16.5 cm)
A tankard and cover on moulded base, the lower part of the body repoussé and chased with acanthus leaves, the slightly domed cover with large flowers, with corkscrew thumb-piece and scroll handle, beneath the base inscribed with scratch weight 28 oz's 12 dwts.
ENGRAVING: (on the handle) the initials S^G^I.
INSCRIPTION: (beneath the base) 'This Tankard bearing the memorable date 1685 was presented to the French Hospital London/ by Sir Henry William Peek. Baronet, Senior Director of the Corporation, July 1893.'
PROVENANCE: Presented to the French Hospital by Sir Henry William Peek, 1893

Fig. 66 Gold badges of the governor and the deputy-governor, Lambert, Jewellers in Coventry Street, 1898, 2⅜ × 1½ in. (8 × 3.8 cm)
A contemporary presentation certificate records that 'The Gold Badges of the Governor & Deputy Governor were presented to this Hospital by Sir Cuthbert Edgar Peek, 2nd Bart. MA FSA, a Director, In Memory of Sir Henry William Peek 1st Bart. A Director 1856–1898 and Deputy Governor 1897–8.'

Fig. 67 Alms-dish, silver-gilt, stamped 'LAMBERT 12 COVENTRY', maker's mark indistinct, London, 1897, 9 in. (22.75 cm)
INSCRIPTION: (on border) 'DOMINUS PROVIDEBIT'; (on base) 'This Dish designed and manufactured by Col. George Lambert F.S.A. was presented by the Deputy Governor to the French Hospital on the occasion of the 170th Anniversary'
PROVENANCE: Given by the deputy-governor, Sir Henry William Peek, 1898

Fig. 68 George Lambert, photograph, Maull & Fox, 187a Piccadilly, London, 7⅝ × 6 in. (19.5 × 15.1 cm)

Fig. 69 Calvin's chair (19th-century copy), oak, 46 × 27 × 31.5 in. (117 × 68.5 × 80 cm)

Fig. 70 Standing cup and cover, sterling silver, German, 1895/6, imported by Berthold Muller, 18¾ × 5 in. (48 × 12.7 cm)
ENGRAVING: The Phené family crest (a coronet with fleur-de-lis and four balls) and the motto 'SAVE NAY'
INSCRIPTION: 'OLD NUREMBERG' around rim and at base 'THE GIFT OF JOHN S. PHENÉ L.L.D. F.S.A. & DIRECTOR OF THE FRENCH HOSPITAL IN THE 60th YEAR OF THE REIGN OF QUEEN VICTORIA 1897'

Fig. 71 Cigarette box, sterling silver, maker's mark JO, London, 1879/80, 6 × 5½ in. (15 × 14 cm)
An cigarette box, the lid cast with the Madonna and Child flanked by Saints George and David, the sides chased with swirling foliage, the interior of the lid engraved with a presentation inscription along the sides of a six-pointed star
INSCRIPTION: 'RICHD·HERVE GIRAUD SECRETARY A GIRAUD BROWNING TREASURER HOPITAL DES PAUVRES PROTESTANTS FRANCAIS Presented to the French Protestant Hospital by the Officers April 1881'

Fig. 72 Cigar box, sterling silver and copper, maker's mark HB, London, 1901/2, width 8¾ in. (22.2 cm)
With fluted ball feet, the lid and front inset with two silvered copper medallions one representing Louis XIV of France. The medal of Louis XIV signed 'J. MAUGER F.' with the legend: 'LUDOVICUS MAGNUS REX CHRISTIANISSIMUS and LUX SPES'
INSCRIPTIONS: (above the medals) 'Edit de Nantes/ 1598–1685'; (beneath the medals) 'Henri' (for Henry IV) and 'Louis' (for Louis XIV); (on the front) 'IIIme CENTENAIRE DE L'EDIT DE NANTES/ 31 MAI/1ER JUIN 2 JUIN 1898' and 'FRENCH HOSPITAL LONDON the gift of ARTHUR GIRAUD BROWNING FSA Deputy Governor 1901.'
PROVENANCE: Gift of Arthur Giraud Browning

Fig. 73 The Browning Memorial bookcase, oak, 1907, 87¾ × 68⅛ in. (223 × 173 cm)
INSCRIPTION: 'BROWNING 1907 MEMORIAL'

Fig. 74 The Library, The French Hospital, Victoria Park, Hackney, photograph, c. 1907. *Huguenot Library*
This photograph appears in an album entitled 'IN MEMORIAM' compiled in memory of Arthur Giraud Browning, FSA, who died 19 October 1907 having served the hospital as director from 1873, secretary from 1875 and deputy-governor from 1898.

Fig. 75 Henry Wagner (1840–1926), oil on canvas, signed 'H Riviere, 1926' (for Hugh Goldwyn Riviere), 31½ × 24¾ in. (80 × 63 cm), in a copy of an 18th-century frame

Fig. 76 Unidentified man formerly called 'Gainsborough Dupont (1754–1797)', oil on canvas, Arthur Devis, 29½ × 23¼ in. (75 × 59 cm)
PROVENANCE: Presented by Mr Arthur Giraud Browning and Mr Henry Wagner, February, 1887

Fig. 77 Peter Le Heup (1699–1777), oil on canvas, John Giles Eckhardt, 1747, 36 × 38¾ in. (91.5 × 98 cm), in a 1770s frame
INSCRIPTION: 'Peter Leheup, junr. Esqr, 1747'
PROVENANCE: Presented by Henry Wagner, 1923
The Le Heup pedigree was compiled by J.H.T. Wood in 1901.

Fig. 78 Clara Le Heup (d. 1773), oil on canvas, John Giles Eckhardt, 1747, 36⅝ × 39½ in. (93 × 100.5 cm)
INSCRIPTION: 'Sarah [*sic*] wife of Peter Leheup ... Eccard, pin(t) 1747'
PROVENANCE: Presented by Henry Wagner, 1923

Figs. 79–80 Silver-gilt cups presented by George Lambert and 'Three Friends', 1892/3 and covers presented by Arthur Giraud Browning, 1907/8, 13½ in. (34.2 cm)
A pair of parcel-gilt cups and covers, each on a circular foot and baluster stem, the bowls decorated with matting and inset with silvered copper medallions on one of William and Mary and on the other of Louis XIV, the covers with baluster finials, each engraved with commemoration and presentation inscription dated 1892, the lids 1907
ENGRAVING: (on the base of second cup) The French Hospital seal
INSCRIPTIONS: (beneath the rim of one cup) 'THE FRENCH PROTESTANT HOSPITAL LONDON DECEMBER 3rd 1892'; (on the base) 'THE GIFT OF LIEUTENANT COLONEL GEORGE LAMBERT, F.S.A. DIRECTOR 1881. PRIME WARDEN OF THE GOLDSMITHS COMPANY, 1886/7'; (on the cover) 'THE COVER OF THIS CUP PRESENTED TO THE FRENCH HOSPITAL ON THE OCCASION OF HIS TENTH ELECTION AS DEPUTY GOVERNOR, 5TH OCTOBER 1907, BY ARTHUR GIRAUD BROWNING, F.S.A.'; (beneath the foot) Lambert coat of arms and motto 'Deo et Principe'
INSCRIPTION: (beneath the rim of the other cup) 'In MEMORIAM The St. Bartholomew Massacre 1572 The Revocation of ye Edict of Nantes 1685 The Gift of Three Friends to the French Protestant Hospital London Christmastide 1892'
PROVENANCE: First cup given by Lt-Col. George Lambert and the second by 'Three Friends'; the covers by Arthur Giraud Browning
EXHIBITED: *The Quiet Conquest*, Museum of London, 15 May–31 October 1985, no. 107
LITERATURE: Murdoch, no. 107, pp. 86, 88

Figs. 81–2 Sketches of residents, pencil, 1881. *Huguenot Library*

Fig. 81 Susannah Ames, widow

Fig. 82 Samuel May, widower, aged 79

Figs. 83–4 Illustrations from the *Graphic*, 26 October 1885

Fig. 83 Looms in use in the men's day-room 5⅞ × 8¾ in. (14.9 × 22.3 cm)

Fig. 84 The women's day-room, The French Hospital 5⅞ × 8⅞ in. (15 × 22.5 cm)

Fig. 85 The laundry, the French Hospital, Victoria Park, Hackney, photograph, c. 1907. *Huguenot Library*
This photograph, like fig. 74, is in the memorial album put together in honour of Arthur Giraud Browning after his death in 1907.

Fig. 86 *Plan of the City of London Cemetery at Little Ilford in the County of Essex*, water-colour, William Haywood Guilshall 1888. *Huguenot Library*
The French Hospital Burial Ground was marked by a monument inset with the seal of the French Hospital and the inscription: 'Here rest many "Children of the Stranger" whose last days were spent at the Hospital or Hospice founded by French Protestant Refugees early in the XVIII Century for the reception and care of the poor and aged among their fellow exiles, and their descendants.'
This is followed by a quotation from Matthew 25: 31–2: 'When the Son of Man shall come in His Glory and all the Holy Angels with Him, then shall He sit upon the Throne of His Glory, and before Him shall be gathered all Nations.'

Fig. 87 View of the French Hospital Burial Ground at Ilford, c. 1907. *Huguenot Library*
The original photograph is mounted in the Arthur Giraud Browning memorial album.

Fig. 88 Communion plate, sterling silver, from All Hallows by the Tower, Thames Street, City of London

An Elizabeth I silver-gilt paten cover, maker's mark a stag's head cabossed, London, 1575/6, diameter 5⅝ in. (14.3 cm)
With spool-shaped foot and reeded rim
INSCRIPTION: (on the top) 'Great Alhallowes in Tham Street, London, 1608'; (on the underside of the foot) '1579'

A James I cup and cover, gilt on the interior; maker's mark FT in monogram, probably for F. Terry, London, 1608/9; 11 in. (27.9 cm)
On circular fluted foot and bracketed spool-shaped stem, the bowl of beaker form engraved with a band of strapwork and foliage round the lip and pendant sprays, the cover fluted and with baluster finial
INSCRIPTION: (on the bowl) 'This Cup And Cover Belongeth To the parish Church of great Alhallowes in Tham Streit London 1608'
The cup is a copy of the 1535 cup at St Michael Paternoster Royal illustrated in Sir C. J. Jackson, *History of English Plate*, fig. 425, as presented by Thomas Kidd [*sic*] for Thomas Kaddy, donor of the accompanying flagon.

A James I cylindrical flagon and cover, maker's mark SO, London, 1608/9, height 13⅞ in. × diameter 6⅜ in. (35.2 × 16.2 cm)
On spreading circular foot with stamped ovolo border and moulding above, the rim and the border to the cover stamped with similar ornament, the cover with raised disc finial, engraved with a coat of arms, and with thumb-piece chased with masks, scrolls and foliage, with elongated scroll handle, the body engraved with the coat of arms of Cadye or Kadye, Gloucester, and with scratch weight 63 oz 16 dwt
INSCRIPTION: (encircling coat of arms on body) 'The. Guift. of. Thomas. Kaddy' (as on the cover's raised disc); 'This Pott belongeth to the Parish Church of great / Alhallows in Thamstret, London, 1608',. The matching flagon is on loan to the Victoria and Albert Museum
LITERATURE: Jackson, p. 111

A James I plain circular paten, maker's mark TA in monogram, mullet below, London, 1608/9, diameter 7½ in. (19 cm)
Of saucer form with upcurved border
INSCRIPTION: 'This Plate Belongeth to the Parish Church of Great Alhallows in Thamstreit London. 1608'
St Michael Paternoster Royal retains a similar paten.

A Charles I standing paten, maker's mark CC a tree between, London, 1634/5, diameter 8 in. (20.3 cm)

On high trumpet-shaped foot with flat border and reeded rim, the centre engraved with a coat of arms and inscription
INSCRIPTION: 'The free guifte of John Hudson unto y[e] parishe of Allhallowes y[e]. greate London Thames Streete'

A George I silver-gilt Britannia rat-tailed straining spoon, London, date letter for 1719/20, no maker's mark, 7⅞ in. (20 cm)
The bowl pierced with scrollwork
INSCRIPTION: (at the end of the stem) 'All Hallowes / The Great / 1719'

LITERATURE: Jackson, p. 111; Edwin Freshfield, *The Communion Plate of the City of London,* 1894, pp. 2–3

Fig. 89 The French Hospital, La Providence, Rochester, 2008, north-western elevation. *Tim Rawle*

Fig. 90 The French Hospital, La Providence, Rochester, 2008, main elevation. *Tim Rawle*

Fig. 91 The French Hospital, La Providence, Rochester, 2008, plaque on main elevation showing Elijah being fed by the ravens. *Tim Rawle*

Fig. 92 Communion cup, sterling silver, maker's mark IT, London, 1631/2, 6⅞ in. (17.5 cm)
Bell-shaped, on a baluster stem and splayed foot
INSCRIPTION: (under base) 'I[B]M A L'eglise vuallonne de Cantorbery 1632'
PROVENANCE: Huguenot congregation of Canterbury
Twelve cups were needed by the Canterbury congregation of a thousand Walloons and Huguenots. Two were stolen in the seventeenth century but a pair is in the Metropolitan Museum of Art, New York, another pair in the Treasury of Canterbury Cathedral and one in the Canterbury Heritage Museum.
A further pair was in the collection of Sir John Noble in 1911. In 1977, the Huguenot Canterbury congregation needed to raise money to restore the organ and sold this cup to the French Hospital.

Figs. 93–100 Stained glass panels, Netherlandish, early 17th century

Fig. 93 Annunciation 9½ × 7⅝ in. (24.5 × 19.4 cm)

Fig. 94 Nativity 9⅝ × 7⅞ in. (24.3 × 20 cm)

Fig. 95 Scourging of Christ 9⅝ × 7⅞ in. (24.4 × 19.3 cm)

Fig. 96 Crucifixion 9¾ × 7⅞ in. (24.5 × 19.5 cm)

Fig. 97 Entombment 9¾ × 7⅞ in. (24.7 × 19.5 cm)

Fig. 98 Resurrection 9⅞ × 8 in. (24.6 × 20 cm)

Fig. 99 Ascension 9¾ × 7⅞ in. (24.7 × 19.4 cm)

Fig. 100 Pentecost 9⅝ × 7⅝ in. (24.5 × 19.5 cm)

The compositions are based on late16th-century Netherlandish prints by Cornelis Cort, Maarten van Heemskerck and Maarten de Vos, illustrating scenes from the life of Christ. The *Scourging of Christ* is based on Cort's engraving of *Ecce Homo* after Etienne du Pérac; the *Annunciation* and the *Entombment* after Maarten de Vos; the *Resurrection* is after Antoine Wierix; the *Ascension* after Hieronymus Wierix published by J. B. Vrints 1584; *Pentecost* or *St Peter Preaching in Jerusalem* is based on an engraving by Maarten van Heemskerck; his drawing of the subject, in Copenhagen, is dated 1571.
The engraved sources are published in *The New Holstein, Dutch and Flemish Etchings, Engravings and Woodcuts 1450–1700; Cornelis Cort*, Part I, Rotterdam, 2000, p. 206 (60/1); Vol. XLIV, *Maarten de Vos*, Rotterdam, 1993, p. 183 (525/1), p. 228(673); *Maarten van Heemskerck*, Part II, Rotterdam, 2000, p. 103 (397/1).
PROVENANCE: Presented by Jacob, 8th Earl of Radnor

Fig. 101 Sundial, brass, supplied by Peter Dollond, c. 1760, diameter 8⅝ in. (22 cm)
INSCRIPTION: 'DOLLOND'
PROVENANCE: Purchased in memory of Jill, Countess of Radnor, 2004

Fig. 102 John Dollond, FRS (1706–1761), mezzotint, J. R. Smith after B. Watson, 15¼ × 11¼ in. (38.8 × 28.5 cm)
INSCRIPTION: 'Who in the Year 1758, invented the ACHROMATIC TELESCOPE, by discovering the difference in the dispersion of the Colours of Light, when the mean rays are equally refracted by different mediums. An important addition to the SCIENCE of OPTICKS, which had been despaired of by the greatest Philosophers in Europe. He died 30th November in the 55th year of his Age'

Fig. 103 Dr Matthew Maty (1718–1776), oil on canvas, Bartholomew Dupan, c. 1750, 27⅛ × 27⅛ in. (69 × 69 cm). *British Museum*

Fig. 104 A pastor of the French Church, Threadneedle Street, pencil drawing, John C. Nixon, (c. 1759–c. 1818), 5½ × 3¾ in. (14 × 9.5 cm)
INSCRIPTION: 'taken at the French Church Lombard S[tr]' and '126' (folio number)
On the reverse is a sketch of a woman in a large brimmed hat and cape.

Fig. 105 *The Huguenot Ancestry of Their Royal Highnesses The Prince William and The Prince Henry*, water-colour and gold leaf on vellum, 1985
Commissioned by the directors and officers of the French Hospital to mark the Huguenot community's continuing loyalty to the monarch on the occasion of the Tercentenary of the Revocation of the Edict of Nantes in 1985, the genealogy was compiled by Royston Gambier, Fellow of the Society of Genealogists and the pedigree was engrossed and illustrated by David N. Chester, FRSA, FSA, Painter-Stainer of London.

Fig. 106 Snuff-box, gold and enamel, maker unknown, Berlin, c. 1750, 3⅛ × 2¼ × ¾ in. (8 × 5.5 × 2 cm)
INSCRIPTION: (on 19th-century parchment label inside the box) 'Snuff box belonging to James Minet, born in Dover in 1698. Died in Berlin in 1774. Said to have been given to J.M by Frederick the Great'

Fig. 107 Hughes Minet (1731–1813), miniature attributed to Samuel Shelley (1750–1808), with hair plaited round the frame and the cipher HM on the reverse, c. 1775, 2¾ × 2½ in. (7 × 5.8 cm)
PROVENANCE: Presented by Paul Minet

Fig. 108 Peter Brissault Minet (1908–1988), oil on canvas, William E. Narraway, 1977, 19½ × 22⅞ in. (49.5 × 58 cm)

Fig. 109 Pocket watch, gold case, maker's mark SG inside the outer case (possibly for Samuel Godbehere, London); verge escapement fuse quarter-repeating, striking on a single bell, Robert Street, c. 1765, 2 1/2 in. (5.5 cm) in diameter
Inscription (replacing the numerals on enamel dial): 'AIME GARNAULT'
Provenance: Donated to the French Hospital by the Ouvry family, 2007

Fig. 110 Aymé Garnault (1704–1782), cut-out miniature in water-colour, 5½ × 4⅜ in. (14 × 11 cm)
Provenance: On loan to the French Hospital from R. Gosling and Miss Gosling

Fig. 111 George II, wax medallion portrait, Isaac Gosset, 4⅜ × 3¼ in. (11 × 8.2 cm)
Provenance: Acquired in 2007 to mark the forthcoming tercentenary of the founding bequest of the French Hospital

Fig. 112 Israel Antoine Aufrère (1677–1758), engraving, Paul van Somer, c. 1700, 6⅞ × 4¾ in. (17.1 × 12.1 cm). *National Portrait Gallery*
Inscription: 'ISRAEL ANTOINE AUFRERE, D en T. Ministre de l'Eglise Françoise de la Savoye a Londres.'

Fig. 113 Peter Anthony Motteux (1660–1718) and family, drawing, Giovanni Antonio Pellegrini, c. 1713, 10¼ × 13⅞ in. (26.1 × 35.3 cm). *British Museum*
Literature: Lindsay Stainton and Christopher White, *Drawing in England from Hilliard to Hogarth*, exh. cat., British Museum, Cambridge, 1987, no. 183, p. 231

Fig. 114 Isaac Gosset (1713–1799), pastel, attributed to Jean-Étienne Liotard, c. 1772, 29¾ × 24⅝ in. (75.5 × 62.5 cm). *Private collection*

Fig. 115 Gideon Saint's trade card, *Metropolitan Museum of Art*
Literature: Morrison Heckscher, 'Gideon Saint, An Eighteenth Century Carver and His Scrapbook', *Bulletin of the Metropolitan Museum of Art*, XXVII, 1969, pp. 299–311

Fig. 116 Pierre Ogier (1711–1775), 1761, oil on canvas, artist unknown, 32⅝ × 22½ in. (83 × 57 cm)

Fig. 117 Hollingworth Magniac (1786–1867), print after portrait, oil on canvas, artist unknown, size not recorded. *National Portrait Gallery*

Fig. 118 Steeple cup and cover, silver-gilt, maker's mark of George Lambert, London, 1898/9, 16¼ in. (41.3 cm)
Inscription: (around the lid) 'Presented to the French Protestant Hospital by George Lambert FSA Decr 3rd 1898'; (around the base of the cup): 'In memory of the late Charles John Shoppee Deputy Governor who died 21st Novr. 1897'
Provenance: George Lambert, 1898

Fig. 119 Ballot box, mid-Georgian 13 in. (33 cm) wide

Fig. 120 Anthony Chamier (1725–1780), oil on canvas, Sir Joshua Reynolds, 1777. *Private collection*

Fig. 121 Sir Robert William Dibdin (1848–1933), photograph

Fig. 122 Tankard, sterling silver, maker's mark of John Langlands, Newcastle, 1760–1768, 8½ in. (21.5 cm)
A covered tankard of shaped outline, on moulded foot, with a rib round the body, open thumb-piece and double scroll handle; the domed cover is unmarked
Inscription: 'Presented to / the French Hospital by / John Dibdin / in memory of his father / Sir Robert William Dibdin, J.P. / Director 1892 / Hon. Secretary & Hon. Solicitor 1896 to 1933.'

Fig. 123 François Duroure (1715–1808), photogravure, Emery Walker, after a wax medallion by Isaac Gosset, 5½ × 4¼ in. (14 × 10.5 cm)
Provenance: Given by Stephen Champion de Crespigny, 1980
Exhibited: *The Quiet Conquest*, Museum of London, 15 May–31 October 1985, no. 317
Literature: Murdoch, no. 317, p. 218

Fig. 124 William Grellier, FRIBA (1847–1934), photograph

Fig. 125 William Pleydell-Bouverie, 3rd Earl of Radnor (1779–1869), engraving, S.W. Reynolds after a drawing by C.A. Du Val, 1843, 13½ × 10¼ in. (34.3 × 26.5 cm)

Fig. 126 Jacob Pleydell-Bouverie, 4th Earl of Radnor (1815–1889), engraving after the portrait by George Richmond, dated 1873, 49 × 39 in. (124.5 × 99 cm)

Fig. 127 William Pleydell-Bouverie, 5th Earl of Radnor (1841–1900), photograph after the portrait by Sir James Jebusa Shannon at Longford Castle, 1897, 10 × 8½ in. (27.7 7/8 × 21.5 cm)

Fig. 128 Arms of Jacob Albert, 1756 (25)

Fig. 129 Arms of Jacques Baudouin, 1718 (43)

Fig. 130 Arms of Jean Bosanquet, 1735 (13)

Fig. 131 Arms of Anthony Chamier, 1780 (22)

Fig. 132 Arms of Pierre Champion de Crespigny, 1718 (35)

Fig. 133 Arms of Thomas Du Bisson, 1731 (9)

Fig. 134 Arms of François Duroure, 1742 (11)

Fig. 135 Arms of Pierre Gaussen, 1741 (45)

Fig. 136 Arms of Thomas Le Heup, 1718 (16)

Fig. 137 Arms of Earl Ligonier, 1748 (49)

Fig. 138 Arms of Jean-Jaques Majendie, 1752 (50)

Fig. 139 Arms of Philippe Ménard, 1718 (46)

Fig. 140 Arms of Sir Paul Pechell, Bt., 1772 (23)

Fig. 141 Arms of Jacob Pleydell Bouverie, 2nd Earl of Radnor, 1770 (36)

Fig. 142 Arms of Moses Pujolas, 1718 (6)

Fig. 143 Arms of William Sanxay (12)

Fig. 144 Philip Champion de Crespigny's book-plate. *Geoffrey Vevers*

Fig. 145 Daniel Olivier's book-plate. *Geoffrey Vevers*

Bibliography

Agnew
D.C.A. Agnew, *Protestant Exiles from France chiefly in the Reign of Louis XIV* (2 vols.), Edinburgh, 1886 (2nd edn, Ticehurst, 2003)

Browning, *Blue Book*
Arthur Giraud Browning: *The Charter and By-Laws*, London, 1892

Browning, 'Communion Plate'
Arthur Giraud Browning, 'Notes on the Communion Plate lately presented to the French Protestant Hospital', *PHS*, V, 4, 1896, pp. 431–40

Browning, 'Early History 1737–1760'
Arthur Giraud Browning, 'The Early History of the French Protestant Hospital (La Providence) continued from 1737 to 1760', *PHS*, VII, 2, 1902, pp. 193–216

Browning, 'History 1760–1801'
Arthur Hervé Browning (Presidential Address), 'History of the French Hospital from 1760 to 1801', *PHS*, XV, 1, 1933, pp. 11–29

Browning, 'Origin and Early History'
Arthur Giraud Browning, 'On the Origin and Early History of the French Protestant Hospital (La Providence)', *PHS*, VI, 1, 1898, pp. 39–80

Dumas
H.C.S. Dumas, 'Huguenot History written in the Portraits and Pictures of the French Hospital', *PHS*, XIV, 1932, pp. 326–32

Faber
R.S. Faber, *Bibliothèque de La Providence, Catalogue of the Library of the French Hospital,* London, 1887, 3rd edn, 1901

Gray
Irvine R.[E.] Gray, 'Institutional Records, The French Protestant Hospital' in *Huguenot Manuscripts: A Descriptive Catalogue of the Remaining Manuscripts in the Huguenot Library, HSQS*, LVI, 1983, pp. 1–103

Howe
E.R.J. Gambier Howe, *Catalogue of the British and American Book-plates bequeathed to the Trustees of the British Museum by Sir Augustus Wollaston Franks K.C.B., F.R.S., P.S.A., Litt. D*, London, 1903–4

Jackson
Sir Charles James Jackson, *English Goldsmiths and Their Marks*, London, 1921

Jones
Edward Alfred Jones, *The Old Silver Sacramental Vessels of Foreign Protestant Churches in England,* London, 1908

Maitland
William Maitland, *History of London*, London, 1739; 2nd edn, 1756

Marmoy, 'French Hospital'
C.F.A. Marmoy, 'More pages from the History of the French Hospital', *PHS*, XXII, 3, 1973, pp. 235–47

Marmoy, *Inmates and Applicants*
C.F.A. Marmoy, The French Hospital. Extracts from the Archives of 'La Providence' relating to Inmates and Applicants for Admission 1718–1957 and to recipients of and applicants for the Coqueau charity 1745–1901, *HSQS*, LII–LIII, 1977, 2 vols.

Marmoy, 'Pest House'
C.F.A. Marmoy, 'The "Pest House", 1681–1717: predecessor of the French Hospital', *PHS*, XXV, 4, 1992, pp. 385–99

Marmoy, 'La Providence'
C.F.A. Marmoy, 'La Providence: the French Hospital during two and a half centuries', *PHS*, XXI, 4, 1969, pp. 335–54

Marmoy, 'La Soupe'
C.F.A. Marmoy, '"La Soupe", La Maison de Charité de Spittlefields [*sic*]', *PHS*, XXIII, 1979, pp. 134–47

Murdoch
Tessa Murdoch (compiler), *The Quiet Conquest: The Huguenots 1685–1985*, exh. cat., Museum of London, 15 May–31 October 1985, London, 1985

Murdoch, *Beyond*
Tessa Murdoch (ed.), *Beyond the Border: Huguenot Goldsmiths in Northern Europe and Northern America*, Brighton, 2008

Smith, 'Financial Aid'
Raymond Smith, 'Financial Aid to French Protestant Refugees, 1681–1727: Briefs and the Royal Bounty', *PHS*, XXII, 3, 1973, pp.248–57

Smith, *Royal Bounty*
Raymond Smith, *Records of the Royal Bounty and Connected Funds in the Huguenot Library*, *HSQS*, LI, 1974, pp. 2–3

Vigne, 'Monument'
Randolph Vigne, '"A Monument of the Piety of Their Ancestors": The Origin and Early History of the French Hospital, London, 1708–1740', *Bulletin of the Huguenot Foundation, 39, Proceedings of the 3rd International Huguenot Conference*, September 2002, pp. 196–207

Vigne, *Poor Relief*
Randolph Vigne, 'Dominus Providebit: Huguenot Commitment to Poor Relief in England' in Anne Dunan-Page, *The Religious Culture of the Huguenots, 1660–1750*, Aldershot, 2006, pp. 70–81

Wagner, *Wills*
Henry Wagner (Dorothy North, ed.), *Huguenot Wills*, 1617–1849, *HSQS*, LX, 2008

Wagner, 'Boislin Trust'
Henry Wagner, 'The Trustees of the Original Administration of the Boislin Trust', *PHS*, VIII, 4, 1908, p. 385

Weiss
Charles Weiss, *History of the French Protestant Refugees*… English edn, Edinburgh, 1854

Index

Page numbers for illustrations are shown in *italic*. All other page references are given in roman.

Adieux de Calas à sa famille, Les, by D. Chodowiecki, *37*
Albert, Jacob: arms of, *102*
All Hallows by the Tower
  communion plate, *74*
alms-box, *40*
alms-dishes
  Clifton, Jonah (attrib.), *39*
  Lambert George, *57*
almshouses: and the City of London guilds, 13; at Dalston (Ironmongers' Company), 13; French Almshouses, Spitalfields, 13 (fig. 4), 36; London Almshouses Committee, 72; Trinity Almshouses, 13. *See also* London Almshouses Committee; National Association of Almshouses
André family, 92
Anglicization, linguistic, 29; English becomes official language at French Hospital, 45; last French-speaking chaplain, *45*
Archer, Thomas, 55
Asylum for Female Orphans, 21
Attlee, J.O., 75
Aubertin, Daniel, 27 (fig. 23), 112
Aubertin, Thomas, 65
Aufrère, Revd Israel-Antoine, 89; portrait by Paul van Somer, *89*
Austen-Leigh, Richard, 65

badges of governor and deputy-governor by George Lambert, *57*
ballot box, *95*
Barnard, Edward and John
  communion flagon, *51*, *53*
Baronneau, Benjamin, 14
Bath Street, 69, 72
Baudouin, Jacques, 12, 14, 16, 31; arms of, *102*
Beckett, Major-General Clifford, 72, 92
benefactions, 30, 39, 42–3
Berchère, Jacques-Louis, 89
Bérenger de Boislin, Lt-Col. Isaac, 30
Bérenger, Isaac, sieur de Boislin, 82
Bethel Hospital, Norwich, 33–4
Bethlehem Royal Hospital, London, 21, 34, 42; as depicted in Hogarth's *Rake in Bedlam*, *33*
Bevault, Thomas
  sugar castors, 28
Blagny, Jacques de La Motte de, 12
Blue Book, 18, 56
Boilly, Louis-Leopold
  Winsor, Frederic Albert (portrait), *49*
Boislin Trust, 82
Bond's Court, Walbrook, 30
Bosanquet, Claude, 90
Bosanquet, Jean, 90; arms of, *102*
Bosanquet, William, 110
Boursin, Edme, 12
Boursin, Madeleine, 12
Bouverie, William, 1st Earl of Radnor, 36; portrait by Thomas Gainsborough, *34*
Browning Memorial bookcase, *60*
Browning, Arthur Giraud, 11, 55; and founding of a book and manuscript purchase trust, 60; and founding of the Huguenot Society, 55; portrait by A. B. Connor, *54*; 'The Inmate's Story', 64
Browning, Arthur Hervé, 65, 68
Brun, Jean David, 112
Buissiere, Constance, 113
Buissiere, Paul, 27, 89
Bulteel, Jean, 78 (fig. 92)
Burn, Dr Stacey S.: donation of Huguenot church records, 84
Busby, T. L.
  Silvester, Sir John (portrait), *34*

Cabibel, Anne-Rose, 37 (figs. 35–6)
Cabibel, Pierre, 12, 30
Cabrier, Charles, 31
  long-case clock, *33*
Calas, Jean, 37 (figs. 35–6), 39
Calvin, John, 8; chair of (copy), *58*
Carcin, Widow, 27, 28, 111, 112
Cardinal Pole Roman Catholic School, 51 (fig. 56), 72
Carmontelle, C. de, *La Malheureuse Famille Calas*, *37*
Carnac, General John, 18
Cazenove Road, 69
cemetery for the City of London at Little Ilford, plan of, *70*
Chaboussant, Jean, 19
chairs
  armchair, carved with C. J. Shoppee's name, *57*
  Calvin's chair (copy), *58*
  library, *36*
Chamier, Anthony, 110; arms of, *102*; portrait by Sir Joshua Reynolds, *96*
Champion de Crespigny, Claude, 31 (fig. 26)
Champion de Crespigny, Philip [Philippe], 30, 31; book-plate of, *107*; portrait, *31*
Champion de Crespigny, Pierre, 89; arms of, *103*
Champion de Crespigny, Stephen, 89
Champion, Claude, sieur de Crespigny, 31
chaplains
  Daubeny, Revd Howard, 78
  Duplessis, Revd François, 19–20
  Duplessis, Revd Jacques, 28, 30–1
  Lescure, Revd Pierre, 39
  Meffre, Revd Joseph Claude, 45
  Ménard, Revd Philippe, 10, 12 n. 1, 13–14, 19, 20, 31; arms of, *104*; portrait, *9*
  Overs, Revd H.W., 72
  Sharp, Canon Maurice, 78
  Stannard, Very Revd R.W., 78
  Young, Canon Geoffrey, 78
Charenton, temple of, 10, 30
charitable institutions, 21
charities. *See* benefactions
Charity Commission, 64, 73, 75
Chauvet, Louis, 91
Chavasse, Rt Revd Christopher Maude, 76
Cheré, Anne, 111
Chester, David, 85
Chodowiecki, D., *Adieux de Calas à sa famille, Les*, *37*
Christie, Lucie, 94
cigar box, *59*
cigarette box, *59*
Clifton, Jonah
  alms-dishes (attrib.), *39*
clock, long-case
  Cabrier, Charles, *33*
Clover, Joseph
  Montolieu, Louis, baron de Saint-Hippolyte (portrait), *17*
Cole, B., *The French Protestant Hospital near Old Street*, *19*
Coligny, Admiral Gaspard de (bust), 81
Colin, Antoine, 24, 112
Collet, Louise, 111
communion plate, 38, *53*
  All Hallows by the Tower, 73, *74*
  French Hospital, *16*, 39, *41*, 42, 51, *53*, 57, 60, *74*, *78*, 89 (fig. 112)
  Hoxton, 42
  Savoy Chapel, *41*
  Walloon congregation, Canterbury Cathedral, *78*
Compton's Lea, Horsham. *See* French Hospital, Compton's Lea
Connor, A. B.: portraits of:
  Browning, Arthur Giraud, *54*
  Hervé, Revd Thomas, *44*
Coqueau, Esther, 30
Court of directors: election to, 95; meetings of, 18, 30, 47, 60, 68, 72, 75
Court prayer, 42, 78, 86
Courtauld, Samuel Augustine, 92
Cripplegate pest-house, 10, 11, 12, 13, 16, 19; demolition of, 22; matrons at
  Bachelier, Anne, n. 16, 12
  La Prade, Mme de, n. 16, 12
  Liège, Madeleine, n. 16, 12
  Sœur Nissole, n. 16, 12
Cuny, Lewis
  communion cups, *41*
  patens, *41*
cups
  communion, *78*
    Cuny, Lewis, *41*
    Hill, Robert, 38
  loving (and covers)
    Lambert, George, 60, *63*, *64*
  standing (with cover), *59*
  steeple (with cover)
    Lambert, George, *93*

Dance, Nathaniel
  Pleydell-Bouverie, Jacob, 2nd Earl of Radnor (portrait), *42*
Dandridge, Bartholomew
  Ligonier, Field-Marshal Sir John [Jean-Louis] (portrait), *32*
Darwin, Jane, 94
Daudé, Pierre: portrait by Joseph Highmore, *31*
Davy, Colonel Robert Manning Matwin, 70
Delmé, Sir Peter, 12
Demedis, Jacques, 29
Denew, James, 12
Desanois, J.
  Roumieu, Robert Lewis (portrait), *50*
Desbouveries, Laurens, 34 (fig. 32)
Desert-Dieu, Pierre-Jacques du, 12
Desmarets, Claude, 26, 111
Devis, Arthur
  'Gainsborough Dupont' (portrait, wrongly identified), *62*
Devisme, Gerard, 110
Dibdin, Sir Robert William (photograph), *96*
Dollond, John
  portrait by B. Watson, *81*
Dollond, Peter
  sundial (attrib.), *81*
Du Bisson, Jean, 35
Du Bisson, Thomas: arms of, *103*; his extensions to French Hospital by, 20, 21

Du Val, C. A.
Pleydell-Bouverie, William, 3rd Earl of Radnor (drawing), *100*
Dufour [Du Four], Paul, 14, 30, 31
Dumas, Judge Hugh, 68
Dumas, Philip Anthony Egerton, 73
Dupan, Bartholomew
Maty, Dr Matthew (portrait), *82*
Dupont
Winsor (the elder), Frederic Albert (lithograph after portrait by Dupont), 50
Duroure, François: arms of, *103*; medallion portrait by Isaac Gosset, *97*
Dutens, Pierre, 91
Dutry, Sir Denis, 12
Duval, David, 36, 45; portrait of, *35*
Duval, Peter James, 36
Duval, Philip Smith: portrait of, *52*
Duval, Revd Dr Stephen P., 69, 72
Duval, Walter John, 72

Eckhardt, John Giles: portraits of:
Le Heup, Clara, *62*
Le Heup, Peter, *62*
Edict of Nantes: Revocation of the, 8; bicentenary of the, 56, 58
Edict of Toleration, 1787, 39
Elijah being fed by the ravens. *See* seal of incorporation
Elliott, Henry, 47
English Committee. *See* Royal Bounty
Esther Coqueau Charity, 82

Fâche, Edward Charles, 69
Fargues, Pierre: early gift of plate, 39
Fauché, Marie, 112, 115
Finsbury, London: hostel for destitute Huguenots, 8
flagons, communion
from All Hallows by the Tower, 74
Barnard, Edward and John, 51, *53*
Fontaine, Revd Jaques, 11
Fontaine, Revd Pierre, 11
Fonteneau, André, 22, 26, 29 n. 13, 116
Fonteneau, Anne, 112
forks
William Scarlett, 27
Foundling Hospital, 21, 29
Fradelle & Young
Shoppee, Charles John (photograph), 56
French Almshouses, Spitalfields, 13 (fig. 4), 36
French Catholic refugees, 41
French Committee. *See* Royal Bounty
French Hospital
founding bequest, 8, 10
property investment, 30; sale of Bath Street site, 52; disposal of property holdings and reinvestment, 73
as repository for Huguenot history, 54, 58
eligibility of applicants, 56; eligibility extended to married couples, 77
as treasury, 39–40
views of:
at Finsbury: by Cole, *19*, 20; anon., *21*
at Hackney: by Roumieu, *51*
at Rochester: by Rawle, *76*, *77*
French Hospital, Compton's Lea (1947–1957)
move to, 72; treasures brought there, 72; library, 73, 75 n. 11; search for more economical premises, 73;
future as almshouse, 72;
search for almshouse-type accommodation, 75
French Hospital, Finsbury (1718–1867)
beginnings at Cripplegate pest-house, 13; leasing of Golden Acre site, 14; building fund appeal, 14; petition to George I for building hospital, 16; incorporation, 16, 18; building at Golden Acre site by Peter Legrant, 19; building dedication, 19; rebuilding of bakehouse wing, 21, 30; rebuilding of brewery, 21; lease for Cripplegate pest-house site, 22; extensions by Du Bisson, 20, 21; extensions by Boulton Mainwaring (1765), 21; gardens, 18, 22; building survey of 1837, 45; life at, 24; administration, 31; board of management, 35; growth of, 30; dwindling numbers of inmates at, 42; deficit, 41; building lease grants, 44; plans and Building Committee for replacement building, 47
French Hospital, La Providence, Rochester (1959–)
official opening, 77;
City Wall development, 79, 82;
Huguenots' Garden, 79;
common room, 79;
Mathematical School development, 79
French Hospital, Victoria Park, Hackney (1867–1941)
plans for a purpose-built hospital, 50; Roumieu designs new building, 50; financing of the building, 51; the search for a new site, 47; Victoria Park site, 50; life at, 64; laundry, *67*; library, 60, *61*, 65 n. 2; day-rooms at, *66*; war years 1914–18, 64–5; war years, 1939–45: building of air-raid shelter, 69; evacuation of inmates to Littlehampton, 69; evacuation of collections, 69; use of, as a day nursery, 70; war damage in 1940, 69; war damage to property held at Finsbury, 71; Littlehampton evacuees, 72; Naboth's vineyard, 68; sale of land to LCC, 69; threat of compulsory purchase, 69; sale to LCC, 72; use of, after the war, 71
French Hospital Burial Ground, Little Ilford, 50, 70, *71*
French Protestant Churches, 11; integration with Anglican churches, 39, 41–2
Église de l'Artillerie, 110
Église des Grecs, Soho, 27, 45
French Chapel Royal, St James's, 10
French Church, Norwich, 43
Hoxton, 16, 38 (fig. 37), 39
Le Carré
Berwick Street, 39; alms-dish from, *39*
Little Dean Street, 39 (fig. 38), 84
Leicester Fields, 39
Sandwich, 84
Savoy Chapel, 41, 43
St Julian's, Southampton, 43
Threadneedle Street, 36: pastor of, 82, *83*
French Protestant School in Westminster, 54 (fig. 59)
French, use of, 18, 43, 46 n. 4, 54 (fig. 59), 60, 78
Fresse, Barthélemy, 31
Fruchard, Philippe, 12
Fyfe, W.
Giraud, Richard Hervé (portrait), *44*

'Gainsborough Dupont' (formerly called): portrait by Arthur Devis, *62*
Gainsborough, Thomas
Bouverie, William Bouverie, 1st Earl of Radnor (portrait), *34*
Galway Street, 44, 69, 72
Galway, Earl of. *See* Massue de Ruvigny, Henri de
Gambier, Royston, 85
Garnault, Aymé, 86; portrait of, *87*
Gastigny Place, 69
Gastigny, Jacques de: bequest of, 8; career of, 9; portrait by circle of Pierre Mignard, 2, 7; signature of, *2;* will of, 10
Gaultier, Jaques, 89
Gaussen, Pierre, 30, 31; arms of, *103*
Gentet, Ester, 111
George II: portrait by Isaac Gosset, *88*
Giraud, Richard Hervé, 45, 50, 51
photograph of bust by J. Lawlor, *49*
portrait by W. Fyfe, *44*
Godbehere, Samuel
watch, pocket (attrib.), *87*
Godin, Jaques, 92
Golden Acre. *See* French Hospital, Finsbury
Gosset, Gideon, 91
Gosset, Isaac, 91; portraits of:
François Duroure, *97*
George II, *88*
portrait by Jean-Étienne Liotard (attrib.), *90*
Gouvernet, marquise de, 14
Grellier, Cecil, 75, 78
Grellier, Christopher, 78, 93
Grellier, Louisa: portrait by George Henry Harlow (circle of), *43*
Grellier, Richard (portrait), *43*
Grellier, William (photograph), *98*
Gribelin, Simon
Trinity Almshouses at Mile End, *13*
Grimwade, Arthur, 73
Guilshall, William Haywood
Plan of the City of London Cemetery at Little Ilford, *70*
Guinand, Jean-Henri [Henri], 26, 30, 36, 83, 111; portrait by circle of John Theodore Heins, *24*
Guy's Hospital, 21, 42

Hackett, L. A., 75
Harlow, George Henry
Louisa Grellier (portrait), *43*
Heins, John Theodore (circle of)
Guinand, Jean-Henri [Henri] (portrait), *24*
Henri IV, 8, 12
Henry of Navarre. *See* Henri IV
Henry, Susanne, 112
Hervart, Philibert d', baron d'Huningue, 30
Hervé, Revd Thomas, 45; portrait by A. B. Connor, *44*
Highmore, Joseph: portraits of:
Daudé, Pierre, *31*
David Le Marchand, *23*
Hill, Robert
communion cups, 38
paten, *16*
Hogarth, William
Rake in Bedlam, The, *33*
Houblon, Sir John, 11
Huguenot ancestry: of TRH Princes William and Henry, 36, 38, 83, *85*; as criterion for French Hospital applicants, 56
Huguenot General Fund, 82
Huguenot Heritage, 83
Huguenot history: revival of interest in, 52
Huguenot Library, 82
amalgamation with French Hospital's holdings, 84
French Hospital records, 7
Maintenance Fund, 83
Huguenot records in Kent, 76
Huguenot Society of London: founding of the, 55; certificate of the, *55*
Huguenots: definition of, 8; *grand refuge*, 8; as refugees in England, 8; hostel for, at Finsbury, 8
Hunt, Frank, 68

Idlewild Trust, 87 (fig. 108)
inmates
Cripplegate pest-house
Boursin, Edme, 12
Boursin, Madeleine, 12
Fourreau, Jean, 12
Haris, Elisabeth, 12
Lemel, Jean, 12
Prestereau, Anne, 12
French Hospital, Compton's Lea
Auvache, Caroline, 78
Beazley, Sarah Alice, 78
Hoinville, Clarissa Emily, 78
Jermy, Eliza, 78
French Hospital, Finsbury
Aubertin, Daniel, 24
Baour, Mathieu, 35
Bauchet, Isaac, 116
Bobin, Nathanael, 22
Buissiere, Constance, 27
Caillon, Marie, 22
Colin, Jean, 24
Coste, David, 22
Couderc, David, 22
Delaunay, Susanne, 116
Delouche, Henri, 30, 112
Desmarets, Jean, 22
Duplessis, Jacques, 30, 112
Fauchet, Magdeleine, 16 (fig. 8)
Fonteneau, André, 29 n. 13
Fonteneau, Anne, 29 n. 13
Fresse, Barthélemy, 31
Fromey, Anne, 70
Ganeron, Madeleine, 22
Gentil, Charles, 50
Giraudeau, Henry, 116
Goudemay, Jacques, 22
Harpin, Jeanne, 27, 29, 116
Kendall (*née* Dambesieux), Elizabeth, 35
L'Heureux, Marie, 22
L'Houmeau, Abraham, 22
Lardant, Jean, 22
Latour, Marie, 27
Le Blond, Pierre, 21
Le Marchand, David, 22
Maniché, Elizabeth, 116
Marchand, Daniel, 70
Margas, Marie, 116
Marmois, Pierre, 94
Peltier, Anne, 35
Pennel (or Pesnel), Jean-Jacques, 22
Ray, Jacques, 21
Raymond, Isaac, 22
Rondelet, François, 22
Rossignol, François, 22
Rousset, Pierre, 21–2
Symons, Sarah, 50
Tabart, Pierre, 89
Tartas, Pierre, 22
Vautier, Marie, 16 (fig. 8)
French Hospital, Rochester
Smart, Florence May, 70
Smart, Grace, 70
French Hospital, Victoria Park, Hackney
Ames, Susannah, *65*
Bond, Mrs Mary, 64
Dabbs, James, 64
Hurlin, James, 70
May, Samuel, *65*
Mignon, Louis De la More, 73
inventories
1742, 22, 26, 111–16
1766, 22
Ironmongers' Company. *See* Worshipful Company of Ironmongers

James II's Brief calling for assistance to the Huguenot refugees, 73
Jamet, Jacob, 91
Janssen, Sir Estienne-Theodore, 91
Jay, Edward
waiter (silver), *47*
Jean, Lieutenant-General Louis de, 18; portrait, *18*
Jolit, Francis, 50; portrait by John Opie, *48*
Jourdain, Nicholas, 91
Jourdain, Revd Ernest Edward, 73
Jourdain, William David, 50

La Chaumette, Lewis Andrew de, 110
La Chaumette, Revd Louis de, 83 (fig. 104)
La Force, duchesse de, 14, 39
La Mare, Francis de, 51
Lambert, George, 60, 94
alms-dish, *57*
badges of governor and deputy-governor, *57*
loving cups and covers, 60, *63*, *64*
photograph by Maull & Fox, *58*
steeple cup with cover, *93*
Lamerie, Paul de, 21: affidavit for Jacques Ray, *20*
Land Committee (Corporation of London), 22
Langlands, John
tankard, *97*
Latour, Marie, 27, 111, 114
Lawlor, J.
Giraud, Richard Hervé (bust of), *49*
Lawrence, Sir Thomas
Romilly, Sir Samuel (portrait), *42*
Layard, Sir Henry Austen, 55; portrait by S.W. Reynolds, *55*
Le Coq de Saint-Leger, Théodore, 30
Le Fanu, William Richard, 82, 84
Le Heup, Clara: portrait by John Giles Eckhardt, *62*
Le Heup, Peter: portrait by John Giles Eckhardt, *62*
Le Heup, Thomas: arms of, *104*
Le Marchand, David, 22–4; portrait by Joseph Highmore, *23*
Lebas, Charles, 89
Legrant, Peter, 19
Lescure, Revd Pierre, 39
Lewis, W.E.A., 75
Lichigaray, Samuel, 110
Ligonier, John [Jean-Louis], Earl Ligonier, 18, 31, 36; arms of, *104*; portrait by Bartholomew Dandridge, *32*; portrait by Philip Mercier, *17*
Liotard, Jean-Étienne
Gosset, Isaac (portrait attrib.), *90*
London Almshouses Committee, 72
London County Council, 68–9; buys Victoria Park building, 72; offers to buy French Hospital buildings, 68
London Hospital, Whitechapel Road, 21, 91
looking-glass with inscription, *29*, 114
Lordell, John, 12
Louis XIV, 8
loving cup ceremony, 60
Lucadou, Jean-Daniel, 42
lunacy, treatment of. *See* mental health care

Magdalen Hospital, 21
Magniac, Hollingworth, 93
portrait, *92*
Mainwaring, Boulton, 21, 92
Maitland, William: *History of London*, 19 (fig. 12), 33
Majendie, Jean-Jaques: arms of, *104*
Malheureuse Famille Calas, La, by C. de Carmontelle, *37*
Marchant, Pierre, 18, 89
Marin, Marie, 113, 116
Marmite, La, soup kitchen, Soho, 10, 30
Marmoy, Charles, 82, 84, 94
Marshall, Joseph Irwin, 64, 71
Massue de Ruvigny, Henri de, Earl of Galway, 12, 14, *15*, 16, 18, 30, 92
Maty, Dr Matthew, 82; portrait by Bartholomew Dupan, *82*
Maull & Fox
Lambert, George (photograph), *58*
Meffre, Revd Joseph Claude, 45
Ménard, Revd Jean, 9 (fig. 1), 10, 14
Ménard, Revd Philippe, 10, 12 n. 1, 13–14, 19, 20, 31; arms of, *104*; portrait, *9*
mental health care, 20, 33, 34; at the French Hospital, 20, 42; cold-water cistern, 21
Mercier, Philip
Jean, Lieutenant-General Louis de (portrait wrongly attrib.), 18
Ligonier, Sir John [Jean-Louis] (portrait), *17*
Middlesex Hospital, 21
Mignard, Pierre (circle of)
Gastigny, Jacques de (portrait), *2*
Minet, Hughes: portrait by Samuel Shelley (attrib.), *86*
Minet, Peter Brissault: portrait by William E. Narraway, *87*
Minet, Susan, 73
Monson, Emma, Lady Monson, 94
Montigny, Jean Remy de, 89
Montolieu, David, baron de Saint-Hippolyte, 18, 30, 92
Montolieu, Louis, baron de Saint-Hippolyte: portrait by Joseph Clover, *17*
Motteux, Peter Anthony: portrait by Giovanni Antonio Pellegrini, *90*
Mounier, Estienne [Stephen], 30, 39; Stephen Mounier Apprenticeship Fund, 82

Narraway, William E.
Minet, Peter Brissault (portrait), *87*
National Association of Almshouses, 75
Nissole, Paul, 19
Nixon, John Colley, 82
A pastor of the French Church, Threadneedle Street, *83*
Norris family, 50

Ogier, Pierre, 92
portrait, *91*
Old Street, 10
Olivier, Daniel Josias, 110; book-plate of, *108*
Ordres et Règlements, 18, 54. *See also* Blue Book
outgifts for specific needs, 78, 82
Ouvry, Ernest Carrington, 65, 69

Pain, Le. *See* Soupe, La
Parker, Owen Fortrie, 69
patens
from All Hallows by the Tower, *74*
Cuny, Lewis, *41*
Hill, Robert, *16*
Peaston, William
salver, *49*
Pechell, Sir Paul: arms of, *105*
Peek, Sir Henry William, 58, 67 n. 4; portrait, *56*
Pellegrini, Giovanni Antonio
Motteux, Peter Anthony (portrait), *90*
Penshurst Road, 82
Perigal, Jean, 89
Pest House Row, 39. *See also* Bath Street
pest-houses, 10. *See also* Cripplegate pest-house
Peter Minet Trust, 87 (fig. 108)
'Petites Maisons', 20, 22, 24 n. 22, 42, 43, 112. *See also* mental health care
petition for admission to French Hospital, *46*
physicians
Maty, Dr Matthew, *82*
Silvester, Sir John-Baptist, 34
Pleydell-Bouverie, Jacob, 2nd Earl of Radnor, 44; arms of, *105*; portrait by Nathaniel Dance, *42*
Pleydell-Bouverie, Jacob, 4th Earl of Radnor: portrait by George Richmond (engraving after), *100*

Pleydell-Bouverie, William, 3rd Earl of Radnor: portrait by C.A. Du Val, *100*
Pleydell-Bouverie, William, 5th Earl of Radnor: portrait by Sir James Jebusa Shannon, *100*
Providence, La: source of name, 18. *See also* French Hospital
Pujolas, Moses: arms of, *105*

Quiet Conquest exhibition at the Museum of London, 83

Radnor, 1st Earl of. *See* Bouverie, William, 1st Earl of Radnor
Radnor, 2nd Earl of. *See* Pleydell-Bouverie, Jacob, 2nd Earl of Radnor
Radnor, 3rd Earl of. *See* Pleydell-Bouverie, William, 3rd Earl of Radnor
Radnor, 4th Earl of. *See* Pleydell-Bouverie, Jacob, 4th Earl of Radnor
Radnor, 5th Earl of. *See* Pleydell-Bouverie, William, 5th Earl of Radnor
Rake in Bedlam, The, William Hogarth, *33*
Rambouillet, Nicolas de, sieur de la Sablière, 12
Rawle, Tim: views of French Hospital at Rochester, *76, 77*
Ray, Jacques, 21; affidavit for, signed by Paul de Lamerie, *20*
Reneu, Hilaire, 12
Reneu, Pierre, 12
residents. *See* inmates
Reynolds, S.W.: portraits of:
 Layard, Sir Henry Austen, 55
 Pleydell-Bouverie, William, 3rd Earl of Radnor (engraving after Du Val drawing), *100*
Reynolds, Sir Joshua
 Anthony Chamier (portrait), *96*
Richmond, George
 Pleydell-Bouverie, Jacob, 4th Earl of Radnor (engraving after Richmond), *100*
Riviere, Hugh Goldwyn
 Wagner, Henry (portrait), *61*
Rochester Cathedral, 76
Rochester, Corporation of, 76
Romilly, Peter, 110
Romilly, Sir Samuel, 44; arms of, 105; portrait by Sir Thomas Lawrence, *42*
Ronjat, Estienne, 39
Roumieu, Adam, 22, 51, 111
Roumieu, Robert Lewis, 51; designs French Hospital at Hackney, 50; portrait by Desanois, J., *50*; water-colour of French Hospital, Hackney (attrib.), *51*
Royal Bethlehem Hospital
 Hogarth, Wiliam
  Rake in Bedlam, The, *33*
Royal Bounty, 11; and the Cripplegate pest-house, 11; definition of, 8; English Committee, 8, 11; French Committee, 8, 11, 12, 16, 36; printed accounts of, *11*
royal charter of incorporation, 16–17, 69, 72, 73; *Charter and By-laws*, 12 n. 18; Supplemental Charter of 1953, 73
Royal Hospital, Chelsea, 21
Royal Hospital, Kilmainham, 21
Royal Naval Hospital, Greenwich, 21
Royrand des Clouseaux, Louis, 19
Ruvigny, Henri de Massue de. *See* Massue de Ruvigny, Henri de

Sabatier, Jean, 91–2
St George's Hospital, 21
Saint, Gideon: trade card, *91*
Saint-Hippolyte, baron de. *See* Montolieu, Louis
St Luke's Hospital (Moorfields, then Old Street from 1786), 34, 42
salver
 Peaston, William, *49*
Santhune, Jaques, 78 (fig. 92)
Sanxay, William
 arms of, *105*
Saurin, Revd Jacques, 14, 18 n. 3; portrait by Thomas Trotter, *14*
Saurin, Revd Louis, 14
Savage and Grellier, surveyors, 45
Savoy Chapel
 communion plate from, *41*
Scarlett, William
 forks, 27
Scott, Joseph, 84
seal of incorporation, 16
 Elijah and the ravens, 68
Shannon, Sir James Jebusa
 Pleydell-Bouverie, William, 5th Earl of Radnor (portrait), *100*
Shelley, Samuel
 Minet, Hughes (portrait attrib.), *86*
Shoppee, Charles John, 58, 94
 photograph by Fradelle & Young, *56*
silk trade: crisis in, 39; as source of inmates at the French Hospital, 45
Silvester, Sir John, 35, 110; portrait by T.L. Busby, *34*
Silvester, Sir John-Baptist, 35, 110
Silvestre, Dr Jean-Baptiste Zacharie, 34–5. *See* Silvester, Sir John-Baptist
Silvestre, Pierre, 40 n. 15
Simon, John
 Massue de Ruvigny, Henri de, Earl of Galway (portrait), *15*
Smith, J.R. (after Watson)
 Dollond, John (portrait), *81*
snuff-box, *86*
Société de Nismes, 43
Société des Parisiens, 10 (fig. 2)
Society for the Propagation of the Holy Gospel, 10
soup kitchens, 10
Soupe, La, soup kitchen, Spitalfields, 10, 12, 30, 43
 Bread House Pensioners, 43
stained-glass panels, Netherlandish, *79–81*
Stephen Mounier Apprenticeship Fund, 82
stewards: records kept by, 22
 Chaboussant, Jean, 19
 Cobden, A.J., 71, 73
 Davies, Leslie, 78
 Elliott, Henry, 47
 Marin, Marie, 27
 Marshall, Joseph Irwin, 64
 Nissole, Paul, 19
 Roumieu, Adam, 22, 26, 51, 111
 Towne, W.E., 78
Street, Robert
 verge escapement for watch, *87*
sugar castors
 Bevault, Thomas, *28*, 113
sundial
 Dollond, Peter (attrib.), *81*
surgeon-apothecaries, 28
 Buissiere, Paul, 27, 89
 Demedis, Jacques, 29

Tabart, Jacques, 89
tankards, 57
 Langlands, John, 97
Teulon, Samuel Sanders, 51
Theobald Square, 76. *See* French Hospital, Rochester
trade suppliers to French Hospital
 Baker, Elizabeth and Martha (glass and ceramics), 26: trade card of, *26*
 Calvert, Francis (oil), 26: bill, *24*
 Hayward, Samuel (linen), 26
 Holt, Joseph (ironmongery), 26: bill, *26*
 Kilpin, Joseph (sugar), 26: bill, *25*
 Knott, Benjamin (linen), 26: bill, *25*
 Leglive & Ardouin (wine and oil), 26
 Perchard, J. (pewter), 26: bill, *25*
Trinity Almshouses, 13; engraving by Gribelin, Simon, *13*
Trotter, Thomas
 Saurin, Revd Jacques (portrait), *14*
Tudert, Louis de, 14, 16 (fig. 9)
Turner, Winifred, 70, 84

Van Sommer, William, 55 (fig. 61)
Viçouse, Guy de, baron de La Court, 12
Victoria Park. *See* French Hospital, Victoria Park, Hackney
Villettes, General William Anne de, 18
Vinter, J.A. (after Dupont)
 Winsor (the elder), Frederic Albert (lithograph after portrait by Dupont), *50*
'visites de la maison', 72, 86
Wagner, Henry, 60, 93
 bequest of Huguenot pedigree material to hospital, 84
 portrait by Hugh Goldwyn Riviere, *61*
waiter (silver)
 Jay, Edward, *47*
Walker, Emery
 François Duroure (portrait), *97*
Walloon congregation, 41 (fig. 40), 78 (fig. 92); communion plate from Canterbury Cathedral, *78*
Walloons
 immigration of, 11
watch, pocket
 Godbehere, Samuel (attrib.), *87*
Watson, B.
 Dollond, John (portrait), *81*
Westminster Hospital, 21
Willen Key Company, 72
Williame, Jeanne, 111
Willis, Mrs Louise, 94
Winsor, Frederic Albert, 50
 portrait by Louis-Leopold Boilly, *49*
Winsor, Frederic Albert (the elder)
 portrait by J.A. Vinter, *50*
Worshipful Company of Ironmongers, 13, 14, 47
 French Hospital land, 14 (fig. 5)
 receipt for, *14*
 French Hospital land lease, 38

Picture credits

The British Library, frontispiece (b)

© Copyright the Trustees of the British Museum, fig. 4, 103, 113

The Huguenot Library, figs. 3, 5, 13, 17–22, 48, 74, 81–2, 85–7

By courtesy of the Kelmarsh Trust. Photograph: Courtauld Institute, Photographic Survey, fig. 26

The Metropolitan Museum of Art, Harry Brisbane Dick Fund, © 2008 The Metropolitan Museum of Art, fig. 115

© National Portrait Gallery, London, figs. 15, 41, 112, 117

Private collection. Photographs: Courtauld Institute, Photographic Survey, figs. 32, 42

Private collection, figs. 114, 120

Tim Rawle, figs. 89–91

Geoffrey Vevers, end-papers, figs. 144–5

V&A Images/Victoria and Albert Museum, fig. 30

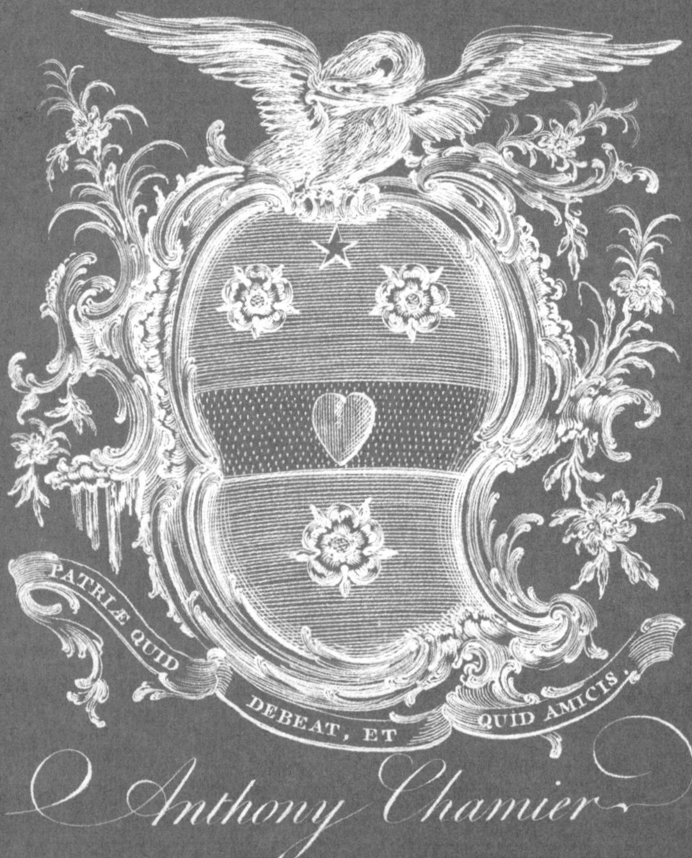
PATRIÆ QUID DEBEAT, ET QUID AMICIS.
Anthony Chamier

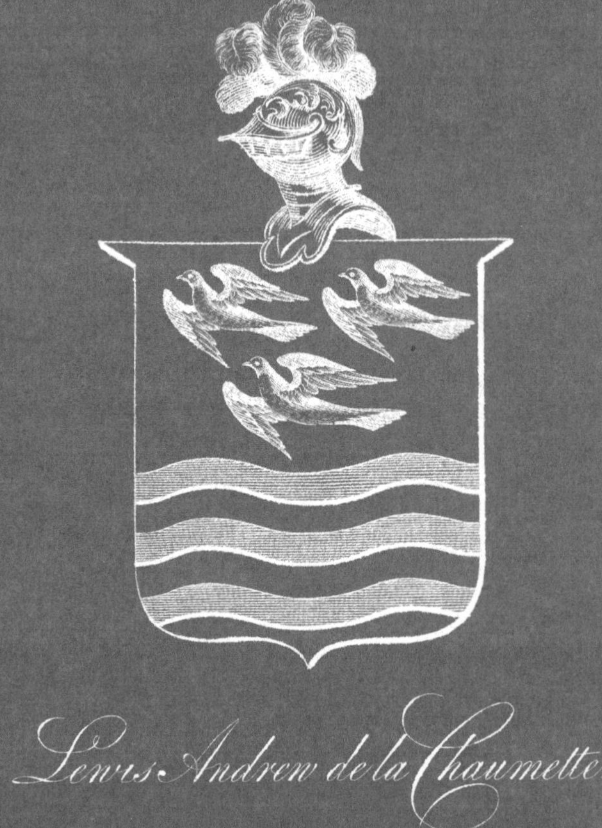
Lewis Andrew de la Chaumette.

Kent Sculp Gutter Lane
Daniel Olivier
LONDON

PERSEVERE
Peter Romilly